Current
Psychiatric
Diagnosis & Treatment

Current Psychiatric
Diagnosis & Treatment

Editors

Lewis R. Baxter, Jr, MD

Kathy Ireland Professor of Psychiatric Research and
Professor of Neurobiology
Department of Psychiatry and Behavioral Neurobiology
University of Alabama at Birmingham School of Medicine
Birmingham, Alabama

Robert O. Friedel, MD

Heman Drummond Professor
Chair
Department of Psychiatry
University of Alabama at Birmingham School of Medicine
Birmingham, Alabama

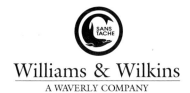

Williams & Wilkins
A WAVERLY COMPANY

BALTIMORE • PHILADELPHIA • LONDON • PARIS • BANGKOK
BUENOS AIRES • HONG KONG • MUNICH • SYDNEY • TOKYO • WROCLAW

Developed by Current Medicine, Inc.
Philadelphia

Current Medicine, Inc.

400 Market Street
Suite 700
Philadelphia, PA 19106

Director of Product Development	Lori J. Bainbridge
Developmental Editors	Scott Thomas Hurd, Deborah Singer
Art Director	Paul Fennessy
Design and Layout	Jerilyn Bockorick
Production Manager	Lori Holland
Production and Marketing Associate	Amy Giuffi
Indexer	Dorothy Hoffman

Current psychiatric diagnosis and treatment / editors, Lewis R. Baxter
and Robert O. Friedel.
     p. cm.
    Includes bibliographical references and index.
    ISBN 1-57340-121-8
     1. Psychiatry. 2. Mental illness—Diagnosis. 3. Mental illness—
Treatment. I. Baxter, Lewis R., 1952– . II. Friedel, Robert O.
1936– .
    [DNLM: 1. Mental Disorders—diagnosis. 2. Mental Disorders—
therapy. 3. Psychotherapy. WM 141C976 1998]
    RC454.C83 1998
    616.89—dc21
    DNLM/DLC
    for Library of Congress   98-39106
                                   CIP

Library of Congress
Cataloging-in-Publication Data

ISSN: 1521-0243
ISBN: 0-683-30772-X

Printed in the United States by Edwards Brothers
10 9 8 7 6 5 4 3 2 1

Although every effort has been made to ensure that the drug doses and other information are presented accurately in
this publication, the ultimate responsibility rests with the prescribing physician. Neither the publisher nor the authors
can be held responsible for errors or for any consequences arising from the use of the information contained herein.
Products mentioned in this publication should be used in accordance with the manufacturers' prescribing information.
No claims or endorsements are made for any drug or compound at present under clinical investigation.

Distributed worldwide by Williams & Wilkins.

Childhood disorders

SECTION EDITOR

Lee I. Ascherman, MD
Associate Professor of Psychiatry
Department of Child and
Adolescent Psychiatry
University of Alabama at Birmingham
Birmingham, Alabama

CONTRIBUTORS

William S. Chitwood, MD
Resident
Department of Psychiatry
University of Alabama at Birmingham
Birmingham, Alabama

Jane L. Daw, MD
Associate Professor of Psychiatry
Department of Child and Adolescent Psychiatry
University of Alabama at Birmingham
Birmingham, Alabama

Kyle Y. Echols, MD
Resident
Department of Psychiatry
University of Alabama at Birmingham
Birmingham, Alabama

Vivian Katzenstein Friedman, PhD
Associate Professor of Psychiatry
Department of Child and Adolescent Psychiatry
University of Alabama at Birmingham
Birmingham, Alabama

Jane M. Gregoritch, MD
Assistant Professor of Human Genetics and Pediatrics
Department of Pediatrics
University of Alabama at Birmingham
Birmingham, Alabama

Elizabeth Lachman, MD
Resident
Department of Psychiatry and Behavioral Neurobiology
University of Alabama at Birmingham
Birmingham, Alabama

Charles M. McInteer, MD
Resident
Department of Psychiatry and Behavioral Neurobiology
University of Alabama at Birmingham
Birmingham, Alabama

Donald A. Paoletti, MD
Associate Professor of Psychiatry
Department of Child and Adolescent Psychiatry
University of Alabama at Birmingham
Birmingham, Alabama

Janice Kay Sandy, MD
Resident
Department of Psychiatry
University of Alabama at Birmingham
Birmingham, Alabama

Margaret Scalise, MD
Assistant Professor of Psychiatry
Department of Psychiatry
University of Alabama at Birmingham
Birmingham, Alabama

Lee Tolbert, PhD
Associate Professor of Psychiatry
Department of Psychiatry and Behavioral Neurobiology
University of Alabama at Birmingham School of Medicine
Birmingham, Alabama

Jon Williamson, MD
Resident
Department of Psychiatry
University of Alabama at Birmingham
Birmingham, Alabama

CONTRIBUTORS

Deliria and other medicopsychiatric disorders

SECTION EDITOR

John Lee Shuster, MD
Associate Professor of Psychiatry
Psychiatric Consultation and Liaison
University of Alabama at Birmingham
Birmingham, Alabama

CONTRIBUTORS

R. Lawrence DePalma, MD
Assistant Professor
Department of Psychiatry and Behavioral Neurobiology
University of Alabama at Birmingham;
Medical/Surgical Psychiatry Program
Birmingham, Alabama

Marc D. Feldman, MD
Associate Professor
Department of Psychiatry and Behavioral Neurobiology
University of Alabama at Birmingham;
University of Alabama at Birmingham Center for
    Psychiatric Medicine
Birmingham, Alabama

Douglas A. Sargent, MD
Professor
Department of Psychiatry and Behavioral Neurobiology
University of Alabama at Birmingham;
University of Alabama at Birmingham Hospital
Birmingham, Alabama

Nathan B. Smith, MD
Associate Professor of Psychiatry
Department of Psychiatry
University of Alabama at Birmingham
Birmingham, Alabama

Adrian Hal Thurstin, MD
Associate Professor
Department of Psychiatry
University of Alabama at Birmingham
Birmingham, Alabama

Dementias

SECTION EDITOR

F. Cleveland Kinney, MD, PhD
Director of Geriatric Psychiatry
Associate Professor
Department of Psychiatry and
Behavioral Neurobiology
University of Alabama at Birmingham;
Center for Psychiatric Medicine
Birmingham, Alabama

CONTRIBUTORS

Marilyn E. Lachman, MD
Senior Resident in Psychiatry
Department of Psychiatry
University of Alabama at Birmingham School of Medicine
Birmingham, Alabama

Alan D. Piha, MD
Assistant Professor of Psychiatry
Department of Psychiatry
University of Alabama at Birmingham School of Medicine
Birmingham, Alabama

Richard E. Powers, MD
Associate Professor
Department of Pathology
University of Alabama at Birmingham
Birmingham, Alabama

Terri S. Steele, MD
Assistant Professor of Psychiatry
Department of Psychiatry
University of Alabama School of Medicine
Birmingham, Alabama

Andree Stoves, MD
Chief Resident in Psychiatry
Department of Psychiatry
University of Alabama at Birmingham School of Medicine
Birmingham, Alabama

Adrian Hal Thurstin, PhD
Associate Professor
Department of Psychiatry
University of Alabama at Birmingham
Birmingham, Alabama

Mood and anxiety disorders

SECTION EDITOR

Jack G. Modell, MD
Professor
  Department of Psychiatry and
    Behavioral Neurobiology
  University of Alabama at Birmingham
  Birmingham, Alabama

CONTRIBUTORS

Shambhavi Chandraiah, MD
Assistant Professor
  Department of Psychiatry and Behavioral Neurobiology
  University of Alabama at Birmingham;
  University of Alabama at Birmingham
    Neuropsychiatry Clinic
  Birmingham, Alabama

R. Lawrence DePalma, MD
Assistant Professor
  Department of Psychiatry and Behavioral Neurobiology
  University of Alabama at Birmingham;
  Medical/Surgical Psychiatry Program
  Birmingham, Alabama

Carl Houck, MD
Assistant Professor
  Department of Psychiatry and Behavioral Neurobiology
  University of Alabama at Birmingham
  Birmingham, Alabama

Marilyn E. Lachman, MD
Senior Resident in Psychiatry
  Department of Psychiatry
  University of Alabama at Birmingham School of Medicine
  Birmingham, Alabama

Charles M. McInteer, MD
Resident
  Department of Psychiatry and Behavioral Neurobiology
  University of Alabama at Birmingham
  Birmingham, Alabama

F. Robert Peluso, DO
Resident
  Department of Psychiatry
  Nova-Southeastern University;
  University of Alabama/Smolian Clinic
  Birmingham, Alabama

Renee Roddam Richeson, MD
Chief Resident
  Department of Psychiatry and Behavioral Neurobiology
  University of Alabama at Birmingham;
  University of Alabama at Birmingham Hospital;
Staff Psychiatrist
  New Life Clinics
  Birmingham, Alabama

William G. Ryan, MD
Associate Professor
  Department of Psychiatry and Behavioral Neurobiology
  University of Alabama at Birmingham;
  University of Alabama at Birmingham Hospital
  Birmingham, Alabama

Douglas A. Sargent, MD
Professor
  Department of Psychiatry and Behavioral Neurobiology
  University of Alabama at Birmingham;
  University of Alabama at Birmingham Hospital
  Birmingham, Alabama

Patricia T. White, MA
Intern
  Department of Psychiatry and Behavioral Neurobiology
  University of Alabama at Birmingham
  Birmingham, Alabama

Neuropsychiatric disorders

SECTION EDITOR

Leon Sebring Dure, MD
Associate Professor of Pediatrics
  Department of Pediatrics
  University of Alabama at Birmingham
  Birmingham, Alabama

CONTRIBUTORS

Lewis R. Baxter, Jr, MD
*Kathy Ireland Professor of Psychiatric Research and
Professor of Neurobiology*
  Department of Psychiatry and Behavioral Neurobiology
  University of Alabama at Birmingham School of Medicine
  Birmingham, Alabama

Jane M. Gregoritch, MD
Assistant Professor of Human Genetics and Pediatrics
  University of Alabama at Birmingham
  Birmingham, Alabama

Anthony Nicholas, MD, PhD
Assistant Professor of Neurology
  University of Alabama at Birmingham School of Medicine
  Birmingham, Alabama

Alan Percy, MD
Bew White Professor of Pediatrics
Professor of Neurology
  Department of Pediatrics
  University of Alabama at Birmingham School of Medicine
  Birmingham, Alabama

Lee Tolbert, PhD
Associate Professor of Psychiatry
  University of Alabama at Birmingham School of Medicine
  Birmingham, Alabama

Merill Wise, MD
Assistant Professor of Pediatrics and Neurology
  Baylor College of Medicine
  Houston, Texas

Ditza Zachor, MD
Assistant Professor of Pediatrics
  Department of Pediatrics
  University of Alabama at Birmingham School of Medicine
  Birmingham, Alabama

Nonschizophrenic and non-mood-related psychoses

SECTION EDITOR

William G. Ryan, MD
Associate Professor
Department of Psychiatry and Behavioral
Neurobiology
University of Alabama at Birmingham;
University of Alabama at Birmingham Hospital
Birmingham, Alabama

CONTRIBUTORS

Jennifer L. Grant, MSW
Instructor
Department of Psychiatry and Behavioral Neurobiology
University of Alabama at Birmingham Community
Psychiatry Program
Birmingham, Alabama

Praveen Jetty, MD, MRC
Resident
Department of Psychiatry and Behavioral Neurobiology
University of Alabama at Birmingham Hospital
Birmingham, Alabama

Meza Kelly, MSW, CSW
Assistant Professor
Department of Psychiatry and Behavioral Neurobiology
University of Alabama at Birmingham;
University of Alabama at Birmingham Hospital
Birmingham, Alabama

Lindsay Ann Levine, MD
Assistant Professor
Department of Psychiatry and Behavioral Neurobiology
University of Alabama at Birmingham;
University of Alabama at Birmingham Center for
Psychiatric Medicine
Birmingham, Alabama

Clemmie Lee Palmer III, MD
Resident
Department of Psychiatry and Behavioral Neurobiology
University of Alabama at Birmingham Hospital
Birmingham, Alabama

Renee Roddam Richeson, MD
Chief Resident
Department of Psychiatry and Behavioral Neurobiology
University of Alabama at Birmingham;
University of Alabama at Birmingham Hospital;
Staff Psychiatrist
New Life Clinics
Birmingham, Alabama

Robert M. Savage, PhD
Assistant Professor
Department of Psychiatry and Behavioral Neurobiology
University of Alabama at Birmingham;
University of Alabama at Birmingham Hospital
Birmingham, Alabama

Paraphilic disorders

SECTION EDITOR

Sheryl R. Jackson, PhD
Assistant Professor
Department of Psychiatry and Behavioral
Neurobiology
University of Alabama at Birmingham
Birmingham, Alabama

CONTRIBUTORS

Warran T. Jackson, PhD
Assistant Professor
Department of Psychiatry and Behavioral Neurobiology
University of Alabama at Birmingham
Birmingham, Alabama

Nicole Siegfried Mason, MS
Psychology Intern
Department of Psychology
University of Alabama at Birmingham
Birmingham, Alabama

Steven A. Montgomery, MD
Psychiatry Resident
Department of Psychiatry and Behavioral Neurobiology
University of Alabama at Birmingham;
University of Alabama at Birmingham Hospital
Birmingham, Alabama

Patricia T. White, MA
Intern
Department of Psychiatry and Behavioral Neurobiology
University of Alabama at Birmingham
Birmingham, Alabama

CONTRIBUTORS

Personality and impulse disorders

SECTION EDITOR

Charles V. Ford, MD
Professor of Psychiatry
Department of Adult Psychiatry
University of Alabama at Birmingham
Birmingham, Alabama

CONTRIBUTORS

Rachael Fargason, MD
Assistant Professor of Psychiatry
University of Alabama at Birmingham School
of Medicine
Birmingham, Alabama

Robert O. Friedel, MD
Heman Drummond Professor
Chair
Department of Psychiatry
University of Alabama at Birmingham School
of Medicine
Birmingham, Alabama

James N. Hall, MD
Staff Psychiatrist
New Life Clinics
Birmingham, Alabama

Nicole Mason, MD
Psychology Intern
University of Alabama at Birmingham
Training Consortium
Birmingham, Alabama

Andree Stoves, MD
Chief Resident in Psychiatry
Department of Psychiatry
University of Alabama at Birmingham School
of Medicine
Birmingham, Alabama

Schizophrenias and related psychoses

SECTION EDITOR

Jacqueline Feldman, MD
Associate Professor
Department of Psychiatry and Behavioral
Neurobiology
University of Alabama at Birmingham;
University of Alabama at Birmingham Hospital
Birmingham, Alabama

CONTRIBUTORS

Lynne S. Goldsmith, MSW
Associate Professor
Department of Psychiatry and Behavioral Neurobiology
University of Alabama at Birmingham;
University of Alabama at Birmingham
Community Psychiatry Program
Birmingham, Alabama

Sue C. Irwin, MSW
Instructor
Department of Psychiatry and Behavioral Neurobiology
University of Alabama at Birmingham;
University of Alabama at Birmingham Community
Psychiatry Program
Birmingham, Alabama

F. Cleveland Kinney, MD, PhD
Director of Geriatric Psychiatry
Associate Professor
Department of Psychiatry and Behavioral Neurobiology
University of Alabama at Birmingham;
Center for Psychiatric Medicine
Birmingham, Alabama

James M. Ledbetter, MSW
Instructor
Department of Psychiatry and Behavioral Neurobiology
University of Alabama at Birmingham;
University of Alabama at Birmingham Hospital
Birmingham, Alabama

Cheryl Patton, LCSW
Program Coordinator
Department of Psychiatry and Behavioral Neurobiology
University of Alabama at Birmingham;
Day Treatment Coordinator
University of Alabama at Birmingham Hospital
Birmingham, Alabama

Robert M. Savage, PhD
Assistant Professor
Department of Psychiatry and Behavioral Neurobiology
University of Alabama at Birmingham;
University of Alabama at Birmingham Hospital
Birmingham, Alabama

Wlliam F. Walker, MD
Medical Social Worker
Department of Psychiatry and Behavioral Neurobiology
University of Alabama at Birmingham;
University of Alabama at Birmingham Community
Psychiatry Program
Birmingham, Alabama

Sexual dysfunctions

SECTION EDITORS

Sheryl R. Jackson, PhD
Assistant Professor

Department of Psychiatry and Behavioral
Neurobiology
University of Alabama at Birmingham
Birmingham, Alabama

Jack G. Modell, MD
Professor

Department of Psychiatry and Behavioral
Neurobiology
University of Alabama at Birmingham
Birmingham, Alabama

CONTRIBUTORS

Jane Forsythe Brown, MA
Associate Professor
Department of Psychiatry and Behavioral Neurobiology
University of Alabama at Birmingham;
Sexual Health Clinic
Birmingham, Alabama

Steven A. Montgomery, MD
Psychiatry Resident
Department of Psychiatry and Behavioral Neurobiology
University of Alabama at Birmingham;
University of Alabama at Birmingham Hospital
Birmingham, Alabama

Substance abuse

SECTION EDITOR

Sandra L. Frazier, MD
Assistant Professor
Department of Psychiatry and Behavioral Neurobiology
University of Alabama at Birmingham;
University of Alabama at Birmingham
Addiction Recovery Program
Birmingham, Alabama

CONTRIBUTORS

William F. Barker, MA
Counselor Substance Abuse I
University of Alabama at Birmingham
Addiction Recovery Program
Birmingham, Alabama

Sharon Douglas, RN
Staff Nurse
University of Alabama at Birmingham
Addiction Recovery Program
Birmingham, Alabama

John R. Encizo, MA
Counselor Substance Abuse II
University of Alabama at Birmingham
Addiction Recovery Program
Birmingham, Alabama

Steve Moore, BSW
Continuing Care Counselor
University of Alabama at Birmingham
Addiction Recovery Program
Birmingham, Alabama

Abbey J. Parris, MA
Program Manager
Addiction Recovery Program
Department of Psychiatry and Behavioral Neurobiology
University of Alabama at Birmingham
Birmingham, Alabama

Kelly E. Wilson, MEd
Counselor Substance Abuse I
University of Alabama at Birmingham
Addiction Recovery Program
Birmingham, Alabama

Adrianne D. Young, MA
Program Coordinator II
University of Alabama at Birmingham
Addiction Recovery Program
Birmingham, Alabama

This *Current Psychiatric Diagnosis & Treatment*, like its companion volumes covering other medical specialties, is not designed to provide detailed knowledge of psychiatric disorders, but rather to help practicing physicians and students remember key points of diagnoses and treatments for entities they might not manage daily. Therefore, it may be useful to nonpsychiatrists as well as to psychiatrists. It also serves to alert all practitioners to recent developments in psychiatric diagnoses and treatment, and notes more in-depth references that are readily available, thus helping the specialist. The format is designed for ease of use by psychiatrists or nonpsychiatrists.

More so in psychiatry than in other fields of medicine, maladies are listed in this and other texts by what is committee-derived as "official" nomenclature—the *Diagnostic and Statistical Manual, edn 4* (DSM-IV), of the American Psychiatric Association. Using DSM-IV terminology does not imply that we believe these are in fact true pathophysiologic entities; we do not, and in some cases have strayed from the DSM-IV headings. DSM-IV does provide a common reference language, however, and is at present the best we have. We hope that future editions of this *Current Psychiatric Diagnosis & Treatment* will employ different categories, reflecting advances in psychopathophysiology.

Lewis R. Baxter, Jr
Robert O. Friedel

CONTENTS

CONTENTS

CONTENTS BY SPECIALTY

CONTENTS BY SPECIALTY

This book provides current expert recommendations on the diagnosis and treatment of all major disorders throughout psychiatry in the form of tabular summaries. Essential guidelines on each of the topics have been condensed into two pages of vital information, summarizing the main procedures in diagnosis and management of each disorder to provide a quick and easy reference.

Each disorder is presented as a "spread" of two facing pages: the main procedures in diagnosis on the left and treatment options on the right.

Listed in the main column of the Diagnosis page are the common symptoms, signs, and complications of the disorder, with brief notes explaining their significance and probability of occurrence, together with details of investigations that can be used to aid diagnosis.

The left shaded side column contains information to help the reader evaluate the probability that an individual patient has the disorder. It may also include other information that could be useful in making a diagnosis (*eg*, classification or grading systems, comparison of different diagnostic methods).

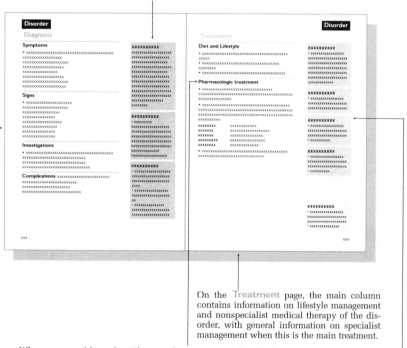

On the Treatment page, the main column contains information on lifestyle management and nonspecialist medical therapy of the disorder, with general information on specialist management when this is the main treatment.

Whenever possible under "Pharmacologic treatment," guidelines are given on the standard dosage for commonly used drugs, with details of contraindications and precautions, main drug interactions, and main side effects. In each case, however, the manufacturer's drug data sheet should be consulted before any regimen is prescribed.

The main goals of treatment (*eg*, to cure, to palliate, to prevent), prognosis after treatment, precautions that the physician should take during and after treatment, and any other information that could help the clinician to make treatment decisions (*eg*, other nonpharmacologic treatment options, special situations or groups of patients) are given in the right shaded side column. The key and general references at the end of this column provide the reader with further practical information.

Diagnosis

Definition
• The essential feature of an adjustment disorder is the development of clinically significant emotional or behavioral symptoms in response to identifiable psychosocial stressor(s). The symptoms must develop within 3 months after the onset of the stressor(s). The clinical significance of the reactions are indicated either by marked distress out of proportion to the nature of the stressor or by significant impairment in social, occupational, or academic functioning [1].
• In acute adjustment disorder, symptoms develop within 3 months of the precipitating stressor and last no more than 6 months beyond its cessation.
• In chronic adjustment disorder, symptoms persist 6 months or longer in association with an ongoing stressor or consequences thereof.

Signs and Symptoms
• Symptom patterns include conduct disorders that occur alone or with anxiety and/or depression.

General
Preoccupation, distraction.

Awareness, self-consciousness about instability: may lack insight and project responsibility for their difficulties upon others.

With depressed mood
Signs: sad facies, tearfulness, irritability, insomnia, mild cognitive impairment, difficulty with decision making.

Symptoms: sadness, morbid preoccupation, irritability, insomnia, and feelings of hopefulness.

With anxiety
Signs: anxious facies, restlessness, jitteriness, tachycardia, exaggerated startle, hyperalertness, and poor concentration.

Symptoms: anxious mood, apprehensiveness, worry, fear of separation from major attachment figures.

With anxiety and depressed mood
• Diagnosis is made when predominant symptomatology is a combination of depression and anxiety.

With disturbance of conduct
Uncharacteristic implosive conduct that violates the rights of others or societal norms: *eg,* fighting, truancy, substance abuse, and driving; appears following the precipitating event.

Mixed disturbance of emotion and conduct
• Diagnosis made when predominant symptomatology includes both emotional and behavioral symptoms.

Investigations
• Query patients about possible self-medication with alcohol or drugs.

Complications
Adjustment disorders: may be provoked by seemingly mild stressors in some individuals because of specific individual sensitivity, especially when the stressor resembles or replicates childhood trauma (*eg,* abandonment, loss, humiliation, etc.); although not dramatically disabling, adjustment disorders that are precipitated by severely traumatic or terrorizing stressors may cause significant suffering and disability.

Increased risk of suicide: in the absence of adequate social support, adjustment disorder is more likely to become overwhelming for the patient.

Differential diagnosis
• The stressor is usually mild to moderately severe in contrast with the usual more severe stressors preceding acute or posttraumatic disorders.
• Distress and disability are not usually severe.
• The diagnosis should not be made in the presence of another Axis I disorder (eg, major depression, bereavement, etc.).
• The primary depressive and anxiety disorders usually have a less specific precipitant or stressor.
• In contrast to a normal response to a stressor, adjustment reactions are characterized by unusually intense or persistent functionally significant responses.
• Unlike personality disorder, onset is fairly acute, and symptoms are uncharacteristic for the patient.

Etiology
• Adjustment disorder is caused by a specific precipitating psychosocial stressor that is exacerbated by individual vulnerability or idiosyncrasy or by preexisting mental disorder.
• Precipitants include any stressful single occurrences or life circumstance that cause an individual marked distress either because the stress is especially disruptive or recurring or because it exacerbates vulnerabilities (eg, family dysfunction, marital distress, job stress, recent loss, pregnancy, individual parturition [especially with bad outcome], and infant care).

Epidemiology
• Adjustment disorders are found in 5%–20% of psychiatric outpatients, although the true incidence in the general population is unknown. Many victims of war or other disasters, short of developing full acute or traumatic stress disorder, may develop adjustment disorders. Morbidity is affected by type, intensity, persistence, and recurrence of stressor(s) as well as by vulnerability to stressor(s) and relief or treatment.

Treatment

General information
• Most adjustment disorders improve as the precipitating stressor resolves. Treatment, however, may shorten the duration and intensity of symptoms as well as decrease the chance for progression to a more chronic condition.

Diet and lifestyle
• Resolve contributing stressors as much as possible.
• Encourage adequate exercise, sleep, and family and social support.

Pharmacologic treatment
• Medications are not generally required unless necessary for short-term management of anxiety (eg, low-dose benzodiazepines [given as necessary]) or insomnia (eg, benzodiazepines, zolpidem, trazodone [occasionally], other antidepressants [infrequently]).

Nonpharmacologic treatment
Psychotherapy
• Both individual and group psychotherapy may be effective.

• Primary goals are 1) to help the individual understand his or her role in the precipitating event(s), if any; 2) to teach ways of avoiding the same situations or mistakes in the future; 3) to make patients see stressor and current problems as positive opportunities for change or improvement; 4) to encourage a balanced perspective of the problems in the context of the individual's life and indicate positive aspects thereof; and 5) to understand the reasons for the patient's particular sensitivity to the stressor.

• Intensive therapies are not usually required for this disorder. The general practitioner can have a very positive impact on symptoms simply by listening to the patient and attending to the above.

Treatment aims
• See Nonpharmacologic treatment.

Prognosis
• Most cases resolve within 6 mo because the stressor wanes, and the patient learns to understand, cope with, and overcome any residual effects of the stressors. Without treatment, the risk of progression to major depression or anxiety disorder increases. Outcome depends on the nature, persistence, and severity of the precipitating stressor; the patient's motivation for improvement; and the degree of family and social support.

Follow-up and management
• Relatively brief psychotherapies are often effective. Occasionally, an individual may wish to continue psychotherapy longer-term, during which time it is recognized that the patient's reactions to the initial stressor were a reflection of more general, underlying conflict that is best understood and resolved to prevent further adverse impact on the patient's emotions and behavior.
• The patient should be instructed that symptoms usually resolve after several weeks to months. If symptoms do not resolve, further evaluation and possible longer-term treatment should be sought.
• Medications for anxiety or insomnia should be gradually tapered and discontinued as symptoms and functional impairment wane.

General references
Diagnostic and Statistical Manual of Mental Disorders, ed 4. Washington, DC: American Psychiatric Association; 1994.

Despland JN, Monod L, Ferrero F: Clinical relevance of adjustment disorder in DSM-III and DSM-IV. Compr Psychiatry 1995, 36:454–460.

Greenberg WM, Rosenfeld DN, Ortega EA: Adjustment disorder as an admission diagnosis. Am J Psychiatry 1995, 152:459–461.

Kaplan HI, Sadock BJ (eds): Adjustment Disorders. In Comprehensive Textbook of Psychiatry, ed 6. Baltimore: Williams & Wilkins; 1995:1418–1424.

Kovacs M, Ho V, Pollock NM: Criterion and predictive validity of the diagnosis of adjustment disorder: a prospective study of youths with new-onset insulin-dependent diabetes mellitus. Am J Psychiatry 1995, 152:523–528.

Diagnosis

Definitions

• Alcohol dependence is a primary, chronic disease with genetic, psychosocial, and environmental factors influencing its development. It is characterized by impaired control over drinking, preoccupation with the drug alcohol, use of alcohol despite adverse consequences, and distortions in thinking (most notably denial).

• Alcohol abuse is the use of alcohol that interferes with a person's overall functioning and usually evolves into dependence.

Symptoms

Preoccupation with drinking.

Gulping the first two or three drinks.

Loss of interest in nondrinking activities.

Increased tolerance.

Repeated attempts to stop drinking.

Blackouts.

Alcohol-related arrests.

Poor hygiene.

Mood swings.

Job problems.

Signs

• Advanced stages of alcoholism (cirrhosis, ascites) are familiar to most physicians. The challenge is in recognizing alcoholism early in its course. Clues include slurred speech, alcohol on the breath, multiple bruises, sedation, untidiness, hypertension, ataxia, peptic ulcers, gout.

Investigations

• Laboratory studies can be helpful but by themselves are not definitive in making a diagnosis of alcoholism. Liver enzymes, mean copuscular volume, uric acid, and triglycerides are often elevated in alcoholics. Likewise, leukocyte count, hemoglobin, and platelet counts are at times decreased in the alcoholic patient.

• A thorough and detailed biopsychosocial history is of primary importance in diagnosing alcohol abuse and dependence. Important areas to cover include the following:

Quantity, frequency, and onset of use.

Marital or relationship problems.

Occupational history.

Legal history.

Financial status.

Family history of alcoholism.

Psychiatric or psychologic history.

Complications

• Alcohol dependence is a biopsychosocial disease; therefore, complications can be seen in all areas of the alcoholic patient's life.

Biologic: liver disease, hypertension, dementia, peripheral neruopathy, pancreatitis.

Psychologic: depression, anxiety, guilt.

Social: divorce, legal problems, motor vehicle accidents, occupational problems.

Differential diagnosis

• Many medical and psychiatric disorders caused by the use of alcohol are treated as primary disorders without discovering their true cause. Alcohol dependence can be the cause of such common disorders as hypertension, peptic ulcer disease, anemia, depression, anxiety, and insomnia. Physicians, therefore, must maintain a high index of suspicion.

Etiology

• The etiology is multifactorial (genetic, environmental, social).
• Males of alcoholic fathers are at highest risk.
• Offspring of alcoholic parents have a fourfold higher risk.
• Comorbid, psychiatric illness increases risk.

Epidemiology

• In the US, 17.8 million abuse alcohol, and 50.5 million are alcoholics.
• Alcohol abuse and dependence costs $130–$140 billion per year.
• Thirty-nine percent of fatal automobile accidents are related to alcohol abuse.
• Sixty-nine percent of drownings are related to alcohol.
• Alcoholism decreases life expectancy by 10–12 y of age.
• Approximately 200,000 deaths per year are related to alcohol abuse.

Treatment

Diet and lifestyle

- The alcoholic patient is encouraged to make lifestyle changes such as establishing an exercise routine and maintaining proper nutrition in order to enhance the recovery process.

Pharmacologic treatment

- After detoxification is complete, some individuals may benefit from short-term trials of medication to increase their likelihood of abstinence.

Disulfram

Standard dosage	125–500 mg daily for 7 days, then 250 mg daily for 1–2 years, to be initiated a minimum of 12 hours after the last drink.
Contraindications:	Not to be given in patients with heart disease, psychosis, pregnancy, chronic liver disease, or cognitive impairment.
Main side effects	Side effects are usually mild and consist of fatigue, somnolence, headache, dizziness, and a garlic-like taste in the mouth. Most of these disappear in 1–2 weeks. An idosyncratic disulfram-induced hepatitis, which is potentially fatal, is rare.
Main drug interactions	May intensify the effects of anesthetics, sedative hypnotics, phenytoin, and coumadin; generally, reducing the disulfram dose to 250 mg three times per week is adequate.
Special points	Reactions to alcohol continue to occur up to 5–7 days after the drug is discontinued.
	Common products containing alcohol (mouth washes, shave lotions, cough medicines) should be avoided.
	The disulfram–ethanol reaction (flushing, nausea or vomiting, headache, and chest pain) is largely treated supportively.

Naltrexone

- Naltrexone is an opiate antagonist that can enhance abstinence.

Standard dosage	50 mg daily for 12 weeks in an opiate-abstinent patient.
Contraindications	Individuals taking opiate medication, individuals with liver disease (hepatitis, elevated liver enzymes, liver failure).
Main side effects	Nausea, vomiting, headache; may be hepatotoxic at high doses.
Main drug interactions	Can precipitate severe withdrawal in persons taking opiate agonists.
Special points	Monitor liver enzymes monthly; simultaneous participation in a treatment program or support group is mandatory.

Nonpharmacologic treatment

- Nonpharmacologic management is the mainstay of treatment for the alcohol-dependent individual. The following options are available: inpatient treatment, outpatient treatment, therapeutic communities, halfway houses, and support groups such as Alcoholics Anonymous and Rational Recovery. Physicians should be aware of local community resources in order to ensure proper access to treatment for the alcoholic patient.

Treatment aims

To maintain abstinence from alcohol.
To develop a support network.
To recognize relapse triggers.

Prognosis

- Recovery is a lifelong process. Individuals who accept this fact and work a daily program of recovery have a good prognosis. Factors that improve prognosis include family involvement in treatment, posttreatment monitoring program (eg, urine drug screening), and a supportive home environment.

Follow up and management

- Because alcohol dependence is a lifelong disease, its treatment is lifelong. Key follow up elements include the following:
Attendance at support group meetings.
Identification of relapse triggers.
Establishment of strong network of support for recovery.
Regular contact with primary care physician.

Alcoholics Anonymous

- Meetings are located throughout the world.
- Local phone directories provide listings.
- Attendance is free.

General references

Aronson MD: Alcoholism: Definition, Epidemiology, and Diagnosis. Alcoholism: Recognition of the Disease and Considerations for Patient Care 1995, 8–13.

Bradley KA: The primary care practitioner's role in the prevention and management of alcohol problems. Alcohol Health Rev World 1994, 18:97–104.

Kaplan HI, Sadock BJ: Disorders associated with alcoholism. Pocket Handbook of Clinical Psychiatry 1990, 50–56.

Kesser C, et al.: Detoxification, principles and protocals. Topics in Addiction Medicine 1995, 1–10.

Milhorn TH: Chemical Dependence. New York: Springer Verlag; 1990:19–21, 124–144.

Diagnosis

Definition

• Alcohol withdrawal syndrome is the development of physical and psychologic signs and symptoms in response to the abrupt reduction or discontinuation of alcohol in an individual in whom dependence is established. It is marked by interpatient variability.

• Detoxification is the process by which an alcohol-addicted person returns to normal physical and mental functioning.

Symptoms

Symptoms of alcohol withdrawal syndrome by stage

Stage*	Time after alcohol consumption, h	Symptoms
1	24–48†	Mild-to-moderate anxiety, tremor, nausea, vomiting, sweating, elevation of heart rate and blood pressure, sleep disturbance, hallucinations, illusions, seizures
2	48–72	Aggravated forms of stage 1 symptoms with severe tremors, agitation, and hallucinations
3	72–105	Acute organic psychosis (delirium), confusion, and disorientation with severe autonomic symptoms

* Stage 1 withdrawal is usually self-limited. Only a small percentage of cases progress to stages 2 and 3. Progression is prevented by prompt and adequate treatment.
† Peak incidence of withdrawal symptoms occurs at 36 h.

Differential diagnosis

Systemic infection.
Seizure disorder.
Psychiatric disorder (psychosis, dementia).
Diabetic ketoacidosis.

Epidemiology

• Grand mal seizures accompany alcohol withdrawal in 10%–15% of patients.
• Delirium tremens is relatively rare.
• The mortality rate associated with delirium tremens is 1%–5%.

Predictors of alcohol withdrawal severity

Prior history of severe withdrawal symptoms.
High blood alcohol level without signs of intoxication.
Withdrawal signs with high blood alcohol level.
Concurrent use of sedative-hypnotics.
Coexisting medical problems.

Investigations

History: if possible, it is important to elicit a detailed alcohol-use history as well as past history of any withdrawal signs and symptoms.

Physical examination: a thorough examination is necessary to diagnose possible underlying medical conditions; because alcoholics are susceptible to subdural hematomas and concussions, focus on identifying signs of trauma.

Laboratory studies: Complete blood count with differential, electrolytes (including magnesium and calcium), liver transaminases, blood urea nitrogen and creatinine, prothrombin time and partial thromboplastin time, vitamin B_{12} and folate levels, urinalysis, urine drug screen, electrocardiogram, chest radiography.

Other possible tests: amylase, ammonia, hepatitis screen.

Complications

Alcohol withdrawal seizures: accompany alcohol withdrawal in 10%–15% of patients; such seizures are generalized tonic-clonic and usually appear within the first 48 hours but may be seen up to 10 days following the last drink; always evaluate for other causes of seizure; long-term treatment with anticonvulsants is not recommended for alcohol withdrawal seizures.

Delirium tremens: delirium, marked autonomic hyperactivity, agitation, tremor, hallucinations; usually begin 72 hours after the last drink.

Wernicke's encephalopathy: ataxia, ophthalmoplegia, and confusion.

Korsakoff's psychosis: irreversible brain damage, mainly loss of recent memory.

Treatment

General information

• All therapies must be individualized to specific patients' needs and adjusted appropriately to their response to treatment. Every means possible should be used to ameliorate withdrawal signs and symptoms. Inadequately treated withdrawal can have a cumulative effect and worsen subsequent withdrawals (a phenomenon known as kindling).

Pharmacologic treatment

Basic guidelines

• Monitor vital signs every 4 hours.

• Give thiamine, 100 mg i.m. initially, then 100 mg orally per day for 2 days. Give thiamine prior to glucose load to prevent precipitation of Wernicke–Korsakoff syndrome.

• Correct electrolyte imbalances.

• Give daily multivitamin.

• Provide medication for adequate sleep.

• Treatment of delirium tremens is usually a medical emergency and requires critical care monitoring.

Benzodiazepines

• Use a cross-tolerant benzodiazepine, *eg*, chlordiazepoxide. (Librium)

Standard dosage	25–100 mg orally every 4–6 hours as needed for increased vital signs, tremors; after stabilized, taper chlordiazepoxide by 20%–25% per day.
Contraindications	Long-acting benzodiazepines are contraindicated in individuals with severe liver dysfunction; only oxazepam and lorazepam are not metabolized by the liver.
Main side effects	Benzodiazepines are relatively safe; the most common side effects are sedation, ataxia.
Main drug interactions	Benzodiazepines are cross tolerant and thus synergistic with alcohol and sedative hypnotics; use with caution in intoxicated individuals or in individuals on high doses of sedative-hypnotics.
Special points	Shorter-acting benzodiazepines should be used in elderly patients and those with liver disease; avoid treatment until blood alcohol level falls below 150%; in medically stable patients with supportive home environments, detoxification can often be conducted on an outpatient basis.

Treatment aims

To provide a safe withdrawal from alcohol. To provide a withdrawal that is humane and that protects the patient's dignity. To prepare the patient for ongoing treatment of his or her dependence.

Prognosis

• Untreated cessation of drinking may result in withdrawal delirium, seizures, marked hyperautonomic signs, or death.
• The mortality rate associated with delirium tremens is 1%–5% and increases with delayed diagnosis, inadequate treatment, and concurrent medical conditions.

Follow-up and management

• After detoxification is complete, the alcohol-dependent patient should be referred to treatment and support groups.
• Disulfram or naltrexone may be helpful in maintaining abstinence.

Examples of structured regimens

Chlordiazepoxide, 50 mg every 6 h for 8 doses, then 25 mg every 6 h for 4 doses; hold any dose for excess sedation. Chlordiazepoxide, 50 mg every 4 h for 6 doses, then 50 mg every 6 h for 4 doses, then 25 mg every 6 h for 4 doses; hold any dose for excess sedation.

Examples of protocols for withdrawal delirium

Lorazepam, 1–4 mg i.v. every 5–15 min until calm, then as needed . Diazepam, 5–20 mg i.v. (maximum, 2.5 mg/min) every 5–15 min until calm, then as needed.

General references

Aronson MD: Alcoholism: definition, epidemiology, and diagnosis. In *Alcoholism: Recognition of the Disease and Considerations for Patient Care* 1992: 8–13.

Bradley KA: The primary care practitioner's role in the prevention and management of alcohol problems. *Alcohol Health Research Worlds* 1994, 18:97–104.

Kaplan HI, Sadock BJ: Disorders associated with alcoholism. In *Pocket Handbook of Clinical Psychiatry*. 1990; 50–56.

Kasser C, et al.: Detoxification: principles and protocols. *Topics in Addiction Medicine* 1995, 1–10.

Milhorn TH: *Chemical Dependence* 1990, 19–21, 124–144.

Diagnosis

Signs and symptoms

• Amnestic disorders are characterized by a predominant (and sometimes isolated) disturbance of memory functioning, with impairments in either the ability to learn new information or the ability to retrieve previously learned information or past events. The memory impairment must be severe enough to cause significant impairment and must not be attributable to other causes of cognitive disturbance (eg, dementia, delirium, intoxication). Some amnestic disorders are acute and transient disturbances of memory (eg, those due to intoxication, transient global amnesia, or mild head trauma), whereas others are chronic and persistent (eg, those due to anoxic injury or stroke).

Investigations

Thorough history: essential, with particular attention to the time course of the development of memory disturbance and any apparent precipitants of the memory disturbance.

Full mental status examination: necessary, especially a comprehensive assessment of cognitive functioning.

Physical examination: should also include a full neurologic exam; the need for other areas of focus in the physical examination, as well as clinical laboratory, neuropsychologic tests, and neuroimaging studies, depends on the suspected etiology of the memory disturbance; a work-up similar to that used for dementia should probably be pursued in most cases of suspected amnestic disorder that does not resolve quickly.

Complications

• The morbidity of significant and persistent memory loss, including effect on quality of life and ability to function without supervision, can be severe. Even for those whose amnesia resolves fairly rapidly, the condition can cause extreme worry about recurrence. Amnestic disorders may be a marker of a recurrent or progressive illness, or may progress to dementia. Specific complications depend on the underlying cause of the amnestic disorder.

Differential diagnosis

• Conditions that can cause a disturbance of memory and may mimic an amnestic disorder include:
Delirium.
Dementia.
Substance intoxication.
Depression.
Dissociative amnesia.
Malingering.
Factitious disorder.
Age-related cognitive decline.

Etiology

• Causes of memory disturbance consistent with an amnestic disorder include:
Acute and chronic sequelae of head injury.
Alcohol-induced persisting amnestic disorder (Wernicke–Korsakoff syndrome) and other substance-induced persisting amnestic disorders.
Alcoholic blackouts.
Benzodiazepines (especially triazolam).
Brain injury from anoxia, carbon monoxide poisoning, hypoglycemia, encephalitis, tumors.
Complex partial epilepsy.
Multiple sclerosis.
Post-stroke amnesia.
Post-electroconvulsive therapy (ECT) amnesia.
Transient global amnesia.

Epidemiology:

• Epidemiologic aspects of amnestic disorders as a category have not been well studied due to several factors, including the wide variety of etiologies of amnestic disorder, the high degree of overlap with other cognitive disorders, noncognitive mental disorders (eg, substance dependence), and the relatively low priority memory disturbance often receives in the settings in which it presents (eg, traumatic amnesia in the setting of multiple other traumatic injuries, amnesia caused by stroke or brain tumor). The most common cause of amnestic disorder is head injury for which ~500,000 people in the U.S. are hospitalized annually. There are an estimated 2.0–2.5 million more head injuries that do not lead to hospitalization in the U.S. each year. As many as 12.5% of all people with alcohol dependence may develop symptoms of Wernicke–Korsakoff syndrome.

Treatment

Diet and lifestyle

- A few causes of amnestic disorder are managed in part by dietary and lifestyle interventions.
- The treatment of Wernicke–Korsakoff Syndrome centers on replacement of thiamine.
- Amnestic disorders related to substance abuse or dependence will likely persist until substance use is reduced or discontinued.
- Lifestyles and recreational activities that place the individual at high risk for head injury may need to be altered or avoided to prevent progressive memory loss.

Pharmacologic treatment

- Little pharmacologic help is available to treat amnestic disorders directly; however the following pharmacologic measures may be quite effective in reducing the burden of memory loss indirectly:

Thiamine replacement: in Wernicke–Korsakoff syndrome.

Discontinuation of benzodiazepines: in benzodiazepine-induced persisting amnestic disorder.

Antiplatelet therapy: after a stroke.

Adequate antidepressant therapy: to minimize the risk that a patient with ECT-induced amnesia will require ECT treatments in the future.

Treatment aims
To detection of the underlying cause of the memory disturbance.
To reverse amnesia (or at least arresting its progress) whenever possible.
To aim rehabilitation at living well with persistent memory loss when reversal is not possible.

Prognosis
- The prognosis varies according to the etiology of the amnestic disorder.

Follow-up and management
- The follow-up and management varies according to the etiology of the amnestic disorder.
- If reversible causes of amnesia are discovered, their reversal should be the focus of initial treatment.
- In other cases, the degree of memory deficit may be fixed, but progression may be preventable through monitoring and therapeutic intervention.
- Periodic follow-up should be scheduled for monitoring of severity of memory disturbance and other associated symptoms.
- Mnemonic strategies, lists, and other reminders can aid the function of a patient with memory impairment.
- In some cases of chronic amnestic disorder, formal rehabilitation therapy aimed at adapting to and partially compensating for memory loss can be beneficial.
- Family members should be engaged in symptom monitoring and treatment over time.

General references
American Psychiatric Association: *Diagnostic and Statistical Manual of Mental Disorders*, ed 4. Washington, DC: American Psychiatric Press; 1994.

Brna TG, Wilson CC: Psychogenic amnesia. *Am Family Physician* 1990, 41:229–234.

Erickson KR: Amnestic disorders: pathophysiology and patterns of memory dysfunction. *Western J Med* 1990, 152:159–166.

Mayes AR: Memory and amnesia. *Behav Brain Res* 1995, 66:29–36.

Wise MG, Gray KF: Delirium, dementia, and amnestic disorders. In *The American Psychiatric Press Textbook of Psychiatry*, ed 2. Edited by Hales RE, Yudofsky SC, Talbott JA. Washington, DC: American Psychiatric Press; 1994:311–353.

Diagnosis

Definition

- The term "amphetamine" is used to refer to a large class of stimulants: amphetamines (black beauties, white bennies), dextroamphetamines (dexies, beans), and methamphetamines (crank, meth, crystal, speed); all are classified as schedule II drugs.

Amphetamine dependence

- Amphetamine dependence is defined as a destructive pattern of amphetamine use leading to significant social, occupational, or medical impairment. It is indicated by the presence of three (or more) of the following:

1. Amphetamine tolerance

2. Amphetamine withdrawal symptoms (sweating or rapid pulse; increased hand tremor; insomnia; nausea or vomiting; physical agitation; anxiety; transient visual, tactile, or auditory hallucinations or illusions; grand mal seizures) or amphetamine being taken to relieve or avoid withdrawal symptoms.

3. Greater use of amphetamine than intended.

4. Unsuccessful efforts to cut down or control amphetamine use.

5. Great deal of time spent in using amphetamine or recovering from its effects.

6. Amphetamine-caused reduction in social, occupational, or recreational activities.

7. Continued use of amphetamine despite knowledge of significant, persistent physical or psychological problems that are likely to have been worsened by amphetamine use.

Amphetamine abuse

- Amphetamine abuse is defined as a maladaptive pattern of use indicated by (1 continued use despite knowledge of having a persistent or recurrent social, occupational, psychologic, or physical problem that is caused or exacerbated by use of the amphetamines; (2 recurrent use in situations in which use is physically hazardous.

- Some symptoms of the disturbance have persisted for at least 1 month or have occurred repeatedly over a longer period of time.

Symptoms and signs

- Both the physical and the psychologic effects of amphetamine use begin within 1 hour after administration and may occur within a few seconds when the drug is administered intravenously or by smoking.

Physical effects

Intoxication: flushing, pallor, cyanosis, fever, headache, tachycardia and palpitations, markedly elevated blood pressure, nausea, vomiting, bruxism, difficulty in breathing, tremor, ataxia and loss of sensory abilities.

Overdose: restlessness, tremors, exaggerated reflexes, panic states, dizziness, confusion, and extreme irritability; patients are hyperalert, talkative, and may have been sleepless for several days.

Psychologic effects

Intoxication: restlessness, dysphoria, logorrhea, insomnia, irritability, hostility, confusion, anxiety, and panic; transient ideas of reference, paranoid ideation, increased libido, and formication (tactile sensation like ants crawling on skin) with high doses.

Withdrawal: anxiety, tremulousness, dysphoric mood, lethargy, fatigue, nightmares, headache, profuse sweating, muscle cramps, stomach cramps, and insatiable hunger; the most characteristic and dangerous symptom is a depression with suicidal ideation.

Investigations

- Completion of a detailed substance use history is recommended.

- Laboratory studies include urine drug screen; in patients suspected of chronic moderate to heavy use, a complete blood count, electrocardiogram, and computed tomography scan should be obtained.

Differential diagnosis

Nonpathologic stimulant use for recreational or medical purposes (refractory obesity, attention deficit disorder, and narcolepsy).
Psychiatric illnesses (eg, depression, insomnia, anxiety disorders, and schizophrenia).
Infection.

Etiology

- Risk factors for amphetamine abuse include the following:
Past history of substance abuse.
Psychiatric illness.
Medical problems treated with amphetamine (ie, obesity).
Family history of substance abuse.

Epidemiology

- Amphetamines were widely used for medical purposes in the 1950s and 1960s to combat depression and cause weight loss.
- Amphetamines are stolen or acquired through "scams" involving physicians and pharmacists. Illicit amphetamines are manufactured in garage or basement labs.
- Amphetamine use and abuse are more prevalent in western states (New Mexico, California).

Complications

Physical: hypertension, cardiac arrhythmias, weight loss or malnutrition, nonhealing ulcers, an exhaustion syndrome (involving an intense feeling of fatigue and need for sleep); injecting amphetamines can lead to infections such as local abscesses, bacterial endocarditis, hepatitis B, and AIDS.
Psychologic: high dose consumption may result in an acute psychosis distinguished by paranoid ideation and delusions, picking at the skin, and auditory and visual hallucinations; depression and suicidal ideation; symptoms of anxiety, panic, and despair.
Social: disruption of interpersonal relationships and impairment of occupational and social functioning; violent and erratic behavior is frequently seen among chronic amphetamine abusers.

Treatment

Diet and lifestyle

• Recovery from amphetamine dependence involves lifestyle changes, such as changing friends, in order to achieve and maintain abstinence. Abstinence from all mood-altering substances is recommended.

Pharmacologic treatment

• Because the amphetamine intoxication and delusional disorder are generally self-limiting, treatment usually requires supportive measures.

• Treatment of daily use or intravenous use of amphetamine may require a period of inpatient hospitalization for depression, suicidal ideation during withdrawal, psychosis, or violence during intoxication. The withdrawal depression may be treated with tricyclic antidepressants for a month or longer.

Amphetamine intoxication

• Treatment consists of decreasing environmental stimuli and giving assurance. For greater degrees of intoxication, agitation, and hyperactivity, a benzodiazepine (*eg*, diazepam 10–20 mg orally or 10 mg i.m. every 3 h) may be given. Tachyarrythmias may be treated with propranolol, 10–20 mg orally every 4 h.

Amphetamine overdose

• Acidification of the urine with ammonium chloride may help with the elimination of amphetamine.

Amphetamine psychosis

• Haloperidol, 2.5–5.0 mg i.m. has been used effectively; however, use haloperidol with caution because it increases the risk of an acute extrapyramidal motor reaction and may lower seizure threshhold.

Nonpharmacologic treatment

• For amphetamine dependence, refer to substance abuse programs or self-help groups (*eg*, Narcotics Anonymous). Physicians should identify substance abuse treatment specialists in their area who can recommend the most appropriate treatment programs for patients based on patient needs, availability, insurance coverage, and cost.

• Referrals to a psychiatrist for depression may also be indicated.

Treatment aims
To identify abstinence as the chief goal of treatment.
To provide education on the disease of addiction and cross-addiction to other chemicals.
To provide support and education to family and other support systems.
To address depressive symptoms following cessation of amphetamine use.

Follow-up and management
Identification and management of relapse signs and symptoms.
Management of psychiatric diagnosis.
Management by physician of medical complications.
Patient participation in aftercare activities or individual therapy for related psycho-logic issues (ie, stress management).

General references
Diagnostic and Statistical Manual of Mental Disorders, ed 4. Washington, DC: American Psychiatric Association; 1994.
Kaplan HI, Sadock BJ: *Synopsis of Psychiatry: Behavioral Sciences/Clinical Psychiatry*; 1991.
The Merck Manual. Merck & Co; 1992.
The Principles of Addiction Medicine. The American Society of Addiction Medicine; 1994.

Diagnosis

Symptoms

Gait and movement disorders: usually ataxia of gait and/or tremulous movement of arms.

Inappropriate laughter, happy demeanor, hand flapping: the combination of this with gait and movement disorders has resulted in this syndrome sometimes being called the "happy puppet syndrome."

Seizures: onset usually <3 years of age; often refractory to conventional therapy.

Marked speech impairment, aphasia, or minimal use of words.

Severe developmental delay and mental retardation: without loss of milestones.

Sleep disorders, abnormal sleep/wake cycles, nighttime wakefulness.

Feeding problems during infancy.

Hyperactivity, short attention span.

Signs

Microcephaly: occurs in >80% of patients by age 2 years.

Prominent jaw, wide mouth, widely spaced teeth, frequent drooling, protruding tongue.

Hypopigmented skin, eyes.

Hyperactive deep tendon reflexes.

Uplifted flexed arms during walking.

Strabismus, myopia, and nystagmus: common.

Investigations

• Approximately 85% of clinically affected individuals have detectable alteration of the PWS/AS (Prader–Willi Syndrome/Angelman Syndrome) gene locus at chromosome 15q11-13.

• Variations include large common deletions (in 70%–75% of patients), chromosome rearrangements leading to absence of the critical 15q11-13 region (2%), paternal uniparental disomy (inheritance of both paternal copies of chromosome 15, no maternal chromosome 15 present; 4%), other rare detectable mutations within the PWS/AS gene locus (4%–6%), unknown (15%).

High-resolution banded chromosome analysis of the blood should be sent for routine and for specific DNA diagnostic studies through a laboratory specializing in diagnosing this syndrome.

Electroencephalograhy: abnormal in >90% of patients; hypoarrhythmia or grand mal seizures.

Computed tomography: scan shows cerebral atrophy in 33% of patients.

Metabolic screening studies, plasma amino, urine organic acids, lactate, pyruvate, ammonia, copper, and ceruloplasmin: should be done in cases in which DNA and chromosome studies are normal.

Ophthalmologic screening.

Differential diagnosis

• Although patients resemble one another markedly, early diagnosis is often difficult due to the nonspecific nature of the early developmental delays.
• Metabolic studies should be done to screen for the possibility of treatable derangements.

Etiology

• In 85% of patients, the cause is an alteration of the PWS/AS gene locus at chromosome 15q11-13. This is an "imprinted" region that requires properly functioning genes from both maternal and paternal lines.
• In 15% of patients, the cause is unknown.

Epidemiology

• Exact incidence is unknown.
• Estimates are between 1:15,000–80,000.
• Male to female ratio is 1:1.

Treatment

Pharmacologic treatment

Anticonvulsant medication: for seizure control.

Melatonin: for nighttime wakefulness; has helped in some patients.

Ritalin: for hyperactivity; a minority of patients have benefited.

Nonpharmacologic treatment

Physical therapy: usually helpful for improving ambulation.

Speech and communication therapy.

Education and developmental training programs.

Ophthalmologic treatment: as needed.

Other treatment options

Genetic counseling: the risk of recurrence is based on the specific category of gene abnormality; prenatal diagnosis is available for at-risk families with abnormal gene studies.

Treatment aims

To address the medical and educational needs of the patient.
To foster family education and support.

Prognosis

• The mental deficiency is nonprogressive but severe.
• Seizures in childhood may stop by adolescence.
• Most individuals can communicate through sign language.
• None are capable of independent living.

Support organizations

National Angelman Syndrome foundation
P.O. Box 12437
Gainesville, FL 32604
Phone: (800) 432-6435
Phone if outside USA: (212) 448-1391
Internet: Angelman Syndrome Information for Families and Professionals at http://www.asclepius.com/angel

General references

Angelman H: "Puppet" children: a report on three cases. *Dev Med Child Neurol* 1965, 7:681–688.

Clayton-Smith J: Clinical research on Angelman syndrome in the United Kingdom: observations on 82 affected individuals. *Am J Med Genetics.* 1993; 46:12–15.

Saitoh S, Harada N, Jinno Y, et al.: Molecular and clinical study of 61 Angelman syndrome patients. *Am J Med Genetics* 1994, 52:158–163

Diagnosis

Definition

• Anorexia nervosa is characterized by extreme concern with body weight, preoccupation with calorie content (especially calorie content from fat), and maintenance of body weight below expected levels. Individuals with anorexia nervosa will often perceive themselves as heavier than they are or overvalue body shape and/or weight in self-assessment. Maintenance of weight <85% of expected for age and height, extreme fears of weight gain or becoming fat, body image distortion, and amenorrhea for 3 consecutive months are the core features of the diagnosis.

Signs and symptoms

Behavioral

Change in eating habits (eg, types of food, frequency of eating); increased exercise; increased frequency of checking body weight; preoccupation with food; change in manner of dress (anorectics often wear oversized garments); wearing multiple layers of clothing (even during warm weather).

Physical

Weight loss below a healthy level; loss of menstrual cycle; change in quality of hair, nails, and skin; constipation or diarrhea; dizziness or fainting; decreased blood pressure, temperature, or pulse rate.

Psychologic

Depressed mood; social withdrawal; irritability; loss of interest in usual activities; anxiety; fatigue.

Investigations

Physical and biomedical

• During the interview, the clinician should address each area identified above that might indicate an eating disorder. If data from history and physical examination suggest anorexia nervosa, consider the following tests:

Electrocardiogram; electrolytes to measure fluid balance and renal function; liver function tests; thyroid function tests; serum calcium and albumin.

Behavioral assessment

Review of dietary intake records and serial monitoring of weight change: noncompliance with record keeping is common and may be a "red flag" for disordered eating behavior.

Inventories

Patient-rated assessment instruments: eg, Eating Attitudes Test, Eating Disorders Inventory, and Eating Questionnaire-Revised; can measure disordered attitudes and behaviors about eating; unfortunately, these instruments may underestimate the problem when the patient is motivated to hide or minimize an eating disorder.

Complications

Mortality: the risk of death from anorexia nervosa is ~5% in the first 5 years after initial presentation, increasing to 10%–15% after 10 years; in patients with comorbid medical conditions, mortality approaches 50%.

Morbidity: eg, cardiac problems (tachycardia, bradycardia, arrhythmia, myocardial infarction), osteoporosis, renal failure, gastrointestinal disorders ("cathartic colon"), infertility, cognitive and personality changes from central nervous system effects of malnutrition, other tissue injury from extreme malnutrition.

Differential diagnosis

Major depression.
Psychosis.
Central nervous system lesions.
Primary gastrointestinal disorders.
Cachexia from cancer or AIDS.

Etiology

• The etiology of anorexia nervosa remains unclear; however, a family history of psychiatric disorder, substance abuse, or maladaptive relationships appears to elevate the risk of developing anorexia nervosa. A history of loss (eg, death of a relative), trauma, or abuse also seem to confer higher risk.

Epidemiology

• Anorexia nervosa is predominantly a disorder of young females, with estimated point prevalences in the range of 0.5%–1.0% among late adolescent and young adult women.
• Sufferers tend to be middle to upper-class women with high achievement orientation.
• Mean age at onset is 17 y.
• The course is extremely variable, with some patients recovering fully after a single, brief episode, and some going on to develop a chronic problem with disordered eating.

Treatment

Pharmacologic treatment

• Pharmacologic treatment is largely focused on antidepressants, which have been shown to be of benefit in the management of anorexia nervosa when combined with psychotherapy. Antidepressant treatment is obviously indicated when anorexia nervosa is comorbid with depression.

Serotonin reuptake inhibitors: especially fluoxetine, which has been most extensively studied for the treatment of anorexia.

Tricyclic antidepressants: especially nortriptyline, which has the most reliable test for serum drug levels.

Nonpharmacologic treatment

Psychotherapies (cognitive and behavioral approaches)

Behavior modification: involves contracting to offer some reward (*eg*, increased ward privileges) in exchange for increased calorie intake; should be used with caution in the outpatient setting because it can lead to increased conflict if family members are required to monitor the patient.

Systematic desensitization: involves gradual increases in caloric intake to overcome phobic avoidance of food.

Cognitive therapy: addresses dysfunctional thoughts and ideas about food ;irrational ideas about food are challenged and modified.

Other treatment options

Feminist therapies: emphasize the conflict between the demands of a patriarchal society and women's natural biologic state, needs, and role expectations.

Experiential therapies: *eg*, music, dance, or art therapy.

Family therapy: to clarify the role of the patient and her illness in the family structure, with the goal of modifying the family's dynamic structure enough to allow recovery.

Follow-up and management

• Follow-up and management should be directed toward achievement of the treatment aims listed above. Of major importance in the management of anorexia nervosa is the decision regarding the safest setting for treatment. The following are general guidelines:

Inpatient treatment: Body weight <80% expected; hypokalemia; impaired renal function; impaired cardiac function; hypoproteinemia; binge eating episodes greater than four times per week; vomiting more than once daily; laxative, diuretic, or exercise abuse; psychosis; suicidal ideation and/or intent; failure to improve with partial hospital therapy.

Partial hospitalization: Body weight <>80% expected; physiologic stability; calories restricted to <500 kcal/d; vomiting less than once daily; binge eating episodes less than four times per week; laxative, diuretic, or exercise abuse; other substance abuse; symptoms of major depression; poor social support system; failure to improve with outpatient therapy.

Outpatient treatment: Body weight >80% expected; physiologic stability; vomiting limited to binge eating episodes; binge eating episodes less than twice per week; episodic laxative or diuretic use; limited exercise activity; no other substance abuse; absence of comorbid psychopathology; stable social support system.

Treatment aims
To achieve abstinence from restrictive or other maladaptive eating patterns;
To regain healthy eating patterns;
To address other psychological and physical issues related to the anorexia.

Prognosis
• Negative prognostic variables include longer duration of disorder prior to treatment, older age at onset, poor family support system, extreme weight loss, bulimia as a behavioral feature, decreased serum albumin or serum calcium, and independent physical illness affecting metabolism (eg, diabetes).

General references
American Psychiatric Association: Practice guideline for eating disorders. *Am J Psychiatry* 1993, 150:212–228.

American Psychiatric Association: *Diagnostic and Statistical Manual of Mental Disorders*, ed 4. Washington, DC: American Psychiatric Press; 1994.

Garner DM, Garfinkel PE (eds): *Handbook of Treatment for Eating Disorders*. New York: Guilford Press; 1997.

Herzog W, Schellberg D, Deter H: First recovery in anorexia nervosa patients in the long-term course: a discrete-time survival analysis. *J Consult Clin Psychol* 1997, 65:169–177.

Kaplan AS, Garfinkel PE (eds): *Medical Issues and the Eating Disorders*. New York: Brunner/Mazel; 1993.

Diagnosis

Definition

• Antisocial personality disorder consists of persistent and pervasive patterns of behavior that begin in childhood or by adolescence and are typified by disregard for the rights of others. Also known as psychopathy or sociopathy, the "sociopath" is characterized by manipulation and deceit in interpersonal relationships and by violation of societal laws and mores.

Symptoms and signs

• Symptoms begin in childhood or adolescence and are typical for conduct disorder (eg, chronic lying, aggression to people or animals, thievery, and disregard of rules). In adult life, the sociopath is characterized by impulsivity, inability to delay gratification, aggressive acts, thievery, sexual promiscuity, substance abuse, and acts of irresponsibility (eg, defaulting on debts, failure to pay child support, the provision of adequate parenting, or reckless driving).

• The sociopath may be superficially charming, even a con artist, but will be unable to maintain occupational or marital stability.

DSM-IV diagnostic criteria

• Antisocial personality disorder is indicated by the presence of three or more of the following:

1. Illegal behaviors.
2. Repeated lying.
3. Impulsivity.
4. Irritability and aggressiveness.
5. Reckless disregard for safety of others.
6. Consistent irresponsibility.
7. Lack of remorse or guilt.
8. Evidence of conduct disorder before 15 years of age.
9. Antisocial behavior is not due to another axis I diagnosis.

Investigations

• The most useful diagnostic aides in these unreliable and deceptive persons is a review of medical, legal, and school records.

Psychological testing: the Minnesota Multiphasic Personality Inventory-2 and the Millon Clinical Multiaxial Inventory-II are valid and reliable for the diagnosis of personality disorders; the Structured Clinical Interview for DSM-IIIR Personality Disorders is a valid and reliable structured interview that provides diagnoses for personality disorders.

Laboratory studies: physiologic studies (eg, levels of central nervous system neurotransmitters and changes of galvanic skin conductivity to conditioned responses) are investigational and not available to clinicians.

Complications

Comorbidity: impulse control disorders, including pathological gambling and intermittent-explosive disorder; features of other cluster B personality disorders; substance abuse/dependence disorders; somatization disorder.

Behavioral outcomes: promiscuity with multiple marriages and relationships; financial problems including bankruptcy; poor work record with multiple jobs; premature death from violent causes, including suicide, homicide, and accidents.

Differential diagnosis

• Other cluster B personality disorders include borderline, narcissistic, histrionic. Schizophrenia. Manic depressive illness. Substance-related disorders. Organic personality disorders (eg, frontal lobe syndromes).

Etiology

• Genetic factors have been shown to be a major contribution to sociopathy; adopted children of persons with antisocial personality are more likely to resemble their biological parents than their adoptive parents.

• Environmental factors include chaotic dysfunctional families, amoral subculture, or inconsistent discipline during childhood.

• Physiologic factors include a decreased capacity to develop conditioned autonomic nervous system responses (eg, sweating) to adverse stimuli such as punishment.

Epidemiology

• The community prevalence of antisocial personality is ~3% for males and ~1% for females. The prevalence rates are higher in substance abuse treatment centers, forensic settings, and prisons.

Treatment

Diet and lifestyle
• In view of the characteristic disorganized lifestyle of these persons, they should be encouraged to increase structure in their life habits (*eg,* sleep, meals, work, and the exercise of financial responsibility).

Pharmacologic treatment
• There is no specific pharmacologic treatment for antisocial personality disorder. Pharmacotherapy should be limited to target symptoms of comorbid axis I disorders such as intermittent explosive disorder.

• The person with antisocial personality disorder is prone to addiction and drug-seeking behaviors; at times to sell drugs obtained through prescriptions. Controlled substances are relatively contraindicated and should be prescribed for specific reasons with a small number of dispensed dosages.

Nonpharmacologic treatment

Psychotherapy
• Individual psychotherapy should be limited to a behavioral model that focuses on personal responsibility and reviews the consequences of impulsive behavior and misbehavior. Traditional insight-oriented psychotherapy is relatively contraindicated because these persons typically use "insights" of the childhood origins of their behavior problems as rationalizations, projecting the blame for misbehavior elsewhere.

• Group therapies are more effective than individual therapies because that the power of group process may serve to confront and socialize the antisocial person's lack of conformity to societal values and lack of remorse for the effects of misbehavior on others.

Other treatment options
• Military service, with its rigorous basic training and the enforcement of a structured lifestyle with firm limit setting, may facilitate the internalization of societal values and also serve to create a sense of responsibility to a social unit. Similarly, civilian "boot camp" or "outward bound" programs may increase self-esteem and bonding to a group.

• Alcoholics Anonymous and similar 12-step programs encourage individual responsibility and obligations to others. Because of the comorbidity of substance abuse, these programs are often ideal for the antisocial person.

Treatment aims
The general treatment aim is to increase compliance with societal values (eg, laws, sexual behavior, substance abuse, and occupational productivity).

Prognosis
• The general prognosis of antisocial persons is poor. Prison and failed marriages and careers are common, as is premature death from a variety of causes (eg, the effects of drug abuse, HIV, and violent deaths from accidents, suicide, and homicide). Some patients, with or without the aid of various treatment modalities, demonstrate increasing maturity. Others remain recalcitrant to any change, and their sadistic predatory behaviors require long-term institutionalization. If they survive beyond 40 y of age, most persons with antisocial personality disorder will spontaneously demonstrate some amelioration of social behavior.

Follow-up and management
• Persons with antisocial personality disorder rarely seek treatment on their own initiative. Treatment and follow-up management is generally mandated by the legal system. Follow-up should include the vigorous encouragement to maintain involvement in programs such as Alcoholics Anonymous.

Pitfalls
• The values and behavior of the sociopath may evoke identification and sympathy with the sociopath's victims and anger in the therapist. Those negative feelings may undercut the therapeutic alliance and defeat the goals of psychotherapy.

General references
Ford CV: *Lies! Lies!! Lies!!!: The Psychology of Deceit.* Washington, DC: American Psychiatric Press; 1996.

Meloy JR: Antisocial personality disorder. In *Treatments of Psychiatric Disorders,* ed 2. Edited by Gabbard GO. Washington, DC: American Psychiatric Press; 1995:2273–2290.

Widiger TA, Corbitt EM, Millon T: Antisocial personality disorder. In *Review of Psychiatry,* vol II. Edited by Tasman A, Riba MB. Washington, DC: American Psychiatric Press; 1992:63–79.

Diagnosis

Symptoms and signs

Significant impairment in reciprocal social interactions: *eg*, lack of ability or desire to interact with peers, lack of appreciation of social cues, socially inappropriate behaviors, and gaze avoidance.

Significantly restricted repertoire of activities, interests, and behaviors: *eg*, obsession with complex specific topics (*eg*, sports statistics, history, music, etc.), routinized/ritualized patterns of daily behaviors, and exclusion of other activities.

Absence of clinically significant language delays or cognitive development: language, although lucid with good grammar, may be stiff, formal, pedantic, repetitive, or have odd prosody or other unusual characteristics.

Pronounced clumsiness or awkwardness in movement.

• Patients whose IQs are not in the retarded range tend to have higher verbal ability scores than performance ability scores, engage in more concrete thought processes (rather than abstract), and lack "common sense."

Investigations

Developmental history: age-appropriate language development (single words by 2 y of age, phrases by 3 y) and self-help skills.

Family history: possibly hereditary, also depression and/or bipolar disorder more common in pedigrees.

High-resolution–band genetic studies: to rule out Fragile X or other genetic abnormalities

Metabolic disorders screen.

Psychometric testing: Wechsler Intelligence Scale for Children-Revised may reflect strengths in verbal ability and troughs on Object Assembly and Coding.

Differential diagnosis
Schizophrenia with childhood onset: usually normal early development.
Autistic disorder: includes significant language delay.
Rett's disorder: typically female, characteristic head-growth deceleration.
Childhood disintegrative disorder: loss of previously acquired skills and likelihood of mental retardation.
Obsessive–compulsive disorder: absence of impairment of social interactions and rituals/compulsions typically ego-dystonic.
Schizoid personality disorder: absence of stereotypic interests and behaviors; better early developmental history; less-impaired social interactions.
Schizotypal personality disorder: absence of early symptoms with later worsening; more chronic unusual ideas or perceptual disturbances.

Epidemiology
• Prevalence rate is 7.1:1000.
• Incidence was 0.55% of boys and 0.15% of girls 7–10 y of age in one study [1].

Treatment

Pharmacologic treatment

• No specific drug treats Asperger's disorder; however psychopharmacologic interventions for "target" symptoms include psychostimulants (for hyperactive and inattentive behavior); benzodiazapines, buspirone, etc. (for anxiety), and selective serotonin-reuptake inhibitors (depression and/or preoccupation's, rituals, compulsions).

Nonpharmacologic treatment

Psychoeducational: individual education plans; parent training and education.

Psychotherapy: behavior modification and individual therapy to address anxiety, depression, and socially

challenged issues.

Treatment aims

Prognosis

• Prognosis is variable; generally productive independent lives may be considered "odd."

• Basic signs and symptoms remain unchanged throughout life; may develop other additional psychiatric disorders, especially anxiety or depression.

Key reference

1. Ehlers S, et al.: Asperger syndrome, autism, and attention disorders: a comparative study of the cognitive profiles of 120 children. J Child Psychol Psychiatry 1993, 34:1327–1350.

General references

Eiserimajer R, et al.: Comparison of clinical symptoms in autism and Asperger's disorder. J Am Acad Child Adolesc Psychiaty 1996, 35:1523–1532.

Volkmar FR, et al.: Asperger's syndrome. J Am Acad Child Adolesc Psychiaty 1996, 35:118–123.

Diagnosis

Signs, symptoms, and DSM-IV diagnostic criteria

Inattention (DSM-IV)

1. Often fails to give close attention to details or makes careless mistakes in schoolwork, work, or other activities.

2. Often has difficulty sustaining attention in tasks or play activities.

3. Often does not seem to listen when spoken to directly.

4. Often does not follow through on instructions and fails to finish schoolwork, chores, or duties in the workplace.

5. Often has difficulty organizing tasks and activities.

6. Often avoids, dislikes, or is reluctant to engage in tasks that require sustained mental effort.

7. Often loses things necessary for tasks or activities.

8. Often easily distracted by extraneous stimuli.

9. Often forgetful in daily activities.

Hyperactivity (DSM-IV)

1. Often fidgets with hands or feet or squirms in seat.

2. Often leaves seat in classroom or when remaining seated is expected.

3. Often inappropriately runs about or climbs excessively.

4. Often has difficulty playing or engaging in leisure activities quietly.

5. Often "on the go" or often acts as if "driven by a motor."

6. Often talks excessively

Impulsivity (DSM-IV)

1. Often blurts out answers before questions have been completed.

2. Often has difficulty awaiting turn.

3. Often interrupts or intrudes on others.

Other DSM-IV criteria

1. Symptoms that have caused impairment have been present < 7 years of age.

2. Symptoms have persisted for at least 6 months and in two or more settings.

3. Three subtypes: predominantly inattentive type, predominantly hyperactive-impulsive type, and combined type.

Associated symptoms

School underachievement; trouble getting along with others; low self-esteem; other comorbid behavior disorders, learning disorders, anxiety and mood disorders.

Developmental patterns of symptoms

In preschool children: temper tantrums, argumentative behavior, aggression, fearless behavior (which leads to frequent accidental injury), boisterous behavior, and sleep problems.

In school-age children: school difficulties, poor peer relationships, and development of comorbid conditions.

In adolescents: internal sense of restlessness, failing to complete independent academic work, poorly organized approaches to school and work, poor follow through on tasks, and risky behaviors.

Investigations

Comprehensive interview with all parenting figures; developmentally appropriate interview with the child and mental status examination; medical evaluation: to assess general health status and to screen for sensory deficits, neurologic problems, or other physical explanations for the difficulties; cognitive assessment of ability and achievement; parent and teacher behavior rating scales; speech and language or motor assessments: as indicated.

Differential diagnosis

• The differential diagnosis must rule out the presence of other psychiatric disorders, developmental disorders, and medical and neurologic disorders and determine whether these are comorbid or whether they are mimicking an attention deficit–hyperactivity disorder (ADHD) syndrome [1].

Age-appropriate overactivity still within the norm.

Developmental delays or specific learning disorders.

Sensory deficits.

Other behavior disorders (eg, oppposition-al-defiant disorder or conduct disorder).

Mood disorders (eg, bipolar disorder or "irritable" depression).

Anxiety disorders (eg, separation anxiety disorder or posttraumatic stress disorder).

Seizures

Etiology

• Genetic factors account for 50% of the explainable variance. Heritability is estimated at .55 to .92. In one study, concordance rate for monozygotic twins was 51 % compared with 33% in dizygotic twins.

• By means of adrenergic mediation, the frontal lobes exert inhibitory influences on striatal structures that are mediated by dopamine. These structures and their projections modulate attention, impulsivity, executive functions, and motor activity. Consequently, norepinephrine and dopamine have been implicated as the primary neurotransmitters involved in ADHD.

Epidemiology

• In the general population, the prevalence of ADHD is 3%–6% in school age children

• Male-to-female ratios range from 3–4:1 in the general population to 6–9:1 in clinically referred samples.

Complications (comorbidity)

Conduct disorder.

Oppositional-defiant disorder.

Mood disorders.

Anxiety disorders.

Specific learning disabilities.

Tourette's disorder.

Treatment

Diet and lifestyle

School interventions

• Goals include 1) improved academic performance, classroom behavior, and peer relationships; 2) structured classroom with predictable, well-organized schedules; 3) child's seat is to be in the front of the classroom close to the teacher to decrease distractions; 4) use of contingency management and daily, teacher-completed report cards showing the child's progress in targeted areas; 5) use incentives and tangible rewards; and 6) assess the need for special education interventions.

Family interventions

• Goals include 1) education about ADHD and referral to support groups; 2) parent management training (eg, contingency management techniques, how to cooperate with schools using the daily report card and point/token-response cost system); and 3) family therapy to address communication, conflicts and distress, and problem solving within the family system.

Individual interventions

• Goals include 1) individual therapy to treat associated symptomatology (eg depression, low self-esteem, or anxiety; 2) social skills training; 3) anger management and impulse control; and 4) cognitive training to help develop reflective, more efficient problem solving skills.

Pharmacologic treatment

Stimulants (70% of children with positive response on the first trial)

Standard dosage	Methylphenidate, 0.2–0.7 mg/kg 2–3 times daily (0.6–2.1 mg/kg/d).
	Dextroamphetamine, 0.1–0.5 mg/kg 2–3 times daily (0.3–1.5 mg/kg/d; maximum 40 mg/d).
	Pemoline, 0.5–4.0 mg/kg/d (maximum of 112.5 mg/d).
Special points	*Pemoline:* liver function monitoring necessary due to risk of chemical hepatitis.

Tricyclic antidepressants

• Hyperactivity and impulsivity respond better to tricyclic antidepressants (TCAs) than does inattention.

Standard dosage	Imipramine, 1–5 mg/kg/d in 2–3 divided doses.
	Desipramine, 1-5 mg/kg/d in 2–3 divided doses.
	Nortriptyline, 0.5–5.0 mg/kg/d in 2 divided doses.
Special points	*Imipramine:* usually requires lower doses than when used to treat depression; combined imipramine/desipramine blood level should be >150 ng/mL.
	Desipramine: can not be recommended for children; in adolescents, it has carried an increased risk of sudden cardiac deaths; blood level should be >150 ng/mL, not to exceed 300 ng/mL.
	Nortriptyline: more sedating than other TCAs; lower doses required than other TCAs; blood level has therapeutic window of 50–150 ng/mL.
	All TCAs: Reduce or discontinue TCA 1) if PR interval >.18 (in patient ≤10 y of age) or >.20 (>10 y); 2) if QRS interval >.12 or widening >50% over baseline QRS interval; 3) corrected QT ≥0.48; 3) or if resting heart rate >110 (≤10 y) or >100 (>10 y).

Prognosis and course

• 20%–30% of ADHD children will no longer manifest symptoms as young adults.
• In one study, two thirds of ADHD children continued to be troubled by at least one of the disabling core symptoms of the original syndrome as young adults.
• ~33% of ADHD children will meet criteria for the full syndrome at 18 y of age.
• 20%–30% of ADHD children develop more serious psychopathology (eg alcoholism, substance abuse, and antisocial personality disorder).

Key reference

1. Cantwell DP: Attention deficit disorder: a review of the past 10 years. *J Am Acad Child Adolesc Psychiatry* 1996, 35:978–987.

General references

Jensen PS, Martin D, Cantwell DP: Comorbidity in ADHD: implications for research, practice, and DSM-V. *J Am Acad Child Adolesc Psychiatry* 1997, 36:1065–1079.

Spencer T, Biederman J, Wilens T, et al.: Pharmacotherapy of attention deficit hyperactivity disorder across the life cycle. *J Am Acad Child Adolesc Psychiatry* 1996, 35:409–432.

Weiss G: Attention deficit hyperactivity disorder. In *Child and Adolescent Psychiatry: A Comprehensive Textbook.* Edited by Lewis M; Baltimore: Williams & Wilkins; 1996:PAGES.

Weiss G, Hechtman LT: *Hyperactive Children Grown Up,* ed 2, CITY: Guilford Press; 1994.

Diagnosis

Definition

- Autistic disorder is included in DSM-IV as one of the pervasive developmental disorders, conditions characterized by severe and pervasive impairment in several areas of development (eg, reciprocal social interaction skills; communication skills; or the presence of stereotyped behavior, interests, and activities). The qualitative impairments are distinctly deviant relative to developmental level or mental age. The pervasive developmental disorders are autistic disorder, Rett's disorder, childhood disintegrative disorder, Asperger's disorder, and pervasive developmental disorder not otherwise specified (PDD-NOS).

Symptoms and signs

- Autistic disorder is characterized by a marked and sustained deviance in development, including the onset of delay or abnormality function before 3 years of age in either social interaction (or language used in social communication or symbolic and imaginative play) together with six or more of the following (at least two from 1–4, one from 5–8, and one from 9–12):

1. Impairment of nonverbal social interaction.
2. Failure to develop appropriate peer relationships.
3. Lack of seeking to share enjoyment, interest, or achievement.
4. Lack of social or emotional reciprocity.
5. Delay or lack of spoken language.
6. Impairment in the ability to sustain a conversation.
7. Stereotyped, repetitive, or idiosyncratic language.
8. Delay or lack of make-believe or social play.
9. Preoccupation with repetitive and restricted patterns of interest.
10. Adherence to nonfunctional routines or rituals.
11. Stereotyped or repetitive motor mannerisms.
12. Preoccupation with parts of objects.

Investigations

Clinical interview and observation.

Physical and neurological examination.

Standardized questionnaires, observations, and interviews: eg, Autism Behavior Checklist, Childhood Autism Rating Scale, Autism Diagnostic Observational Scale, and Autism Diagnostic Interview; may be helpful.

Chromosome analysis: including fragile X.

Psychometric and language assessments.

Electroencephalography (EEG), computed tomography (CT), and magnetic resonance imaging (MRI).

Genetic counseling.

Audiological assessment.

Assessment for associated general medical condition: may include EEG, CT, or MRI; chromosomal analysis; and specific investigations in which a particular condition is suspected.

Complications

Mental retardation: in 75% of patients.

Increased incidence of epilepsy: 25% in adolescence.

Associated psychiatric disorder.

Self-injurious or aggressive behavior.

Distress to others in social network (eg parents, siblings).

Differential diagnosis

Rett's disorder: multiple specific deficits after normal development for 5–48 months; occurs only in girls.

Childhood disintegrative disorder: marked regression in multiple areas of functioning after at least 2 y normal development, followed by loss of language, social, motor skills and bowel or bladder control.

Asperger syndrome: social and behavioral abnormalities similar to autistic disorder, without delay in language or cognitive development, self-help skills, adaptive behavior.

PDD-NOS: abnormalities characteristic of autistic disorder but insufficient to meet criteria because of late age and atypical or subthreshold symptomatology.

Expressive language disorder: abnormalities in social interaction and restrictive or repetitive patterns of behavior not present.

Selective mutism: communicative and social skills apparent in some contexts; no evidence of restricted or repetitive patterns of behavior.

Uncomplicated mental retardation: social, communicative, and behavioral skills appropriate to intellectual level.

Schizophrenia with childhood onset.

Sensory impairment: some degree of social isolation, echolalia, and pronoun reversal are present.

Severe abuse or neglect: language delay, abnormal social behavior, and unusual habits and motor stereotypies.

Etiology

- No evidence that minor environmental stresses or parenting abnormality causes autism. The etiology is probably biologic—various abnormalities have been noted, but no specific neuropathologic mechanism has been identified. Genetic contribution is significant. Elevations in peripheral serotonin levels are consistent but not specific to autism. Cerebellar anomalies may be important.

Epidemiology

- Prevalence is 2–5:10,000 for strictly defined autistic disorder, with a male-to-female ratio of 4–5:1. Rett's and childhood disintegrative disorder are probably less common. Subthreshold conditions (eg, PDD-NOS) are probably much more common, especially in populations of mentally retarded individuals, in which the rates may be as high as 1:20. There is a male predominance (except in Rett's, which is confined to girls).

Treatment

Diet and lifestyle
• Megavitamin supplementation has not been supported by systematic research.
• Autistic disorder is a lifelong disabling condition.

Pharmacologic treatment
• Pharmacologic treatment is supplementary to other treatment options and probably has little effect on the underlying (unknown) disease process. Specific problems and symptoms should be targeted; medications may include stimulants (usually ineffective) or α-2 agonists, selective serotonin-reuptake inhibitors and tricyclics, low-dose antipsychotics, mood stabilizers, and opiate antagonists.

Nonpharmacologic treatment
• Clear recommendations supporting early intensive intervention cannot be made at present. The mainstay of treatment is educational and behavioral programming. Common features of successful programs include structure, with emphasis on individual needs; family involvement; language and communication therapy; and the fostering of vocational skills, adaptive skills, and independence.

Treatment aims
To minimize associated deficits and maximize skills; aim for independence and skills of daily living.

Prognosis
• Outcome is guarded and depends on 1) the degree to which the child is affected, 2) associated mental retardation, and 3) presence of associated behavioral problems.
• Social, behavioral, and language deficits tend to persist, although improvement may be apparent,
particularly in high functioning individuals. Only approximately half develop speech. The majority of adults with autistic disorder are significantly handicapped, many need residential placement, and only a minority succeed in working independently; marriage is rare.
• Intellectual level and communicative competence are predictors of prognosis. An IQ <50, mutism, and the presence of seizures and severe behavioral problems indicates a worse outcome; presence of communicative speech by 5 y of age predicts a better outcome. Individuals with Asperger syndrome and PDD-NOS diagnoses do better; Rett's and childhood disintigrative disorder do worse.

General references
Rutter M, Lord C: Autism and pervasive developmental disorders. In *Child and Adolescent Psychiatry: Modern Approaches*. Edited by Rutter M, Taylor E, Hersov L; CITY: Blackwell; 1994.

Volkmar FR: Autism and the pervasive developmental disorders. In *Child and Adolescent Psychiatry: A Comprehensive Textbook*. Edited by Lewis M. Williams & Wilkins; 1991.

Volkmar FR, Klin A, Marans WD, McDougle CJ: Autistic disorder. In *Psychoses and Pervasive Developmental Disorders in Childhood and Adolescence*. Edited by Volmar FR; 1997.

AVOIDANT PERSONALITY DISORDER

Diagnosis

Definition
• The individual with avoidant personality disorder (APD) perceives himself as inadequate in relation to others, with resulting hypersensitivity to criticism or ridicule and socially inhibited behaviors.

Symptoms and signs
Timid, introverted, awkward, inhibited, pessimistic; views others as disapproving: misinterprets innocuous comments as derogatory, has inferiority complex, exaggerates obstacles or somatic complaints to justify avoidance.

Anxious preoccupation
Fears of embarrassing oneself, being shamed in front of others, criticism, rejection, losing control; longs for acceptance, feels personally unappealing.

Childhood history
Often shy, with severe stranger anxiety and insistence on routine: symptoms worsen in adolescence when social pressures increase.

Occupational dysfunction
Makes career sacrifices to avoid risk of embarrassment: *ie,* pass up promotion or new responsibilities, avoids group-oriented activities, stays in dead-end job, resists public speaking.

Social dysfunction
Avoids social contact, especially group settings; lives constricted lifestyle due to need for certainty or security; has few friends; lacks social support network; keeps emotional distance in intimate relationships: hides feelings for fear of being exposed; **easily injured by marginally critical comments, ingratiating to "protect" against negative responses from others; symptoms worse in new situations or with strangers:** but decrease inversely with familiarity.

DSM-IV diagnostic criteria
• Beliefs and behaviors are pervasive and inflexible to a degree that causes social dysfunction or marked distress.
• The patient must suffer from at least four of the following on a long-term basis:

Behavioral symptoms: avoids personal risk or new activities due to fear of embarrassing himself; avoids occupational activities with significant interpersonal contact; resists involvement with people unless positive reaction guaranteed; shows excess reserve in intimate relationships; acts inhibited in new interpersonal situations.

Subjective symptoms: worries excessively about being criticized or rejected in social situations; is preoccupied in social contexts with feeling inferior, inept, or unappealing to others.

Investigations
History
Assess developmental issues: *eg,* history of trauma, parental rearing style, social behavior as child and adolescent; **explore educational and occupational history and behavior in work and social settings; inquire about fears and preoccupations; attain additional data if possible from parents, employers, significant others; observe behavior toward interviewer.**

Questionnaires and tests
Minnesota Multiphasic Personality Inventory and Millon Clinical Multiaxial Inventory: when administered by a psychologist can suggest clustering of avoidant personality traits.

Physician-rated questionnaires: Structured Clinical Interview for DSMIII-R Personality Disorders (SCID-II) and the Personality Disorder Examination are valid and useful.

Other questionnaires: the patient-rated Personality Diagnostic Questionnaire-Revised and the SCID-II self-report questionnaire.

Differential diagnosis
Social phobia, generalized type, is more specific to social situations, with less global impairment, avoidance, distress.
Rule out panic disorder with agoraphobia, personality disorders due to a general medical condition such as traumatic brain injury, or due to substance use; rule out dependent and schizoid personality disorders.
Consider situationally related avoidance, *ie,* language or cultural barriers.

Etiology
Unknown; believed to be combination of the following:
Biological factors.
Genetic factors.
Constitutional factors: anxious, self-conscious temperament.
Environmental factors: dysfunctional parenting, poor role models, cultural factors.
Experiential factors.

Epidemiology
• The degree to which social avoidance is abnormal may be culturally defined.
• The prevalence rates in the general population are 0.5%–1.0%; in outpatient mental health settings, 10%.

Complications
Comorbidity
• There is an increased risk for major depression and eating disorders.
• A large minority of patients suffer comorbid anxiety disorders, particularly social phobia and panic disorder.
• May coexist with other personality disorders, particularly dependent personality disorder but also borderline, paranoid, schizoid, and schizotypal personality disorders.
• Avoidant personality disorder may exacerbate the course of comorbid conditions.

Behavioral
• Alcohol, drugs, and prescription medications such as benzodiazepines may be misused as coping measure to avoid experiencing negative affects and anxiety; substance dependence may develop.
• Intimate relationships are highly valued once formed; when these relationships are disrupted or other stressors overwhelm coping mechanisms, patient is at increased risk for self-injury or psychiatric complications.

Treatment

Diet and lifestyle management
• Improve social functioning and increase risk-taking.
• Reach full potential occupationally.

Pharmacologic treatment
• Avoidant personality disorder is one of the few personality disorders that responds to medications. The outcome is better when medication and therapy are used conjointly.
• Select pharmacologic agents specifically address the most distressing aspects of syndrome. The following agents are effective for social phobia and also reduce avoidant behaviors and social anxiety in APD:

Monoamine oxidase inhibitors: *eg*, phenelzine and tranylcypromine (often in low doses).

Benzodiazepines: *eg*, clonazepam, alprazolam.

Beta-adrenergic blockers: *eg*, propanolol, address physiologic symptoms of anxiety present in "performance" situations (*ie*, tremor, palpitations, sweating, blushing); this can break the negative cycle of physiologic symptoms aggravating anxiety that exacerbates physiologic symptoms, and so on.

Selective serotonin reuptake inhibitors: *eg*, fluoxetine, decrease rejection hypersensitivity, increase stress tolerance, and improve overall mood.

Nonpharmacologic treatment
• Combination of therapy to address cognitive distortions and exposure techniques to address avoidant behaviors is particularly effective.

Psychotherapy
• Short- and long-term psychodynamic therapies are particularly helpful in addressing deep fear of shame and exposure in patients with intimacy problems.

Cognitive therapy
• Cognitive therapy addresses maladaptive thought processes leading patient to distorted perception that he is viewed negatively by others.

Behavioral therapy
Relaxation training, social skills training, assertiveness training, systemic desensitization, graduated exposure therapy, flooding.

Group therapy
• Many of given therapies may be done in group format, which provides a safe, predictable environment in which to try new behaviors.
• APD patients will resist group settings due to self-consciousness; can benefit greatly once engaged.
• Self-help groups (*eg*, Toastmasters) are also available.

Family therapy
• Family therapy encourages supportive atmosphere for patient and prevents over-coddling or over-aggressive pushing of the anxious patient.

Pitfalls
• Due to negative self-evaluation, patients may fail to acknowledge their treatment gains (even when clear progress is occurring) and fail to sustain improved functioning. Clinician must continue to help patient see situations more objectively.
• When painful issues are addressed, these patients may characteristically avoid treatment (drop out, miss sessions); outreach to patient and interpretation of this process can keep patient in treatment.

Treatment aims
To correct distorted self-perceptions.
To teach acceptance or management of painful affects (in place of avoidance).
To reduce social inhibition or avoidance.

Prognosis
• Disorder tends to improve naturally as patient ages and encounters and successfully masters previously avoided situations.
• Clear and sustained symptom reduction results from combination cognitive-behavioral therapies or medications.
• Outcome is worse when comorbid axis I disorder present.

Follow-up and management
For the acute phase
• Due to patients' fear of clinician's disapproval, adopting a supportive, approving stance helps establish positive rapport and engage resistant patient.

For the continuation phase
• Brief therapy may be adequate for less severely affected patients; more severely impaired patients require ongoing treatments; can eventually taper down or off medications; some patients relapse on discontinuation. Discontinuation of monoamine oxidase inhibitors after many years may be difficult.

General references
American Psychiatric Association: *Diagnostic and Statistical Manual of Mental Disorders*, ed 4. Washington, DC: American Psychiatric Association; 1994.

Fahlen T: Personality traits in social phobia, II: changes during drug treatment. *J Clin Psych* 1995, **56:**569–573.

Pederson NC, Plowin R, McClearn GE, et al.: Neuroticism, extraversion, and related traits in adult twins reared apart and reared together. *J Pers Soc Psychol* 1988, **55:**950–957.

Sutherland SM, Frances A: Avoidant personality disorder. In *Treatments of Psychiatric Disorders*, ed 2. Edited by Gabbard GO. Washington, DC: American Psychiatric Association; 1995:2345–2353.

Diagnosis

Definitions

• Mood disorders are classified into unipolar and bipolar disorders. The presence of hypomania or mania classifies a mood disorder as bipolar because most patients with mania will develop depressive episodes at some point in their lives.

• A manic syndrome consists of a distinct period of elevated, expansive, or irritable mood lasting at least 1 week (or less if hospitalization is required). A hypomanic episode is a period of at least a few days of mild elevation of mood, sharpened and positive thinking, and increased energy and activity levels, typically without the impairment caused by mania.

• According to DSM-IV, patients with bipolar I disorder have had at least one episode of mania. Bipolar II is defined as a depressive episode with at least one hypomanic episode [6].

Symptoms and signs

Presence of elevated, expansive, or irritable mood lasting >1 week; along with the presence of at least three of the following:

1. Elevated self esteem and or grandiosity.

2. Decreased need for sleep.

3. Pressured speech.

4. Flight of ideas.

5. Distractibility.

6. Psychomotor agitation.

7. Recklessness.

8. Lability of mood.

9. Impulsivity.

10. Financial extravagance.

11. Sexually inappropriate behavior.

12. Delusions or hallucinations.

• The term rapid cycling is used when a patient experiences four or more occurrences in 1 year. These patients share many of the same symptoms with patients who have mixed episodes (exhibiting both manic and depressive states in one episode).

Investigations

Full psychosocial history: necessary from different and collateral sources.

Bagnetic resonance imaging: consider for first episode to rule out space-occupying lesions causing mania.

Electroencephalography: to rule out partial complex seizures.

Drug screen: to rule out possibility of substance-induced mood disorder.

Complete blood count.

Liver function tests: for Tegretol and Depakote toxicity.

Renal function.

Thyroid-stimulating hormone: annually for lithium toxicity

Free thyroxine tests, rapid plasma reagin test: to rule out central nervous system (CNS) syphilis as a cause; not for medication toxicity.

Psychologic projective and personality tests: may be of some value if diagnosis is unclear.

Complications

Suicide: high risk (~15%).

Alcohol and substance abuse: high prevalence (sometimes used to self-medicate).

• Possible stressors that the patient may experience throughout the course of this illness include sexually transmitted diseases; legal problems; debts incurred; and possible loss of employment, marriage, or family support.

Differential diagnosis

• Although the psychiatrist should first determine if a patient meets the criteria for bipolar I or II, the following diagnoses mimic this disorder:
Substance-induced mood disorder (including prescription drugs, eg, corticosteroids).
Schizoaffective disorder.
Personality disorders (eg, borderline, narcissistic, antisocial, and histrionic; these may coexist with bipolar disorder).
Schizophrenia.
Attention deficit–hyperactivity disorder in adolescence.
Mood disorder due to general medical condition (eg, hyperthyroidism, CNS syphilis, AIDS, Cushing's disease).

Etiology

• A family history of mood disorder is the most important risk factor for developing bipolar disorder. Results of controlled family studies of probands with bipolar disorder show a significantly increased risk (3.8%–17.5%) among first-degree relatives when compared with controls [2]. The rate of unipolar depression in families of bipolar probands shows a twofold increase compared with controls, whereas in unipolar proband families, there is no increase in incidence of bipolar disorders. Rates of bipolar disorders among first-degree relatives of bipolar probands were approximately twice those of second-degree relatives. There is no single mode of genetic transmission. Although environmental stressors play a very important role in bipolar disorder, their specific significance is still unclear.

Epidemiology

• The lifetime prevalence of bipolar I disorder in community samples varies from 0.4%–1.6%. Community studies suggest a lifetime prevalence of bipolar II at ~0.5%. Bipolar I disorder affects both men and women equally; however, the prevalence for bipolar II is higher for women. There is no increased prevalence of bipolar I or II disorder in any one racial group.
• Studies indicate a mean age of onset in the early twenties. Fewer than 5% of the population studied had onset of mania before 10 y of age. Male patients will typically experience manic first episodes, and female patients will experience depressive first episodes. The apparent earlier onset of bipolar disorder seen in male patients may reflect earlier recognition.

Treatment

Pharmacologic treatment

• Lithium, valproate, and carbamazepine have been studied and used in the treatment of bipolar disorder not only in acute episodes of mania but also in the prevention of future episodes.

• *Note*: In pregnant women who are manic, depressed, or psychotically depressed, the safest and most effective treatment is usually electroconvulsive therapy [3] (*see* Nonpharmacologic treatment). Psychiatrists will need to discuss the benefits, risks, and alternatives with women who are pregnant or planning to conceive.

Lithium

• Lithium has been the traditional and primary mood stabilizer used in the treatment of bipolar disorder, for both depressive and manic episodes. Lithium is used for acute and preventive treatment.

Standard dosage	600–1200 mg/d, with serum trough levels ranging from 0.5–1.2 mEq/L.
Contraindications	Pregnancy and the postpartum state. First-trimester exposure is associated with increased risk of birth defects [3].
Main drug interactions	Drugs that will increase lithium levels (*eg*, diuretics and nonsteroidal anti-inflammatories).
Main side effects	Prominent hand tremor, significant weight gain, lethargy, hair loss, and gastrointestinal difficulties (nausea, diarrhea, or vomiting).
Special points	Levels should be taken every 2–3 months to monitor for toxicity (more often on initiation of drug). Lithium is not metabolized and is fully water soluble; thus, a major change in fluid intake will change serum levels. making them unreliable.

Valproate

• Valproate studies indicate higher efficacy for mixed bipolar patients and rapid cyclers (patients who have four or more occurrences in 1 y, including both depressive and manic episodes).

Standard dosage	500–2000 mg/d, with therapeutic serum levels ranging from 50–125 µg/mL.
Contraindications	Same as for Lithium.
Main drug interactions	Valproate is metabolized by the liver and highly protein bound; therefore, watch for interactions with other medications that are also protein bound, possibly causing toxicity.
Main side effects	Usually minimal but may include sedation, tremor, gastrointestinal difficulties, liver toxicity, and hair loss.

Carbamazepine

• Carbamazepine studies show good maintenance response when used in conjunction with lithium or valproate. However, studies are inconclusive as to its efficacy when used alone. Carbamazepine is metabolized through the liver.

Standard dosage	400–1600 mg/d, with serum levels 4–12 µg/mL.
Contraindications	Same as for Lithium.
Main side effects	Diplopia, blurred vision, fatigue, ataxia, agranulocytosis, and a decrease in sodium levels [3].
Main drug interactions	Carbamazepine will decrease the plasma levels of many medications also metabolized by the liver (*eg*, antipsychotics, tricyclics, benzodiazepines, and hormonal contraceptives) [3]. Medications such as selective seritonin–reuptake inhibitors, calcium channel blockers, and erythromycin can increase carbamazepine serum levels [3].

Treatment aims [3]

To enhance treatment compliance.
To monitor psychiatric status.
To maintain and establish a therapeutic alliance.
To promote health activity and sleep hygiene.
To promote understanding and adaptation to the psychosocial effects of bipolar disorder.

Prognosis

• Long-term prognosis is variable. However, some patients will do quite well when the above treatment aims are met.

Follow-up and management

• A relapse rate of 50% (within 1 y) is largely due to noncompliance with medications and being poorly informed of the chronicity of the illness.

Nonpharmacologic treatment

Electroconvulsive therapy.
Psychotherapy.

Key references

1. *Diagnostic and Statistical Manual of Mental Disorders*, ed 4. Washington, DC: American Psychiatric Association; 1994:350–355.

2. Keck PE, Strakowski SM: Psychopharmacological treatment of bipolar disorder across the life span. In *Review of Psychiatry*, vol 16. Edited by McElroy SL. Washington, DC: American Psychiatric Press, Inc.; 1997:7–30.

3. American Psychiatric Association: Practice guidelines for the treatment of patients with bipolar disorder. *Am J Psychiatry* 1994, 151(suppl):12.

General references

Dieperink ME, Sands JR: Bipolar mania with psychotic features. *Psychiatr Ann* 1996, 26:633–634.

Janicak PG, Davis JM, Preskorn SH, Ayd FJ: Treatment with mood stabilizers. In *Principles of Practice of Psychopharmacotherapy*. Washington, DC: Williams & Wilkins Press; 1997:403–470.

Goodwin FK, Ghaemi SN: Understanding manic depressive illness. *Arch Gen Psychiatry* 1998, 55:23–25.

Diagnosis

Definition
• Borderline personality disorder is a pervasive pattern of instability in affects, interpersonal relationships, and self-image. Marked impulsivity and conceptual impairment are present most commonly under stress.

Symptoms and signs
Somatic complaints: headaches, abdominal pain, malaise.

Autonomic instability: cold hands, nausea, vomiting, diarrhea, etc.

Tendency to demonstrate factitious illnesses (Munchausen's syndrome and Munchausen's syndrome by proxy): leads to overuse of medical resources and needless surgeries.

Commonly present in individuals demonstrating multiple personalities: dissociative identity disorder.

DSM-IV diagnostic criteria
• The disorder is indicated by the presence of five or more of the following:

1. Frantic efforts to avoid real or imagined abandonment (does not include suicidal or self-mutilating behavior, which is covered in the fifth criterion).

2. A pattern of unstable and intense interpersonal relationships characterized by alternating between extremes of idealization and devaluation.

3. Identity disturbance (markedly and persistently unstable self-image or sense of self).

4. Impulsivity in at least two areas that are potentially self-damaging, eg, spending, sex, substance abuse, reckless driving, binge eating (does not include suicidal or self-mutilating behavior, which is covered in the fifth criterion).

5. Recurrent self-mutilating or suicidal behavior, gestures, or threats.

6. Affective instability due to a marked reactivity of mood (eg, intense episodic dysphoria, irritability, or anxiety usually lasting a few hours and only rarely more than a few days).

7. Chronic feelings of emptiness.

8. Inappropriate, intense anger or difficulty controlling anger (eg, frequent displays of temper, constant anger, recurrent physical fights).

9. Transient, stress-related paranoid ideation or severe dissociative symptoms.

Investigations
Psychologic testing: distinct patterns on Minnesota Multiphasic Personality Inventory and other psychologic tests indicating behavioral instability and impulsivity; subpopulations demonstrate a variety of disturbances on neuropsychologic tests, especially those involving complex attentional functioning.

Laboratory studies: preliminary research reveals disturbances in central nervous system dopaminergic (hyperreactive), serotonergic (hyporeactive), and cholinergic (hyperreactive) responses to chemical challenge tests.

Screening tests: Millon Clinical Multiaxial Inventory III.

Complications

Comorbidity
Mood disorders, substance-related disorders, panic and anxiety disorders, eating disorders (especially bulimia), posttraumatic stress disorders, attention deficit–hyperactivity disorder, other personality disorders.

Behavioral outcomes
Interrupted education, frequent job changes and losses, broken marriages; bankruptcy; physical handicaps from self-inflicted abuse; premature death from suicide.

Differential diagnosis
• Mood disorders (major depressive disorder and bipolar disorder) demonstrate less affective lability and impulsivity; more stable relationships.

• Other personality disorders include the following:

Histrionic: distinguished by less self-destructiveness, angry disruptions in relationships, and persistent feelings of loneliness and emptiness.

Schizotypal: psychotic symptoms are less transient and interpersonally driven; less desire for interpersonal intimacy.

Narcissistic and paranoid: relative stability of self-image and less self-destructiveness; impulsivity and concerns over abandonment.

Antisocial: manipulative to gain profit, power, or material gratification rather than the concern of caretakers.

Dependent: more stable and less intense relationships; response to fear of abandonment characterized by appeasement, submissiveness, and seeking of replacement relationships.

• Personality change due to a general medical condition: traits arise as a direct result of a medical condition or chronic substance abuse on the central nervous system.

Etiology
• Biologic investigations suggest impairment of neuropsychologic function and specific neurotransmitter, neurohumoral, and electrophysiologic dysfunction.

• Psychosocial studies reveal high prevalence of childhood trauma (especially physical and sexual abuse), early separation or loss, and abnormal parenting.

Epidemiology
• The prevalence in the general population is 2%; in psychiatric outpatients, 10%; in psychiatric inpatients, 20%; in all personality disorders, 30%–60%.

• Occurrence is more common in women than in men (3:1 ratio).

Treatment

Diet and lifestyle
- Decrease or eliminate alcohol and recreational drug use.
- Develop routine diet, work, sleep, and recreational habits and patterns.

Pharmacologic treatment
- Enhance mood stability, decrease impulsivity, and improve cognitive performance by using low-dose neuroleptics, valproic acid, lithium, and newer antidepressants (eg, selective serotonin reuptake inhibitors and venlafaxine).
- The concomitant use of a mood-stabilizing agent will usually be required to prevent paranoid or dissociative episodes and reduce dysphoria, which may be produced by antidepressants or stimulants when used alone.

Standard dosage	High-potency neuroleptics (eg, thiothixene, trifluoperazine, risperidol, olanzapine) 1–10 mg/d.
	Other mood-stabilizing agents may also be effective in doses less than commonly used for mood disorders.
	Newer antidepressants may reduce impulsivity and stabilize mood when used in moderate to high dosages.
Contraindications	Allergy to medication.
	Neuroleptics: symptoms of or factors predisposing to tardive dyskinesia.
Main drug interactions	Multiple medication use (eg, neuroleptics, antidepressants [especially buproprion], and stimulants) may significantly reduce seizure threshold.
Main side effects	*Neuroleptics*: sedation and akithisia.
	Other mood stabilizers: sedation, weight gain, and toxicities specific to each.
	Antidepressants: excitation, nervousness, sedation, weight gain, sexual dysfunction, paranoid and dissociative episodes.

Follow-up and management

For the acute phase
- Hospitalization may be required during periods of acute decompensation to prevent self-destructive behaviors and to stabilize patient. Medications such as mood stabilizers (eg, neuroleptics) and antidepressants (bupropion, venlafaxine) may be indicated for major depressive disorder or dysthymic disorder.
- Supportive therapy may be required 2 or 3 times per week to stabilize mood, maintain control over self-destructive behaviors, assure medication compliance, and provide counsel on reducing situational stresses.
- Family counseling can determine stresses and interventions to reduce stress and provide information on the nature, management, and expected course of the illness.

For the continuation phase
- Educate patient on appropriate titration of mood stabilizer to accommodate fluctuations in stress levels and to minimize total body burden of medication. Psychotherapy should develop stable working relationship with patient; provide safe holding environment to reduce maladaptive, impulsive behaviors during evaluation and management of patterns of situational stresses; provide continued education on the nature, course, and management of the disorder; and establish new, adaptive behaviors that result in more stable interpersonal relationships and improved vocational and social functioning. As therapy progresses, frequency of treatment declines.
- Group therapy reduces sense of isolation by recognizing the disorder in others, by improving strategies for control of emotional lability and impulsive and self-destructive maladaptive behaviors in response to situational stresses, and by developing additional support for acute situational stresses.

Treatment aims

Short-term
To provide crisis stabilization and situational support to prevent or reduce self-destructive behaviors and rapidly enhance functioning.

Long-term
To enhance the consistency of adaptive psychosocial functioning and stress tolerance.

Prognosis
- Depends on severity of the disorder and other predictive factors.
- Predictors of positive outcome include high intelligence, artistic talent, physical attractiveness, education, absence of transgenerational sexual or physical abuse, lack of substance abuse, and no history of being jailed.
- Predictors of negative outcome are converse of positive predictors.

Nonpharmacologic treatment
Supportive psychoeducational therapy: most common form of therapy used; designed to enhance understanding of specific manifestations, and to develop less impulsive and emotionally overreactive and more adaptive responses.
Dynamic therapy: useful in a limited group of patients.
Cognitive-behavioral therapy and biofeedback: may be particularly helpful for control of headaches and symptoms of panic or anxiety disorders and autonomic instability.
Group therapy: recent evidence suggests effectiveness in select populations.

General references
Coccaro EF: Clinical outcome of psychopharmacologic treatment of borderline and schizotypal personality disordered subjects. *J Clin Psychiatry* 1998, 59 (suppl 1):30–35.

Linehan M, Heard H, Armstrong H: Naturalistic follow-up of a behavioral treatment for chronically parasuicidal borderline patients. *Arch Gen Psychiatry* 1993, 50:971–974.

Paris J: The etiology of borderline personality disorder: a biopsychosocial approach. *Psychiatry* 1994, 57:316–325.

Quaytman M, Sharfstein SS: Treatment for severe borderline personality disorder in 1987 and 1997. *Am J Psychiatry* 1997, 154:1139–1144.

Diagnosis

Symptoms and signs
• At least one primary symptom must be present. Symptom(s) must be present minimum of 1 day but less than 1 month. Patient's cultural context must be taken into account. Some culture-bound syndromes mimic symptoms of psychosis (*eg*, amok, koro, wihtigo).

Primary
Delusions.

Hallucinations.

Disorganized speech.

Grossly disorganized or catatonic behavior.

Secondary
Overwhelming confusion.

Emotional turmoil.

Suicidal ideation.

Rapid affective shifts.

Impaired insight and judgment.

Specifiers
With marked stressor(s): symptoms often develop shortly after and in response to an event or events that would be markedly stressful to most anyone in similar circumstances within the same cultural context.

Without marked stressor(s): symptoms may not be in response to an event or events that would be markedly stressful to most anyone in similar circumstances within the same cultural context.

With postpartum onset: noted if symptoms occur within 4 weeks postpartum.

Investigations
• A number of medical conditions may cause symptoms of psychosis and must be ruled out using the following assessments:

Complete psychiatric and general medical history.

Mental status examination.

Physical examination with neurological evaluation.

Chemistry panel.

Complete blood count.

Toxicology screen.

Thyroid function test.

Syphilis serology.

• Perform other tests as clinically indicated (*eg*, HIV antibody screen, heavy metals screen, computed tomography or MRI, tuberculin skin test).

Complications
Impaired psychosocial functioning.

Increased incidence of suicide.

Decreased insight and judgement.

Possible symptoms of posttraumatic stress disorder or mood disorder: if diagnosis occurs in relation to marked stressor.

Differential diagnosis
Psychotic disorder due to a general medical condition.
Substance-induced psychotic disorder.
Malingering or factitious disorder.
Mood disorder with psychotic features.
Schizoaffective disorder.
Schizophrenia.
Seizure disorder.
Delirium.
Personality disorder.

Etiology
• The cause of brief psychotic disorder (BPD) is not clear.
• A preexisting personality disorder has been found in 63%–87% of patients with transient psychosis.
• Mood disorder is associated with BPD. Marked psychosocial stress is associated with some, but not all, incidences of BPD.

Epidemiology
• There is a marked absence of studies on epidemiologic aspects of BPD, but the incidence rate is believed to be rare.
• Among military recruits, 1.4:100,000 met DSM-IIIR diagnostic criteria [1]; however, the rate is believed to be higher with DSM-IV criteria.
• BPD may be more common in younger and low socioeconomic-status patients.

Clinical course
• There are no prodromal symptoms.
• Onset is abrupt.
• Must be asymptomatic with return to premorbid level of functioning within 1 month.

Treatment

Diet and lifestyle

• As with all illnesses, care must be taken to assure appropriate rest, diet, exercise, avoidance of substance dependence and stress.

Pharmacologic treatment

• Antipsychotic medications (neuroleptics and atypical and antipsychotics) are indicated for treatment of acute symptoms of psychosis.

Risperidone

• Risperidone is used for acute symptoms of psychosis [2].

Standard dosage	2–10 mg/d (6 mg/d is the most effective dose [2]).
Contraindications	Cardio- and cerebrovascular disease, pregnant or nursing mothers, history of seizure disorder.
Main drug interactions	May enhance hypotensive effects of other drugs with this same potential. May antagonize effects of dopamine agonists and levodopa. Long-term use of carbamazepine or clozapine may interfere with resperidone clearance.
Main side effects	Extrapyramidal symptoms (*eg*, tremor, dystonia, hyperkinesia, hypertonia, ataxia), dizziness, somnolence, nausea, elevated prolactin levels, tardive dyskinesia.
Special points	Cost may exclude use by low socioeconomic-status patients.

Haloperidol

• There is substantial clinical confidence in the use of haloperidol from decades of clinical use and research [2].

Standard dosage	2–20 mg/d orally for symptoms of acute psychosis.
Contraindications	Comatose states, Parkinson's disease, toxic central nervous system (CNS) depression.
Main drug interactions	May block vasopressor activity of epinephrine, may interfere with effects of anticoagulants, potentiates CNS depressant effect.
Main side effects	Extrapyramidal symptoms (*eg*, Parkinson-like symptoms, akathesia, dystonia), insomnia, agitation, lethargy, tardive dyskinesia.
Special points	Initial high dosing (>16 mg/d) is no more effective than moderate dosing (10–14 mg/d) [3].

Other drugs

• Olanzapine (Zyprexa) [4] and Quetiapine (Seroquel) may be useful.

• Benzodiazepines are indicated as possible adjunct to antipsychotics for agitation, anxiety, and tension. Lorazepam is commonly prescribed [2].

Nonpharmacologic treatment

Crisis intervention: for initial presentation of acute psychotic symptoms and secondary symptoms.

Cognitive-behavioral and psychoeducational interventions: for stress reduction/management and coping skills strengthening may be indicated.

Family therapy: for strengthening family support for patient.

Psychotherapy: for mood disorder, personality disorder, or posttraumatic stress disorder, if present.

Treatment aims

To alleviate and reduce symptoms to return patient to baseline role functioning.

Prognosis

• By definition, patient should be asymptomatic within 1 mo.
• Symptoms may resolve in 2–3 d.
• No further psychiatric symptoms were experienced by 50%–80% of patients in European follow-up studies.

Follow-up and management

• Post 1-mo follow-up should include evaluation for mood disorder and suicidal/homocidal ideation.
• If suspected, patient should be evaluated for personality disorder.
• If marked stressor was associated with patient's BPD diagnosis, patient should be evaluated for posttraumatic stress disorder.

Key references

1. Beighly PS, Brown GR, et al.: DSM-III-R brief reactive psychosis among Air Force Recruits. *J Clin Psychiatr* 1992, 53:283–288.
2. American Psychiatric Association: Practice guidelines for the treatment of patients with schizophrenia. *Am J Psychiatr* 1997, 154(suppl):1–63.
3. Baldessarini RJ, Cohen BM, et al.: Significance of neuroleptic dose and plasma level in the pharmacological treatment of psychosis. *Arch Gen Psychiatry* 1988, 45:79–90.
4. Tollefson GD, Beasley CM, Tran PV, et.al.: Olanzapine versus haloperidol in the treatment of schizophrenia and schizoaffective and schizophreniform disorders: results of an international collaborative trial. *Am J Psychiatr* 1997, 154:457–465.

General reference

Diagnostic and Statistical Manual of Mental Disorders, ed 4 (DSM-IV). Washington, DC: American Psychiatric Association; 1994.

Diagnosis

Definition
• Bulimia nervosa is an eating disorder characterized by periods of significant overeating (binging) and purging.

Signs and symptoms

Behavioral
Surreptitious behavior: *eg*, hiding food, long periods in the bathroom with vague excuses.

Outwardly restrictive meal patterns or overconcern with dieting and nutrition: but with little change in weight or appearance.

Dissatisfaction with body size and shape.

Physical
Decaying teeth, dehydration, fatigue, swollen salivary glands, scars on dorsum of hand (Russell's sign).

Psychologic
Depressed mood, low self-esteem, high achievement orientation, "people pleasing" tendencies.

DSM-IV diagnostic criteria
1. Recurrent episodes of binge eating (eating an amount larger than most people would eat during a similar period of time and a sense of lack of control over eating during the episode).

2. Compensatory behavior in order to prevent weight gain (e.g., self-induced vomiting; misuse of laxatives or diuretics; fasting or excessive exercise).

3. These behaviors occur at least twice a week for 3 months, on average.

4. Body shape and weight unduly influence self-evaluation and self-esteem.

Investigations
• Laboratory studies may be helpful to identify the degree of electrolyte imbalance caused by frequent purging and to determine the individual's nutritional status and state of overall health. If purging behaviors are frequent, laboratory profiles should be followed serially to monitor fluid balance and detect hypokalemia.

Complications

Comorbidity
Depression, anxiety disorders, borderline personality disorder, anorexia nervosa.

Behavioral outcomes
Impairment in social network due to lying to friends, social isolation, and poor social skills.

Impairment in financial status due to money spent on food and laxatives.

Impairment in family relationships due to concealment and lying.

Medical complications
Gastric distress or bleeding, esophagitis, dental erosion, cardiac complications (*eg*, arrhythmia, tachycardia), muscle cramping due to electrolyte imbalance, renal failure.

Differential diagnosis
Binge eating disorder: characterized by binging but with no purging.
Anorexia nervosa: may involve binges and purges, but individual must be 25% below ideal (healthy) body weight.
Digestive disorders: some bowel dysfunction and gastrointestinal dysfunction; may have vomiting or diarrhea that is either self-induced or not used to lose weight.

Etiology
• Etiology of bulimia is unclear. Hypothesized risk factors for the disorder include:
Biologic risk factors (dysregulation of the serotonergic system).
Familial risk factors (families of individuals with bulimia have been shown to be more chaotic and less cohesive than non-bulimic families).
Sociocultural risk factors (acceptance of societal standards of thinness and beauty is associated with bulimia).
Psychologic risk factors (individuals with low self-esteem and depressive symptomatology are at higher risk for bulimia).

Epidemiology
• The prevalence of bulimia nervosa is between 3%–5%, with a higher prevalence in women than in men. Prevalence rates for bulimic symptoms in college-aged women have been reported as high as 19%.

Treatment

Diet and lifestyle

• It may be helpful for the individual with bulimia to see a dietitian in order to learn nutritional eating patterns and to restructure beliefs about food as energy rather than as something "bad" or "good."

Pharmacologic treatment

• Antidepressants have been used in the treatment of bulimia with encouraging results. Selective serotonin-reuptake inhibitors (SSRIs) are usually favored over tricyclic antidepressants (TCAs) because SSRIs have fewer and less severe side effects.

Standard dosage	SSRIs: fluoxetine, 20–80 mg/d orally.
	TCAs: desipramine, 150–300 mg/d orally, or imipramine, 150–300 mg daily.
	Bupropion, 150–450 mg/d orally.
Main side effects	*SSRIs*: agitation, anxiety, sleep disturbance, tremor, sexual dysfunction (primarily anorgasmia), headache.
	TCAs: increased heart rate, anticholinergic effects (*eg*, dry mouth, blurred vision, constipation, urinary retention), sedation, weight gain.
	Buproprion: appetite suppression, potential for emergence of psychotic symptoms, seizures (individuals with bulimia appear to have a somewhat higher risk than other patients for developing grand mal seizures from this medication)

Nonpharmacologic treatments

Cognitive-behavioral therapy: has four distinct phases: 1) history and self-monitoring (detailed information about psychologic, emotional, and behavioral functioning is assessed through a clinical interview and through self-monitoring of nutritional intake, binging, and purging behaviors); 2) dietary intake is normalized (patients are educated in healthy, regular eating patterns and encouraged to resume or begin eating healthily); 3) cognitive restructuring (cognitive distortions about food, thinness, achievement, and assertiveness are examined and restructured to be more adaptive); and 4) relapse prevention (therapy is slowly tapered down; signs of relapse are discussed; preventive strategies are emphasized).

Behavioral techniques: exposure plus response prevention; based on anxiety and phobic avoidance involved in the binge-purge cycle, individuals with bulimia are exposed to feared foods either gradually or through a binge and then prevented from purging; as the anxiety decreases with the repeated exposure without the compensatory behaviors, the individual becomes less fearful of eating.

Relaxation training: *eg*, progressive muscle relaxation; individuals are taught alternative means to deal with negative emotions such as anxiety; has been used successfully with bulimic patients.

Stimulus control: antecedent and consequential behaviors associated with binging and purging are examined and restructured to prevent binges and purges from occurring.

Other treatment options

Family therapy: individuals whose family dynamics contribute to or exacerbate bulimic symptomatology may benefit from family therapy.

Group therapy: individuals who demonstrate particularly poor social skills and who appear particularly susceptible to group or societal pressures toward thinness may benefit from group therapy targeted at bulimia recovery.

Feminist therapy: individuals who demonstrate overidentification and internalization of sociocultural standards of thinness for females may benefit from therapy that restructures beliefs about societal influences and empowers women to become more independent and assertive.

Treatment aims

To achieve abstinence from binging and purging.
To regain healthy eating patterns.
To address other psychological issues related to the bulimia.

Prognosis

• ~30% of individuals with bulimia benefit from pharmacologic treatment alone; however, as many as 70% of individuals with bulimia benefit from the combination of medication and cognitive-behavioral interventions. Thus, the combination of cognitive-behavioral and pharmacologic interventions appears to be the treatment of choice for bulimia.

Follow-up and management

• Self-help groups or support groups (eg, Overeaters Anonymous) may be helpful for individuals with bulimia.
• Booster sessions to review healthy eating patterns and coping skills may be beneficial.
• Regular moderate exercise may be helpful for individuals to deal with the expected weight fluctuations as their bodies adjust to their new healthy eating patterns.

General references

Agras WS: Treatment of eating disorders. In *Textbook of Psychopharmacology.* Edited by Schatzberg AF and Nemeroff CB. Washington, DC: American Psychiatric Press; 1995.

American Psychiatric Association: Practice guideline for eating disorders. *Am J Psychiatry.* 1993, 150:212–228.

American Psychiatric Association: *Diagnostic and Statistical Manual of Mental Disorders,* ed 4. Washington, DC: American Psychiatric Press; 1994.

Fairburn CG, Agras WS, Wilson GT: The research on the treatment of bulimia nervosa: practical and theoretical implications. In *The Biology of Feast and Famine: Relevance to Eating Disorders.* Edited by Anderson GH Kennedy SH. New York: Academic Press; 1992.

Thurstin AH, Mason NS: Behavioral, physical, and psychological symptoms of eating disorders. In *Eating Disorders: A Reference Source Book.* Edited by Lemberg. Phoenix, AZ: Oryx Press; in press.

Diagnosis

Definition

• Cocaine problems are classified into two types based on decreasing severity: dependence and abuse.

Cocaine dependence

• Cocaine dependence is indicated by the presence of the following:

Physical tolerance.

Withdrawal symptoms.

Use of drug for longer periods and in greater amounts than intended.

Persistent desire or unsuccessful attempts to cut down or control use.

Large portion of time spent in activities relating to the acquisition and use of drug.

Reduced participation in occupational, recreational, and social activities due to use.

Use of substance despite negative consequences, including legal, medical, physical, financial, and family dysfunction.

Cocaine abuse

• Cocaine abuse is defined as:

Recurrent use resulting in a failure to fulfill major role obligations at school, work, and home.

Recurrent use in physically hazardous situations or despite legal consequences or interpersonal problems.

Symptoms and signs

Intoxication: perspiration or chills, tachycardia, pupillary dilation, elevated blood pressure, nausea, tremor, chest pain, arrhythmia, fever, convulsions, anorexia or weight loss, dry mouth, impotence, hallucinations, hyperactivity, irritability, aggressiveness, paranoid ideation.

Withdrawal: dysphoria, fatigue, sleep disorder, agitation, and craving.

• A "yes" response to two or more of the following questions would indicate a need for thorough assessment for dependence or abuse:

1. Do you frequently feel down and wish you could quickly put yourself into an "up" mood?

2. Do you place a high value on the feeling of euphoria?

3. Do you often feel worn out or tired enough to want a stimulant to get you going?

4. When you see other people having "fun" with cocaine, do you feel the need to experience the same fun?

5. Do you feel insecure about sex and relationships and wish you could raise your self-confidence by the use of a drug?

6. Have you ever thought of using cocaine just to get through a day of work?

7. Do you use cocaine to raise your confidence and be a success at work or in social situations?

8. Have you driven a car while under the influence of cocaine?

9. Have you felt you should cut down on your use?

10. Have people annoyed you by criticizing your use?

11. Have you ever felt guilty or bad about your use?

12. Have you wondered if you had a problem with cocaine?

Investigations

• A deatiled drug and alcohol history is essential for patients suspected of cocaine abuse or dependence. The following areas are to be included:

Family history of drug and alcohol problems; amount and frequency of use; concomitant substance abuse; legal history related to use; family problems; urine drug screens.

Differential diagnosis

• Consequences and results of cocaine use are often mistaken for primary rather than secondary problems (eg, insomnia, depression).

• The marked mental disturbances should be distinguished from the symptoms of schizophrenia (paranoid type), bipolar and other mood disorders, generalized anxiety disorder, and panic disorder.

Etiology

• Risk factors for cocaine use include the following:

Drug use in teenage years.

Psychiatric illness.

History of antisocial behavior.

Family history of drug abuse or dependence.

Epidemiology

• Approximately 10% of casual cocaine use becomes abuse or dependence, according to studies conducted on the general population.

• Approximately 142,410 cocaine-related emergency room episodes were reported in 1994.

• In 1994, ~22 million Americans ≥12 y of age had tried cocaine at least once in their lifetimes, ~3.7 million had used cocaine during the past year, and ~1.3 million had used cocaine in the past month.

Complications

Physical: preterm labor, abruptio placentae, mycardial infarction, intravenous use can increase risk for AIDS, hepatitis, septicemia, venous thrombosis; intranasal use can lead to perforated septum, impotence.

Social: isolation, disruption of social structure, job loss, divorce, suicide attempts.

Psychologic: erratic behavior, paranoid ideation, auditory hallucinations in a clear sensorium, and tactile hallucinations that the user recognizes as the effects of use.

Treatment

Diet and lifestyle
• A balanced diet and nutritional plan can help the recovery process.

Pharmacologic treatment
• Antidepressants, dopamine agonists, and anticonvulsants have been used but have not proven effective for cocaine withdrawal.

Nonpharmacologic treatment
• Referral to treatment program or a 12-step program (*eg*, Cocaine Anonymous) is the preferred course of treatment. Practitioners should identify a colleague (counselor, social worker, addictions counselor specialist) who can evaluate and recommend the best course of action or the level of care most appropriate.

Prognosis
• In 1990, 238,071 patients entered treatment identifying cocaine as the drug of choice.
• One report indicates that 30%–90% of abusers remaining in outpatient programs cease cocaine use.

Follow-up and management
• Relapse prevention is primary goal of follow-up.
• Family programs offer education on healthy support and identify dysfunction.
• Periodically assess need for maintenance counseling or continued care.

General references
Dennison SJ, White CF: Cocaine use and associated cardiovascular risks. *Resident and Staff Physician* 1990, 36:49–52.

Falvo DR: *Medical and Psychological Aspects of Chronic Illness and Disability*. Gaithersburg, MD: Aspen Publishers; 1991.

Mehl D: *The High Road*. Park Ridge, IL: Parkside Publishing Corporation; 1988.

Miller NS, Gold MS: Cocaine: recognition of abuse and pharmacologic responses. *Family Practice Recertification* 1990, 12:86–98.

Diagnosis

Symptoms and signs

General communication disorder

Speech dysfluency: characterized by frequent repetitions of individual sounds, syllables, or monosyllabic words; there may be pauses within a word or pauses between words (which may be audible or silent), interjections, an excess of physical tension in word production, or word substitutions to avoid difficult words; the dysfluency must be of sufficient severity to interfere with academic, occupational, or social functioning; if a neurologic disorder or speech-motor deficit is present, the dysfluency must be in excess of that expected with the underlying disorder; performance anxiety may increase the severity of symptoms; **stuttering:** may diminish or remit in situations such as singing, reading aloud, or talking to pets or objects; **tics or other unusual movements:** may be associated with stuttering.

Expressive language disorder

Limited speech or vocabulary, word-finding difficulties, delays in acquiring new vocabulary, shortened or limited sentences or grammatical structures, odd syntax, slow rate of language development, nonlinguistic cognitive functioning usually within normal limits for age.

Mixed receptive–expressive language disorder

Difficulties associated with expressive language disorder; difficulties comprehending words or sentences.

• A pure receptive language disorder is almost never seen in children because expressive language is dependent upon receptive language acquisition

Phonological disorder

Failure to use speech sounds that are developmentally appropriate to the speaker's age and dialect: difficulties may include omission of sounds, substitution of one sound for another, or failure to produce a speech sound correctly; **lisping and reversal of sound order within a word:** common forms of phonological disorder; **failure to pronounce sounds acquired late in the speech sequence (eg, th, ch, l, s, r, z).**

Investigations

General communication disorder

Assessment by a speech pathologist: to determine if the dysfluency is of sufficient severity and deviation from norms to warrant the diagnosis.

Expressive and mixed receptive–expressive language disorder

Standardized tests of expressive language development: usually administered by a speech pathologist or psychoeducation specialist.

Phonological disorder

Assessment by a speech pathologist: taking into account the individual's culture, dialect, or bilingual home environment.

Complications

General communication disorder

Low self-esteem; limited career choice and advancement: in adults.

Expressive language disorder

Phonological disorder and dysfluencies; developmental coordination disorder, enuresis, attention deficit–hyperactivity disorder, and social withdrawal, and atypicalities on neurodiagnostic tests and neurologic examination; significant limiting of academic performance.

Mixed receptive–expressive language disorder

Inattentive or oppositional behavior; difficulty in acquiring age-appropriate conversational and social skills.

Phonological disorder

Impairments in academic, occupational, and social functioning.

Differential diagnosis

General disorder

• Dysfluencies occur normally in young children and typically resolve as language development advances. A speech-motor deficit or sensory deficit (eg, hearing impairment) should be ruled out in cases in which stuttering exceeds developmental norms.

Expressive disorder

Mixed expressive–receptive language disorder, pervasive developmental disorders, selective mutism, acquired aphasia.

Mixed disorder

Pervasive developmental disorder, selective mutism, acquired aphasia.

Phonological disorder

• Speech problems limited to rhythm or voice are classified as stuttering or communication disorder not otherwise specified. If a comorbid condition exists (eg, mental retardation, hearing impairment, environmental deprivation, speech-motor deficit), the speech deficit must be in excess of that usually associated with those problems.

Etiology

General disorder

• Genetic factors have been implicated in studies of twins and families who stutter, with a threefold increase in risk in first-degree relatives.

Expressive disorder

• There are two types—developmental and acquired. The developmental type is usually recognized by 3 y of age and may slowly resolve by late adolescence, although long-lasting deficits persist in 50% of affected children. Brain lesions, head trauma, or stroke occurring at any age may result in the acquired type; resolution is dependent on the age at which the brain insult occurs and upon the course of the underlying process. Environmental deprivation, mental retardation, hearing impairment or other sensory deficit, and speech-motor deficits may all influence language development. Impairment must be in excess of that expected with these disorders in order to make the diagnosis of expressive language disorder.

Treatment

Diet and lifestyle
• No special precautions are necessary.

Pharmacologic treatment
• No specific pharmacologic treatment is recommended; however, treat any existing comorbid conditions.

Nonpharmacologic treatment
• Usually, no intervention is recommended for preschool children because 85% will improve spontaneously. After 6 year of age, speech therapy once or twice weekly as well as language enrichment in the educational program are usually effective. Parents may assist by providing supplemental experiences in the home, as guided by the speech pathologist or special educator.

Treatment aims
To restore expressive language to age-appropriate level with concomitant improvement in social, academic, and occupational functioning.

Mixed disorder
• There are two types: developmental and acquired. The developmental type is usually evident by 4 y of age unless it is extremely mild, in which case it may not be noted until elementary school. The prognosis is worse than for expressive language disorder. The acquired type is associated with head trauma, brain lesions, or other medical condition. An extremely rare entity (Landau–Kleffenr syndrome) appears between the ages of 3–9 y of age, is associated with an abnormal electroencephalogram, and may have a variable course.

Phonological disorder
• Causes include hearing impairment, environmental deprivation, cognitive limitations, neurologic problems, and disorders of the oral speech-motor mechanism.

Epidemiology

General disorder
• The prevalence rate is ~1% in children, with a slight decrease by adolescence. Affected boys outnumber girls 3:1.

Expressive disorder
• The developmental type affects 3%–5% of children and is more common in boys. The acquired type is more rare.

Mixed disorder
• The developmental type is more prevalent in boys than in girls and affects up to 3% of the population. There is evidence of familial aggregation of the developmental type.

Phonological disorder
•The prevalence of the functional or developmental type in preschool children is at least 2.5%. Boys are more commonly affected, and some forms show a familial pattern.

General references
Cantwell DP, Baker L: Psychiatric and learning disorders in children with speech and language disorders: a descriptive analysis. *Adv Learn Behav Disabil* 1985, 4:29–47.

Diagnosis

Definition
• Compulsive buying is an increasingly recognized syndrome that consists of repetitive, intense, and excessive impulses to buy, resulting in personal, familial, and financial distress.

Symptoms and signs
• Compulsive buying impulses are frequently in the context of mild-to-moderate depression, and the actual spending of money is associated with a transient "buzz" or sense of well-being. This transient euphoric state is often followed by guilt, recrimination, and secretive behaviors to hide knowledge of the purchases from others, such as a husband. Typical purchases include clothing, cosmetics, jewelry, or collectibles. Articles are rarely bought because they are needed or advantageously priced. Once purchased, they may be used or, over half the time, returned to the vendor (never removed from packaging), given away, or even thrown away.

DSM-IV diagnostic criteria
• There are no specific DSM-type criteria, in that compulsive buying is not as yet a recognized specific disorder; presently it is classified as an "Impulse disorder not otherwise specified."

• McElroy et al. [1] proposed the following diagnostic criteria for compulsive buying:

Maladaptive preoccupations with buying or shopping, or maladaptive buying or shopping impulses or behavior, as indicated by at least one of the following: 1) frequent preoccupation with buying or impulses to buy that are experienced as irresistible, intrusive, or senseless; or 2) frequent buying of more than what can be afforded, frequent buying of items that are not needed, or shopping for longer periods of time than intended.

• The buying preoccupations, impulses, or behaviors cause marked distress, are time-consuming, significantly interfere with social or occupational functioning, or result in financial problems (eg, indebtedness or bankruptcy).

• The excessive buying or shopping behavior does not occur exclusively during periods of hypomania or mania.

Investigations

Psychologic testing
• The Minnesota Impulsive Disorders Interview is an instrument designed for exploration of a variety of impulse control disorders, including compulsive buying. In view of the significant comorbidity of compulsive buying with obsessive-compulsive disorder, affective disorders, and addictive disorders, psychologic tests (eg, the Minnesota Multiphasic Personality Inventory, the Millon Clinical Multiaxial Inventory, the Beck Depression Inventory, and the Mandsley Obsessive-Compulsive Inventory) may also prove to be useful adjuvants to diagnosis.

Laboratory studies
• No specific laboratory studies have been reported for compulsive buying.

Differential diagnosis
• The primary diagnoses to exclude are those of mania or hypomania and personality disorders.

Etiology
Specific etiologic factors presently have not been identified. The following factors have been proposed as important in at least some patients: 1) social and cultural attitudes that promote spending behaviors, eg, advertising and the widespread distribution of credit cards; and 2) compulsive buying as a symptom of one or more of the following: obsessive-compulsive disorder, depression, impulse control disorder, and addictive behaviors.

Epidemiology
• The prevalence of compulsive buying behavior in the general population is 1%–5% (dependent on stringency of diagnostic criteria). There is a marked preponderance of women (80%–90%) and the modal patient is in her 30's.

Complications

Comorbidity
• The overwhelming majority of patients will be comorbid for at least one axis I disorder, and over one half will meet criteria for a personality disorder. Comorbid conditions include the following:
Affective disorders.
Substance abuse or dependency.
Anxiety disorders.
Other impulse control disorders.
Eating disorders.
Personality disorders.

Behavioral outcomes
• Patients with maladaptive buying behaviors may also have the following:
Guilt.
Substantial debt, risk of bankruptcy.
Interpersonal marital conflicts, risk of divorce.
Criminal legal proceedings.

Treatment

Diet and lifestyle
• Persons with compulsive buying are frequently comorbid for impulse-driven lifestyles. They should be encouraged to increase structure and routine in their lives, particularly in the realm of shopping for essentials. They may also require help from financial advisors or responsible family members to control the financial aspects of their lives. The possession of multiple credit accounts must be discouraged.

Pharmacologic treatment
• All comorbid psychiatric disorders that are responsive to psychotropic agents should be treated. Affective disorders, including bipolar affective disorders, are very common and should receive needed attention. Fluvoxamine has been demonstrated, in an open label study, to significantly reduce compulsive buying. The presumptive method of therapeutic action is to increase mood and decrease impulsivity; other selective serotonin reuptake inhibitors may be similarly effective.

Standard dosage:	Fluvoxamine, 50–300 mg 4 times daily in divided dosage.
Contraindications	Persons with a known hypersensitivity to the drug and persons who are taking a monoamine oxidase inhibitor, terfenadine, astemizole, or cisapride.
Main side effects	*Fluvoxamine:* nausea, somnolence, dizziness, and delayed ejaculation; may also precipitate mania.
Main drug interactions	*Fluvoxamine:* this potent P450 3A4 inhibitor is likely to reduce metabolism of the benzodiazepines alprazolam, midazolam, and triazolam; will significantly raise blood levels of theophylline, warfarin, carbamazine, clozapine, and methadone.
	Lithium may enhance the serotonergic effects of fluvoxamine; the combination should be used with caution.
Special points	Best tolerated when prescribed at an initial low dosage and gradually increased to a therapeutic range.

Nonpharmacologic treatment
Psychotherapy
• Insight-oriented psychotherapy has not been shown to be effective.

• Behavioral therapy may play an important therapeutic role in helping patients identifying triggers for buying behaviors and by providing alternative, less destructive behaviors.

Treatment aims
To facilitate the capacity to make reasonable purchases and to use credit in a responsible manner.

Prognosis
• Compulsive buying, although long recognized, has only recently received scientific and clinical attention. No long-term follow-up data are available. It is likely that, similar to other impulse-driven disorders, symptoms will diminish spontaneously with age and maturity.

Other treatment options
• As public awareness of compulsive buying increases, it is likely that there will be the emergence of self-help groups similar to "Over-Eaters Anonymous." Such adjuvant therapy may be of therapeutic benefit.

Follow-up and management
For the acute phase
• Patients require regular follow-up visits to monitor dosage of medication, side effects, and efficacy. Behavioral therapy requires regularly scheduled visits (eg, weekly) over a period of several months.

For the continuation phase
• Long-term medication management will require periodic (every 3–6 mo) visits to reevaluate the need to continue pharmacotherapy. Periodic "touch-up" visits to reinforce behavioral therapy techniques are often useful.

Key reference
1. McElroy SI, Keck PE, Pope HG Jr, et al.: Compulsive buying: a report of twenty cases. *J Clin Psychiatry* 1994, 55:242–248.

General references
Black DW, Monaham P, Gabel J: Fluvoxamine in the treatment of compulsive buying. *J Clin Psychiatry* 1997, 58:159–163.

Christenson G, Faber RJ, deZwaan M, et al.: Compulsive buying: descriptive characteristics and psychiatric co-morbidity. *J Clin Psychiatry* 1994, 55:5–11, 1994.

Lejoyeux M, Adis J, Tapain V, Solomon J: Phenomenology and psychopathology of uncontrolled buying. *Am J Psychiatry* 1996, 153:1524–1529.

Diagnosis

General information

• There are two types of conduct disorders, childhood-onset type (at least one characteristic evident prior to 10 years of age) and adolescent-onset type (absence of any characteristics prior to 10 years of age).

Symptoms and signs

In preschool children

Aggression against other children.

Aggression at home.

Deliberately destructive.

Temper tantrums and defiance.

In grade-school children

Aggressive behavior.

Verbal aggression.

Deliberate cruelty: to people and animals.

Stealing in and outside the home.

Lying.

Classroom disruption.

Truancy.

Fire setting: uncommon

Investigations

Diagnostic assessment.

Interview of the child or adolescent.

Family history.

School information.

Standard parent and teacher rating scales.

Psychologic testing.

Physical evaluation.

Complications

School failure, suspensions.

Legal problems.

Injuries: due to fighting, retaliation.

Accidents.

Sexually transmitted diseases.

Drug addiction.

Suicide.

Differential diagnosis

• *Note:* conduct disorder is a descriptive diagnosis with high rates of comorbidity of other psychiatric disorders and neurologic findings. Attention to comorbid disorders is critical.
Oppositional defiant disorder.
Attention deficit–hyperactivity disorder (ADHD).
Isolated act of antisocial behavior.
Depression.

Etiology

Individual factors

Boys more susceptible.
Genetic predisposition.
Abnormal need for stimulus seeking.
Low intelligence and associated lower impulse control, communication abilities, and self-esteem.

Psychosocial factors

Psychopathology in parents.
Alcoholism.
Antisocial behavior.
Poor parental supervision.
Parental neglect, abuse, and passivity.
Excessive, harsh parental discipline.
Family discord.
Socioeconomically disadvantaged.
Neighborhood or school influence.
Crowded, urban area.

Epidemiology

• Prevalence is 10% in the general child and adolescent population.
• There is a male predominance.

Treatment

Pharmacologic treatment

Psychostimulants: for comorbid ADHD.

Lithium for severe aggression.

Antidepressants.

Anticonvulsants.

Propranolol.

Antipsychotics: for severe aggression linked to psychotic disorders, vulnerability to paranoid perceptions.

Nonpharmacologic treatment

Family interventions: parental guidance, training, and therapy.

Individual and group psychotherapy.

Peer interventions.

Alliance with Juvenile Justice System.

Social welfare agencies.

Community support resources.

Job training.

Residential and day treatment programs.

General references

Jaffe SL, et al.: AACAP Practice Parameters for the Assessment and Treatment of Conduct Disorders, September 1991.

Synopsis of Psychiatry. Edited by Hales R, Yudofsky S. DC: American Psychiatric Press; 1996.

Comprehensive Textbook of Psychiatry, ed 5. Edited by Kaplan H, Saddock B. Baltimore: Williams & Wilkins; 1989.

Diagnosis

Symptoms and signs

• Conversion disorder is diagnosed if 1) there is a presence of symptoms or deficits (*see* below) affecting voluntary motor or sensory functions that suggest a medical or neurological condition; 2) after appropriate medical and neurologic evaluation, the symptom or deficit cannot be fully explained by any known medical or neurologic disorder or pathophysiologic process; and 3) psychologic factors are judged to be associated with initiating the symptom or deficit, which is regarded as not intentionally produced or feigned by the patient.

• Conversion disorder is not diagnosed if a symptom is fully explained by culturally sanctioned behavior or experience.

Symptoms and deficits

Motor: paralysis, weakness, aphonia, falling, astasia-abasia, abnormal gait, involuntary movements, tics, seizures.

Sensory: anesthesia, paresthesia, blindness, tunnel vision, double vision, deafness, visceral, psychogenic vomiting, Globus hystericus, difficulty swallowing, syncope, urinary retention.

Associated characteristics [1]

• Factors judged to be useful in diagnosis of conversion disorder include the following:

Useful: prior history of somatization, a precipitating stressor, a model for the symptom, nonphysiologic findings.

Partially useful: secondary gain, concurrent psychiatric or neurological disorders.

Not useful: La belle indifference (relative lack of concern about the symptoms), hysterical personality disorder, symbolism.

Investigations

• The first step is to conduct an appropriate investigation to determine if a neurologic or medical condition exists and to rule out medication or substance induced causes.

• There are no known routine laboratory tests to confirm the disorder.

• Collateral information about the nature and onset of symptoms, as well as current stressors, need to be included in the assessment.

• Be alert for possible abuse. Victims of physical or sexual abuse may present with conversion symptoms.

Complications

• Although symptoms may resolve or be modified by suggestion or other cues, this is not specific to conversion disorder because this may also occur in patients with medical or neurologic conditions.

• Patients with conversion disorder may also have similar medical or neurologic conditions (a patient with pseudoseizures may also have a seizure disorder).

• Caution should be used with making the diagnosis of conversion disorder. Dramatic remission of nonphysiologic symptoms does not rule out the possibility of underlying disease [2].

• Dependency and adoption of the sick role may be fostered in the course of treatment.

• Persistent symptoms may lead to the development of secondary medical problems (*eg*, disuse atrophy).

Differential diagnosis

Medical and neurologic conditions

Multiple sclerosis, myasthenia gravis, periodic paralysis, brain tumor, optic neuritis, Guillain–Barré syndrome, Parkinson's disease, subdural hematoma, AIDS, degenerative diseases of basal ganglia or peripheral nerves, pregnancy, medication effects, effects of alcohol and other substances.

Psychiatric conditions

Mood Disorder, schizophrenia or other psychotic disorder, somatization disorder, body dysmorphic disorder, pain disorder, dissociative disorders, factitious disorder, malingering.

Etiology

• Likely biologic factors include brain hemispheric dysfunction and abnormal interhemispheric relations, with lateralizing symptoms more commonly experienced on the left side of the body.

• Limited data suggest conversion symptoms are more frequent in relatives of individuals with conversion disorder.

• Psychosocial factors include recent or chronic stressors as well as psychodynamic and cognitive factors.

Epidemiology

• Ages range from childhood to old age.

• Conversion disorder appears to be more common in women than in men, with reported ratios ranging from 2:1 to 10:1. It is also more common in rural populations, in individuals of lower socioeconomic status, and in individuals who are less knowledgeable about medical and psychologic concepts.

• Prevalence of conversion symptoms is 0.3% or less in the community-based populations, 1%–3% of outpatient referrals to mental health clinics, 1.2%–11.5% of psychiatric consultations to medical and surgical patients, and 1%–3% of neurologists' patients.

Treatment

Pharmacologic treatment
• Although not a treatment of the disorder, in acute situations, parenteral amobarbital or lorazepam may reduce anxiety and allow some patients to engage more effectively in treatment.

Nonpharmacologic treatment [3]
• Many conversion symptoms remit either spontaneously or after behavioral treatment. Suggestion of recovery and a supportive environment are often sufficient to initiate a recovery process.

• Elements of successful treatments include nonconfrontational approach, discouraging retention of symptoms, and manipulating the patients environment to decrease stressors.

• Most approaches work when symptoms are not reinforced and when the patient and his or her psychosocial plight is the focus of attention.

• Not all symptoms resolve in hours or days. Although relatively uncommon, persistent conversion symptoms may require inpatient psychiatric or rehabilitation treatment, utilizing behavioral modification techniques and physical therapy.

Treatment aims
To obtain remission of the disorder.
To promote more effective management of psychosocial stressors.

Prognosis
• Favorable prognosis is associated with acute and recent onset, readily identifiable stressor at onset, and absence of other major psychological and physical illnesses.
• Pending legal or disability issues usually complicate recovery.

Follow-up and management
• Acute conversion symptoms often present to hospital emergency departments. Adequate follow-up care is essential to ensure that appropriate medical and neurologic diagnostic evaluations are conducted.
• Referral for psychiatric evaluation is indicated for patients with possible comorbid conditions or those with persisting symptoms.
• Victims of physical or sexual abuse require appropriate protective action.
• Persistent conversion symptoms require less focus on precipitating factors and more attention toward the reinforcing behaviors of the patient, family, and environment.

Key references
1. Ford CV: Conversion disorder and somatoform disorder not otherwise specified. In *Treatments of Psychiatric Disorders*, ed 2. Edited by Gabbard G. Washington, DC: American Psychiatric Press; 1995:1783–1801.
2. Fishbain D, Goldberg M: The misdiagnosis of conversion disorder in a psychiatric emergency service. *General Hospital Psychiatry* 1991, 13:177–181.
3. Guggenheim F, Smith GR: Somatoform disorders. In *Comprehensive Textbook of Psychiatry/IV*. Edited by Kaplan SI, Saddock BJ. Baltimore: Williams & Wilkins; 1995:1251–1270.

General reference
American Psychiatric Association: *Diagnostic and Statistical Manual of Mental Disorders*, ed 4. Washington, DC: American Psychiatric Press; 1994.

Diagnosis

Definition
• Cyclothymia is a chronic mood disorder of at least 2 years' duration manifested by episodes of hypomania and mild depression. (In children and adolescents, the duration must be at least 1 y.)

Symptoms and signs
• Cyclothymic patients have hypomanic and dysphoric periods that are not severe enough to qualify as bipolar disorder or major depression. The patients' "highs and lows" do not usually merit hospitalization.

Hypomanic symptoms and signs
Inflated self-esteem or grandiosity.

Decreased need for sleep.

More talkative than usual or feels pressure to keep talking.

Flight of ideas.

Distractibility.

Increase in goal-directed activity or psychomotor agitation.

Excessive involvement in pleasurable activities that have a high potential for painful consequences.

Depressive symptoms and signs
Depressed mood.

Diminished interest or pleasure in usual activities.

Change in weight or appetite.

Insomnia or hypersomnia.

Psychomotor agitation or retardation.

Fatigue or loss of energy.

Feeling of worthlessness or guilt.

Diminished ability to think or concentrate.

Recurrent thoughts of death.

Investigations
Screening for cyclothymia.

Laboratory and imaging studies: not necessary.

Semistructured interviews: for depression and mania.

Screening instruments: *eg*, Beck Depression Inventory and Mania Rating Scale; may help identify cyclothymia among patients who are at risk.

Complications
Suicide: rate is unknown but seems to be much lower than that associated with major or bipolar depression.

Impaired judgment and decision making.

Social, academic, and occupational impairment.

Differential diagnosis
Medical and substance-related causes of depression (eg, seizures, stimulants).
Personality disorders (eg, borderline antisocial, histrionic, narcissistic).
Attention deficit–hyperactivity disorder.
Bipolar II disorder (eg, major depression, hypomanic episodes).

Etiology
• Specific causes are not known.
• Risk factors for cyclothymia include family history of bipolar disorder (~30% of all cyclothymic disorder patients have positive family histories for bipolar I disorder).
• Cyclothymia is frequently associated with interpersonal loss.

Epidemiology [2]
• Lifetime prevalence in the general population is ~1%.
• Cyclothymia frequently coexists with borderline personality disorder.
• Female-to-male ratio is 3:2.
• Approximately 50%–75% of all patients have onset between 15–25 y of age.

Treatment

Diet and lifestyle
• Avoid alcohol, stimulants, hallucinogens, etc.

Pharmacologic treatment
• Mood stabilizers are the first line of treatment for patients with cyclothymia.

• Standard dosages of antimanic drugs are generally recommended by clinical psychiatrists.

Standard dosage	Lithium, 300–600 mg 2–3 times per day; levels ranging from 0.6–1.0 mEq/L are usually used for long-term treatment.
	Valproic acid, 15 mg/kg/d increased by 5–10 mg/kg/d at weekly intervals. Most patients attain therapeutic plasma levels (50–100 mg/mL) or a dose between 1200–1500 mg/d in divided doses.
	Carbamazepine, 200 mg twice daily increased to 800–1200 mg/d. Therapeutic goal is 4–12 µg/mL.
Contraindications	*Lithium*: use cautiously in patients who are dehydrated or sodium-restricted or who have renal impairment or a preexisting thyroid disease; pregnancy rating D.
	Valproic acid: substantial hepatic dysfunction, pregnancy rating D.
	Carbamazepine: bone marrow depression, pregnancy rating C.
Main drug interactions	*Lithium*: diuretics, nonsteroidal anti-inflammatory agents, digoxin, antipsychotics (possible idiosyncratic neurotoxic interaction); prolongation of muscle paralysis has been reported in lithium-treated patients who have been given pancuronium and succinyl-choline as muscle relaxants during the course of anesthesia.
	Valproic acid: may potentiate the effects of monoamine oxidase inhibitors and other antidepressants; may increase phenobarbital level; chlorpromazine decreases the clearance of valproic acid.
	Carbamazepine: may enhance the antimanic effect of lithium; phenytoin may decrease plasma level; calcium channel blockers may inhibit its hepatic metabolism; warfarin decreases its level.
Main side effects	*Lithium*: gastrointestinal complaints, tremor, polyuria/diabetes insipidus, acne, hypothyroidism, weight gain, edema.
	Valproic acid: gastrointestinal complaints, sedation, ataxia , nystagmus , tremor, dysarthria.
	Carbamazepine: gastrointestinal complaints, ataxia, confusion, drowsiness, nystagmus, blurred vision, headache, rash.

Treatment aims
To obtain remission and prevent relapse of cyclothymia.

Other treatment options
Psychosocial treatment: to deal with losses and to develop coping strategies for this chronic mood disorder.

Prognosis
• Approximately one third of all cyclothymia disorder patients develop a major mood disorder (most often bipolar II disorder); specific time period is unknown.

Follow up and management

For the acute phase
• Administer antimanic drugs. Follow-up office visit 1 wk after initiating therapy, with phone availability in the interim.

For the continuation phase [3]
• Check pertinent laboratory studies and serum level of the medication used. Lithium, electrocardiography, blood urea nitrogen, creatinine, thyroid-stimulating hormone, calcium, glucose, complete blood count (CBC) with differential every 6–12 mo. Valproic acid: LFTs, platelets every 4 mo. Carbamazepine: CBC, platelets, liver function tests (LFTs), sodium every 4 mo.

Key references
1. Howland R, Thase M: A comprehensive review of cyclothymic disorder. *J Nerv Ment Dis* 1993, 181:485–492.

2. Kaplan H, Sadock B, Grebb J: *Kaplan and Sadock's Synopsis of Psychiatry.* Baltimore, MD: Williams & Wilkins; 1994.

3. Maxmen J, Ward N: *Psychotropic Drugs: Fast Facts.* New York: WW Norton & Co.; 1995.

Diagnosis

Definition
• In DSM-IV, delirium is classified as a cognitive disorder, along with dementia and amnestic disorders. Delirium is a disturbance in consciousness and cognition which develops over a short period of time.

DSM-IV diagnostic criteria
1. Alteration ("clouding") of consciousness with a reduced ability to focus, sustain, or shift attention.

2. Alterations in cognitive and cortical functioning similar to those seen in other cognitive disorders (eg, memory disturbance, language disturbance, perceptual disturbance).

3. Development over a short period of time (hours to days).

4. Evidence of a general medical condition as a cause of the delirium.

Signs and symptoms
• Delirium is a transient organic mental syndrome of acute onset, characterized by global impairment of cognitive functions, a reduced level of consciousness, attentional abnormalities, increased or decreased psychomotor activity, and a disordered sleep-wake cycle [1].

• Delirium usually develops in the setting of a serious physical illness. Symptoms worsen as illness, metabolic imbalances, or other toxicities affecting cerebral function worsen. Symptoms are commonly more severe at night and can be worsened by overstimulation or understimulation of the delirious patient.

Investigations
• Initial detection of delirium is usually straightforward, especially with a characteristic rapid development of symptoms in the setting of significant physical illness. "Quiet" (nonagitated) delirious states are more difficult to detect. The severity (or even the presence) of the classic signs and symptoms of delirium commonly fluctuates over the course of the day, further complicating detection in some cases.

• Confirmatory evaluation requires demonstration of diffuse cognitive disturbance of relatively sudden onset

Instruments: eg, Mini-Mental State Exam or the Trail Making Test; may be helpful at the bedside; other screening instruments (which are more precise but place more burden on the patient and rater) include the Delirium Symptom Interview, the Confusion Assessment Method, the Delirium Rating Scale, and the Memorial Delirium Assessment Scale.

Electroencephalogram: generalized slowing can confirm the presence of delirium when diagnosis is unclear after initial examination.

• A search for the cause of delirium is required after delirium is detected. The investigational approach depends on the known or suspected underlying cause.

Complications
Paranoid ideation, agitation, combativeness, and fluctuations in arousal: ranging from hypervigilance and restlessness to coma.

Morbidity and mortality of the underlying disease or diseases: untreated delirium impairs the patient's ability to comprehend his condition or comply with recommended treatment and, thereby, places the patient at risk for self-injury.

Differential diagnosis
Amnestic disorders.
Brain injury (especially to frontal lobe).
Dementia.
Depression (with agitation or psychotic features).
Extreme anxiety.
Pain, dyspnea, and other extreme physical distress.
Psychosis.
Seizure or preepileptic neuroelectrical disturbance.
Substance intoxication or withdrawal.

Etiology
• Delirium is generally a consequence of an underlying physical disorder, metabolic disturbance, or drug side effect. Any condition that adversely effects cerebral perfusion, oxygenation, or metabolism can cause delirium. Multifactorial etiology is the rule, not the exception. Etiologic differential diagnosis of delirium is very broad, but categories of problems that commonly cause delirium include:
Central nervous system (CNS) infections.
CNS trauma.
CNS tumors.
Electrolyte disturbances.
Hepatic failure.
Hypoglycemia.
Hypotension or extreme hypertension.
Hypoxia.
Intoxication and withdrawal.
Medications (eg, anticholinergics).
Seizures.
Stroke.
Uremia.
Vitamin deficiencies.

Epidemiology
• Delirium is very rare in community samples. The presence and severity of delirium are positively correlated with the presence and severity of physical illness. Elderly patients or patients with multiple physical illnesses are at higher risk for developing delirium. Approximately 10%–15% of all general medical inpatients are delirious. Reported prevalences of delirium approach or exceed 50% in settings such as critical care units, burn units, or cardiovascular surgical units. Delirium occurs in up to 85% of terminally ill patients in the last days of life.

Treatment

General information
• The key to the management of delirium is to treat the underlying cause. Delirium resolves most quickly when the etiologic condition or conditions can be found and reversed. Pharmacologic measures (*see* below) are useful to control symptoms (*eg*, agitation, sleeplessness) and to hasten the resolution of delirium while underlying causes are treated.

Diet and lifestyle
• Other than the maintenance of adequate nutrition, dietary interventions have little role in the treatment of delirium.

• A calm and soothing environment with as many familiar items and people as possible can be very helpful in controlling the agitation that often complicates delirium. Delirious patients need gentle reassurance and calm reorientation to their environment. A setting that avoids overstimulation and understimulation should be sought in order to minimize agitation and fearfulness, respectively. Delirious patients need close observation to prevent inadvertent self-injury, removal of intravenous lines, or wandering.

• Education of patients and families about delirium and its treatments is essential to full and rapid recovery from delirium.

Pharmacologic treatment
• Even when deliriogenic physical conditions cannot be found or reversed, pharmacologic treatment can provide substantial relief. Initial pharmacologic measures should include discontinuation of any potential pharmacologic causes of delirium, which may be the only pharmacologic approach necessary.

High-potency antipsychotics
• The most effective pharmacologic interventions for delirium is low-dose administration of a high-potency antipsychotic drug. These agents are rapidly calming and reliably effective in reducing symptoms of delirium. Extrapyramidal side effects are common with these drugs, but are rarely troublesome with the doses and brief time course of treatment usually required to control delirium.

Standard dosage	Haloperidol, 0.5–2.0 mg twice daily (initial dose, depending on the severity of agitation); can be rapidly titrated to effect, with dose range of 15–20 mg per 24 hours (maximum usually administered via oral or i.m. routes).

• For severe or refractory agitated delirium, intravenous haloperidol, dosed from 2.0–10.0 mg initially, may be administered on an escalating schedule by doubling the previously administered dose every thirty minutes until response is achieved (high doses may be required). Once an effective dose is determined for an individual delirious patient, the time to symptom recurrence gives the dosing interval. Calculating the initial 24-hour dose requirement allows determination of a divided dose schedule or hourly rate for continuous infusion. By the intravenous route, haloperidol is well tolerated at higher doses with less liability for extrapyramidal symptoms and can provide relief from agitation without causing extreme sedation or respiratory suppression.

Other useful agents
Standard dosage	Thiothixine, 2.0–30.0 mg/d orally in divided doses.
	Risperidone, 1.0–6.0 mg/d orally in divided doses.
	Olanzapine, 5.0–10.0 mg/d orally at bedtime.

• Benzodiazepines (primarily lorazepam) can be beneficial adjuncts to antipsychotic therapy but do not usually have beneficial effect for the treatment of delirium other than providing sedation. Some delirious patients develop increased agitation on benzodiazepines. Some delirious states (*eg*, due to hepatic failure) are worsened by benzodiazepine administration. For delirium due to alcohol or sedative-hypnotic drug withdrawal, however, benzodiazepines are a first-line treatment.

Treatment aims
To detect and monitor the delirious state. To reverse underlying cause of delirium (if possible). To control the delirious symptoms. To restore baseline cognitive functioning (usually possible if underlying cause of delirium can be reversed).

Prognosis
• The prognosis after delirium largely depends on the severity and reversibility of the underlying illness(es). Delirium has long been recognized as a marker of serious illness or acute deterioration. A substantial proportion of delirious patients progress to death or to a chronic state of cognitive impairment, requiring supervision such as that provided in a nursing home. The great majority of patients who are delirious from an acute illness quickly return to their premorbid levels of cognitive functioning once the underlying problems are fully resolved, although full recovery of cognitive function may take hours to days (a similar time course to the onset of acute delirium).

Follow-up and management
• Once delirium fully resolves, recurrence is primarily related to recurrence of severe physical illness; therefore, follow-up specifically for delirium is not usually required once the acute episode clears.

Key reference
1. Lipowski, ZJ: *Delirium: Acute Confusional States.* New York: Oxford University Press; 1990.

General references
American Psychiatric Association. *Diagnostic and Statistical Manual of Mental Disorders*, ed 4. Washington, DC: American Psychiatric Press; 1994.

Breitbart W, Marotta R, Platt MM, et al.: A double-blind trial of haloperidol, chlorpromazine, and lorazepam in the treatment of delirium in hospitalized AIDS patients. *Am J Psychiatry* 1996, 153:231–237.

Shuster JL: Delirium, confusion, and agitation at the end of life. *J Palliative Med* 1998, in press.

Wise MG, Trzepacz PT: Delirium (confusional states). In *The American Psychiatric Press Textbook of Consultation-Liaison Psychiatry.* Edited by Rundell JR, Wise MG. Washington, DC: American Psychiatric Press, Inc.; 1996:259–274

Diagnosis

Symptoms

• There must be evidence from history, physical examination, and laboratory investigations that the delirium and dementia are due to HIV.

Delirium

Rapidly developing cognitive decline.

Attention deficit.

Learning deficit.

Difficulty learning new information.

Orientation with decline or fluctuation of alertness: clouding of consciousness, disorganized thinking.

Increase or decrease in psychomotor activity.

Dementia

Memory impairment: inability to learn and recall new material.

Cognitive disturbances (at least one): aphasia (language disturbance), apraxia (impaired ability to carry out motor activities despite intact motor functions), agnosia (failure to recognize or identify objects despite intact sensory function), disturbance in executive function (plan, organize, sequence).

Impairment in social or occupational function: representing a significant decline from previous level of function.

Investigations

Laboratory studies: complete blood count, electrolytes, liver function tests, etc.

Blood tests: cultures, HIV, metals, vitamin B_{12} and folate, rapid plasma reagin.

Urine: culture, toxicology, metal screen.

Electrography: electroencephalography, etc.

Cerbrospinal fluid.

Radiography: computed tomography (CT), magnetic resonance imaging (MRI), positron-emission tomography, etc.; head CT and MRI usually show diffuse cerebral atrophy with enlarged ventricles and wide sulci.

Complications

• Success of treatment may depend on correctly identifying the nature of the changes in the patient's mental status. Failure to due so could result in morbidity and mortality.

Differential diagnosis

• In both delirium and dementia, the following need to be considered:
Infection.
Neoplasms.
Pharmacological toxicity.
Metabolic imbalances.
Substance intoxication.
Substance withdrawal.
Delirium or dementia due to a medical condition other than HIV.

Etiology

• Aside from the direct effects of HIV itself, secondary complications (eg, *Pneumocystis carinii* infection) and treatment drugs may contribute to deliria and dementias seen in these patients

Delirium

Systemic illness.
Drugs including withdrawal.
Multiple causes simultaneously.
Other unknown organic problems.

Dementia

Decreased neurotransmitters: acetylcholine, dopamine, γ-aminobutyric acid, serotonin, somatostatin, substance P.

Epidemiology

• Research is lacking on the epidemiology of dementia and delirium in HIV.
• One study reported 13.5% were delirious on hospitalization and 3.3% became delirious during hospitalization.
• AIDS dementia may occur in as many as 15% of AIDS patients with CD4 counts <200.

Treatment

Diet and lifestyle
• Patients should comply with HIV medications, have regular checkups with CD4 and viral load counts, eat a nutritious well-rounded diet, and get plenty of exercise and rest.

Acute pharmacologic treatment
• Treat symptoms.

• Administer Haloperidol (1–5 g orally, i.m., or i.v.), Thiothixene (2–5 g orally), Droperidol (5 g i.m. or i.v.).

Other treatment options
Psychosocial: family members and sitters may be necessary.

Environmental: dark rooms should be lit; keep clocks, calendars, and other familiar objects near to avoid temporal confusion; frequently orient and remind patient of whereabouts.

Treatment aims
Primary treatment aim: to provide support for the patient and the family or care providers in such a way as to minimize the confusion, frustration, and hardship placed on the patient and family.

To correct any underlying and precipitating factors for dementias or deliria that are correctable.

To use appropriate medications in appropriate doses

To use environmental and psychosocial influences in an organized systematic fashion

Prognosis
• HIV-associated dementia and delirium have a grave prognosis.

Follow-up and management
• Symptomatic medical management is essential.

• Psychosocial and environmental counseling and planning is essential.

• Support systems must be established for the patient and the care providers.

General references
Hahn R, Albers L, Reist C (eds): *Psychiatry, Current Clinical Strategies.* Laguna Hills, CA: CCS Publishing; 1997.

Hill CD, Risby E, Morgan N: Cognitive deficits in delirium: assessment over time. *Psychopharmacol Bull* 1992, 28:401–407.

Kaplan HI, Sadock BJ (eds): *Comprehensive Textbook of Psychiatry.* Baltimore: Williams & Wilkins; 1995.

Kunik ME, Yudofsky SC, Silver JM, *et al.*: Pharmacologic approach to management of agitation associated with dementia. *J Clin Psychiatry* 1994, 55(suppl S2):13–17.

Peiperl L (ed): *Manual of HIV/AIDS Therapy*, ed 2. Current Clinical Strategies Publishing; 1995.

Simpson DM, Tagliati M: Neurological manifestations of HIV infection. *Ann Intern Med* 1994, 121:769–785.

Tomb D (ed): *Psychiatry, House Officer Series.* Baltimore: Williams and Wilkins; 1995.

Wise M, Rundell J (eds): *Consultation Psychiatry*, ed 2. DC: American Psychiatric Association; 1994.

Diagnosis

Signs and symptoms

Presence of nonbizarre delusions: lasting ≥1 month that are unreal but possible.

Few or absent psychopathologic features beyond the delusional system.

Intact cognitive functioning.

Unique feature: patients can shift between a calm, neutral, capable normalcy and a driven, preoccupied, hypervigilant delusional state.

Delusional subtypes (in order of prevalence)

Persecutory: self-perceived victim of conspiracy, harassment, injustice, etc.; often seeks legal action.

Somatic: three types (olfactory, infestation, body dysmorphic); intensive search for medical care.

Erotomanic: delusions of love from another, usually of higher status; found more in women.

Grandiose: belief of unrecognized talent, insight, or major discovery (more common); belief of association with a prominent person (less common).

Jealous: intense belief of infidelity by spouse or partner.

Mixed: more than two subtype characteristics with no predominant theme.

Nonspecific: more than one type of delusion.

Investigations

Toxicology screening and routine lab work.

Neuropsychologic testing: Electroencephalography or computed tomography scan if cognitive impairment or lesions are suspected.

• Assess for persistence (transient delusions suggest a medical cause), systemization (pervasiveness and intellectual capacity), and impact on behavior (danger to self or others) [1].

Complications

Potential for violence: more likely in jealous and erotomanic subtypes, especially with men.

Lack of insight into delusions: can lead to resistance and noncompliance to treatment.

Frequent involvement with police, attorneys, or nonpsychiatric medical professionals.

Depression: common comorbid condition [2].

Social withdrawal: typical.

• Delusional disorder is often undiagnosed or misdiagnosed.

• Gradual onset can resemble a Cluster A personality disorder [3].

Differential diagnosis

Delirium, dementia.
Psychotic disorder due to a general medical condition.
Substance-induced psychotic disorder, Iatrogenic disorder.
Schizophrenia or schizoaffective or schizophreniform disorder.
Mood disorder with psychotic features.
Psychotic disorder not otherwise specified.
Hypochondriasis.
Somatoform disorders.
Malingering.
Factitious disorder.

Etiology

• The cause is unknown.
• Risk factors include advanced age, social isolation, immigration, sensory isolation, and family history of psychiatric illness.
• Onset may be induced by organic illness or injury.
• Lesions in the limbic system or basal ganglia may be associated.

Epidemiology

Onset: gradual or acute.
Range of onset age: 18–80 y; mean age, 35–45 y (women are usually older).
Prevalence: 24–30:100,000
Incidence: 0.7–3.0:100,000
Male-to-female ratio: 0.85:1.
Common features: premorbid personality disorders [3], widowhood (women), celibacy (men), history of substance abuse or head injury (men) [3].

Treatment

Pharmacologic treatment
- Relevant data are limited.
- Antipsychotic drugs are the treatment of choice.
- Compliance is difficult due to denial of a psychotic illness.
- Start with the lowest dose and increase slowly.
- In emergencies, extremely agitated patients can be given an antipsychotic intramuscularly
- Antidepressants, lithium, or anticonvulsants may be necessary if antipsychotics are not effective.
- Most clinical trials have been with pimozide.
- Most recent trials have found success with the atypical antipsychotics (eg, risperidone, clozapine) [4].

Pimozide
Standard dosage	2–16 mg/d.
Contraindications	Use with caution if hypersensitive to antipsychotics; prolongs the QT interval.
Main side effects	Tardive dyskinesia, extrapyramidal reactions.
Main drug interactions	Avoid administering with other medications that prolong the QT interval.
Special points	Three trials have confirmed success with treating the somatic subtype [5].

Risperidone
Standard dosage	2–6 mg/d.
Contraindications	Do not use if hypersensitive to this medication.
Main side effects	Orthostatic hypotension (especially during initial dose titration), tardive dyskinesia, somnolence (in high dose patients 16 mg/d).
Main drug interactions	Prescribe with caution if combined with other central nervous system (CNS) active drugs and alcohol
Special points	Expensive but on most indigent drug/patient assistance programs; covered by Medicaid.

Clozapine
Standard dosage	Up to 900 mg/d (partial remission of somatic delusions has been obtained with 325 mg/d [4]).
Contraindications	Myeloproliferative disorders, uncontrolled epilepsy, clozapine-induced agranulocytosis, severe granulocytopenia, severe CNS depression, comatose states.
Special points	Leukocyte count at baseline every week throughout treatment and for 4 weeks after discontinuation of treatment.
Main drug interactions	Caution is advised if used in combination with other CNS active drugs.
Main side effects	Agranulocytosis, seizures, orthostatic hypotension (especially during initial dose titration), CNS effects (sedation, vertigo, headache, tremor), effects on the autonomic nervous system (excessive salivation, sweating, visual disturbances).

Treatment aims
Essential element: to establish rapport. To modify or neutralize delusional thinking. To develop more effective coping skills and support system.

Prognosis
- Prognosis is best with early and acute onset.
- Approximately 33%–50% of patients improve after 10–15 y [1].
- Of patients reviewed in the literature, 80.8% show total or partial recovery [5].
- Only minimal improvement is seen in the most chronic, severe cases.

Other treatment options
Individual psychotherapy: may be more effective than group psychotherapy. Insight-oriented supportive, cognitive, behavioral, and family therapies. Hospitalization: if patient is a danger to self or others.

Follow-up and management
- As delusional symptoms subside, depressive symptoms may develop, and they can be severe.
- Reassess potential for violence to self or others, especially in patients with intense emotional responses to their delusional system.

Key references
1. Manschreck TC: Delusional disorder: the recognition and management of paranoia. J Clin Psychiatry 1996, 57(suppl 3):32–38.
2. Manschreck TC: Delusional disorder: a not-so-rare psychotic disorder. J Psychotic Disorders 1997, 1:8–9.
3. Munro A: The classification of delusional disorders. Psychiatric Clinics N Am 1995, 18:199–212.
4. Songer DA, Roman B: Treatment of somatic delusional disorder with atypical antipsychotic agents. Am J Psychiatry 1996, 153:578–579.
5. Munro A, Mok H: An overview of treatment in paranoia/delusional disorder. Can J Psychiatry 1995, 40:616–622.

Diagnosis

General information
• Dementia due to a general medical illness is a syndrome of acquired, persistent impairment in intellectual function that is a direct consequence of a medical condition. Its age of onset, gender distribution, presenting symptoms, and clinical course vary according to its specific etiology.

Signs and symptoms
• Signs and symptoms depend on the underlying etiology.

DSM-IV diagnostic criteria
• For criteria A and B, *see* Dementia of the Alzheimer's type.

Criterion C: there is evidence from the history, physical examination, or laboratory findings that the disturbance is the direct physiologic consequence of one of the following general medical conditions: normal-pressure hydrocephalus, hypothyroidism, brain tumor, vitamin B_{12} deficiency, intracranial radiation.

Criterion D: the deficits do not occur exclusively during the course of a delirium.

Investigations
Psychologic testing
• Psychologic testing is useful in distinguishing mild dementia from normal aging and from the effects of low intellectual or educational level; also can give quantitative information to help distinguish the types of dementia or to follow progress or treatment response.

Laboratory studies
• Laboratory studies are useful primarily to rule out reversible causes such as toxic, metabolic, endocrine, or infectious. Screening tests include the following:

Serum chemistry (electrolytes, liver function tests [LFTs], glucose); thyroid-stimulating hormone; B12 and folate; erythrocyte sedimentation rate; FTA; complete blood count (CBC); tests based on presentation, symptoms, or history; urine and serum drug screens; electroencephalography (EEG); HIV; heavy metals; disease-specific tests.

Other investigations
Mini mental status examination.

Neuroimaging: especially in patients with acute onset or young age.

Complications
Comorbidity
Depression: common, especially in the early stages of dementia.

Substance abuse.

Behavioral outcomes
Severe stressor for families: often results in financial hardships, emotional conflicts; however, family support is essential.

Increased suicide rate: possible in patients who are capable of following through.

Differential diagnosis
Delirium, amnestic disorder, substance intoxication or withdrawal, schizophrenia or other psychotic disorders, major depressive disorders, malingering or factitious disorders, age-related cognitive decline.

Etiology
• DSM-IV specifically excludes Alzheimer's dementia, vascular dementia, and substance-induced persisting dementia from this classification. After these exclusions, ~10%–30% of dementias are due to other etiologies.

Epidemiology
• Age of onset, gender distribution, and presenting signs and symptoms vary based on etiology.

Pick's disease: ~20% of frontal lobe dementias; prevalence, 24:100,000 (female > male); onset, middle adult life (50–60 y of age); duration, 2–15 y from onset to death.

Wilson's disease: prevalence, 10:100,000 (male = female); autosomal-recessive inherited disorder of copper metabolism; onset, adolescence and young adulthood.

Huntington's disease: prevalence, 19:100,000 (male = female); autosomal-dominant inheritance, single gene of short arm chromosome 4; onset, usually 35–45 y of age, although juvenile (3%) and late-onset (>80 y of age) variants exist.

Subacute sclerosing panencephalitis: male > female; rural > city; onset, ~10 y of age; caused by an aberrant measles virus (?).

Creutzfeldt-Jacob disease: prevalence, ~0.5:1,000,000 worldwide (male = female); onset, usually sixth decade (rare); postulated to be caused by an infectious protease-resistant protein particle (prion), which causes spongiform degeneration of the brain; rapidly progressive to death within 6 mo–2 y.

Parkinson's (PD) disease: prevalence, 133–200:100,000 (male > female); 20%–60% of PD patients develop dementia (most are <50 y of age); 40% of PD patients who are >70 y of age will have some degree of dementia, although it is unclear whether it is due only to the PD processes.

Neurosyphilis: prevalence, ~10% of patients with late syphilis (male = female in untreated cases).

Normal-pressure hydrocephalus: fifth leading cause of dementia.

Treatment

Diet and lifestyle
- Maintain nutritional status.
- Maintain familiar routines and surroundings.
- Early in the course, provide cues to maintain temporal orientation (clocks, calendars)
- Avoid alcohol.
- Maintain sleep hygiene

Pharmacologic treatment
- Aggressively treat coexisting medical conditions with a close attention to avoiding or minimizing use of drugs that may adversely affect cognitive or motor function.
- Target specific behavioral symptoms with appropriate psychotropic drugs in minimally effective doses, especially in the elderly.

For psychotic symptoms (low-dose high-potency antipsychotics)
Standard dosage   Haldol, 0.5 mg orally twice daily,

Risperdal, 0.5–1.0 mg/d, or

Zyprexa, 2.5 mg/d.

For agitation or mood lability
Low-dose benzodiazepines (especially short-acting)

Standard dosage   Ativan, 0.25 mg 2–3 times daily or

Serax, 5–10 mg 2–3 times daily.

Some patients may require longer-acting agent to avoid rebound, Clonazepam is preferred over those requiring extensive liver metabolism (*eg*, diazepam).

Mood stabilizers

Standard dosage   Valproic acid, start at 250 mg twice daily (adjust dose to effect; therapeutic levels; monitor LFTs and serum ammonia) or

Carbamazepine, start at 200 mg/d in divided doses (adjust dose to effect; therapeutic levels; monitor CBC and electrolytes).

For insomnia
Standard dosage   Trazodone, start at 25–50 mg every bedtime,

Ambien, 2.5–10.0 mg every bedtime,

Restoril, start at 7.5 mg every bedtime, or

Serax, 5–10 mg every bedtime.

For depression
See Major depressive disorder.

Contraindications
- Note: many medications have significant anticholinergic effects, and their use should be closely monitored (amitriptyline, diphenhydramine) or avoided in the elderly. Antipsychotics may exacerbate movement disorders in Parkinson's disease and Lewy body dementia.

Nonpharmacologic treatments
Psychotherapy: supportive therapy may be of use early in selected processes.

Alternative therapies: strengthening the social support system may be crucial in extending the time the patient can remain at home, thereby delaying or preventing institutionalization.

Treatment aims
To treat the underlying medical condition: imperative because some conditions are at least partially reversible or arrestable.
To slow the progression of cognitive decline.
To treat comorbid psychiatric conditions (eg, depression).
To treat specific symptoms that may affect the patient's safety, ability to maintain basic activities of daily living, and ability to remain at home.

Prognosis
Depends on etiology and stage at initiation of treatment; can vary widely from months to years.

Follow-up and management
Acute phase: family education and modification of home environment (to minimize danger of accidents and falls); medical treatment as indicated by specific disorder.
Chronic phase: many patients ultimately require institutionalization.

General references
American Psychiatric Association: Practice guidelines for the treatment of patients with Alzheimer's disease and other dementias of late life. *Am J Psychiatry* 1997, 154(suppl):PAGES.

Clinical Handbook of Psychotropic Drugs, ed 6. Edited by Bezchlibnyk-Butler ??, Jeffries ??, Hogrefe ??, Huber ??. CITY: PUBLISHER; 1996.

Comprehensive Textbook of Psychiatry, vol 2, ed 6. Edited by Kaplan ??, Saddock ??. CITY: PUBLISHER; 1995.

Diagnostic and Statistical Manual of Mental Disorders, ed 4. Washington, DC: American Psychiatric Association; 1994.

Psychiatry, vol 1. Edited by Tasman ??, Kay ??, Lieberman??. Philadelphia: WB Saunders Co.; 1997.

Textbook of Consultation-Liaison Psychiatry. Edited by Rundell ??, Wise??. CITY: American Psychiatric Press; 1996.

Diagnosis

Symptoms and signs

Clinical determinants

• The clinical manifestations of dementia from TBI are affected by the following:

Nature of damaging force applied to brain: *eg*, closed head injury versus gun shot wound; **location of damaged brain tissue; extent of additional brain damage caused by medical complications of injury:** *eg*, hypoxia, hypotension, infection; **age of patient; premorbid intellectual function; premorbid psychiatric illness; emotional reaction to injury; development of epilepsy; environmental, social, and family factors; expected compensation of legal issues; professional risk:** *eg*, boxers with dementia pugilistica.

Stages of neuropsychiatric symptoms

Acute: loss of consciousness followed by symptoms of delirium.

Intermediate: fluctuating cognitive, psychiatric, and behavioral symptoms that slowly improve.

Persistent: fixed neuropsychiatric deficits.

Symptoms and signs of dementia from TBI

Cognitive: Amnesia, impaired visual and verbal memory, impaired verbal performance, similarities; the neuropsychiatric deficits depend on type of lesion (*ie*, focal [*eg*, contusion] versus diffuse [*eg*, diffuse axonal injury]).

Psychiatric: depression, anxiety, and psychosis are common.

Behavioral: apathy, irritability, and impulsivity are common.

Physical: symptoms depend on extent of injury.

Neurologic: variable, from none to multiple deficits (*eg*, hemiparesis).

DSM-IV diagnostic criteria

• Diagnostic features of postconcussive dementia include the following:

1. Nonprogressive cognitive loss.
2. History of significant traumatic brain injury (TBI).
3. Temporal relationship between injury and onset of symptoms.
4. Patient >18 y of age.
5. Patient has sufficient time to recover cognitive and functional abilities

Investigations

Structural imaging

Acute: computed tomography (CT) and magnetic resonance imaging (MRI) can demonstrate contusions, lacerations and hematomas.

Late: CT and MRI can demonstrate atrophy, ventriculomegaly, and reduction of white matter, but brain imaging will not identify patients with dementia.

Functional imaging

Single photon emission computed tomography (SPECT): can demonstrate hypometabolism from damage and increased perfusion with recovery of function; SPECT scan results will not identify patients with dementia.

Electroencephalography (EEG): variable correlation between degree of EEG abnormality and severity of head trauma.

Lumbar puncture: only useful to exclude infection.

• *Note:* Diffuse axonal injury and mild to moderate anoxic encephalopathy are poorly visualized with imaging techniques.

Complications

Loss of autonomy: *eg*, job, self care, etc.; **family disruption; legal problems:** *eg*, loss of driver's license; **suicide; substance abuse; physical impairments; financial:** *eg*, loss of income or job; Alzheimer's disease.

Epidemiology

Incidence and prevalence

• In the US, 132–367:100,000 per year have TBI.

• Increased risk of head injury seen in young (16-25 y) and elderly (>75 y).

• There are 2 million reported head injuries per year; 500,000 patients require hospitalization; 70,000–90,000 patients lose function.

• Approximately 2% of patients with serious TBI develop dementia.

• TBI causes 2% of dementia in adults.

Causes of injury that produces significant TBI

Motor vehicle accidents, 37%; falls, 28%; assault, 11%; redestrian injury, 10%; motor-cycle accidents, 9%; gunshot wounds, 1%.

• No specific cause of injury produces dementia.

Pathology

• Types of pathology associated with TBI include the following:

Direct trauma

Extracranial hemorrhages (epidural hematoma, subdural hematoma, subarachnoid hemorrhage); focal cerebral lesions (contusions, lacerations, hematomas); diffuse subcortical lesions (diffuse axonal shearing, cerebral edema).

Damage from medical complications of trauma

Anoxic encephalopathy; hypotensive brain injury; marrow or fatty embolic; secondary infections.

Glasgow Coma Scale

Eye-opening response, score
Open spontaneously, 4
Open to verbal command, 3
Open to pain, 2
No response, 1

Best motor response, score
Obeys verbal command, 6
Localizes painful stimuli, 5
Flexion withdrawal, 4
Flexion abnormal (decorticate rigidity), 3
Extension (decerebrate rigidity), 2
No response, 1

Best verbal response, score
Oriented and converses, 5
Disoriented and converses, 4
Inappropriate words, 3
Incomprehensible sounds, 2
No response, 1

Treatment

General information

For acute disease
• Manage acute trauma, medical complications, and cerebral edema.

For long-term disease
• Avoid additional brain damage (*eg*, reinjury, hypoxia, central nervous system infections).

• Maximize medical care for health problems.

• Advise physical rehabilitation and cognitive reteaching or retraining.

• Control seizures

• Support family caregiver

• Treat substance abuse

Pharmacologic treatment
• For depression, selective seritonin-reuptake inhibitors or tricyclic antidepressants are effective.

• For psychosis, administer atypical or standard antipsychotics.

• For mania and impulsivity, prescribe lithium, Tegretol, or Valproic acid.

• *Note:* use benzodiazepines and narcotics with caution and avoid use of antihistamines and anticholinergics.

Nonpharmacologic treatment
• For apathy, institute behavioral interventions (few medications lessen apathy).

Prognosis

Clinical features that predict poor outcome
Glasgow Coma Scale score <8 (see Diagnosis page).
Length of coma >1 h.
Duration of posttraumatic amnesia >24 h.

Cognitive complaints at 5 y after severe TBI
Memory, 71%
Word finding, 67%
Concentration, 60%
Comprehension, 35%

Psychiatric complaints at 5 y after severe TBI
Irritability, 66%
Depression, 56%
Anxiety, 53%
Impulsivity, 44%

Natural history
• The natural history of TBI is as follows:
Month 6: physical recovery
Month 12: maximal cognitive recovery
Month 24: behavioral recovery
• Some patients, especially children, may continue to improve after 2 y.

General references
Hillier SL, Hiller JE, Metzer J: Epidemiology of traumatic brain injury in South Australia. *Brain Injury* 1997, 11:649–659.

Olver JH, Ponford JL, Curran CA: Outcome following traumatic brain injury: a comparison between 2 and 5 years after injury. *Brain Injury* 1996, 10:841–848.

Diagnosis

Definition

Alzheimer's disease is a degenerative disorder of the central nervous system that typically has a slow, insidious onset and involves all areas of cognition (*eg,* memory, judgment, language, spatial, mathematical abilities, etc.).

Symptoms and signs

• DSM-IV emphasizes that an inability to retain new information or to recall previously learned material should be present; deficits are in long- and short-term memory. In addition, one of the following cognitive disturbances should be present:

1. Aphasia (language disturbance).
2. Apraxia (impaired motor abilities despite intact motor pathways).
3. Agnosia (inability to identify objects or to recognize objects despite intact sensory pathways).
4. Disturbance in executive functioning (*ie,* planning, organizing, sequencing, abstracting).

• The cognitive impairments above result in significant social and occupational functioning and represent a significant decline from the previous functioning level.

• The cognitive decline in Alzheimer's disease cannot be due to other degenerative disorders of the central nervous system (*eg,* Pick's disease, Parkinson's disease, vascular dementia).

• DSM-IV also codes Alzheimer's disease with either early onset (<65 y of age) and with late onset (>65 y of age).

• Alzheimer's disease may be noted as delirium, delusions, or depressed mood, or it may be uncomplicated.

Investigations

Neuroimaging: (preferably magnetic resonance imaging) used to rule out disorders of the central nervous system (*eg,* stroke, tumor, and normal pressure hydrocephalus); patients with dementia of the Alzheimer's type most typically have generalized cortical atrophy (narrowed gyri and widened sulci), which affects all lobes of the telencephalon.

Neuropsychologic testing: most commonly reveals cognitive decline in all spheres of higher intellectual functioning (*eg,* abstract thinking, visuospatial abilities, language abilities); neuropsychologic testing can be especially helpful in distinguishing between dementia of the Alzheimer's type and vascular dementia.

Single photon emission computed tomography and positron emission tomography scans: reveal decreased regional cerebral metabolism and blood flow to the posterior temporal lobes and to the adjacent parietal lobes bilaterally; this finding may be present in very early dementia of the Alzheimer's type.

Laboratory investigations: (*eg,* serum B_{12} level, thyroid function tests, serum folate level, rapid plasma reagin test, ANA) to rule out autoimmune central nervous system vasculitis.

Mini-Mental State examination: score of ≤23 is usually indicative of a dementing illness.

Electroencephalography: may be normal in early dementia of the Alzheimer's type, but as the disease progresses, it most commonly becomes generally slowed bilaterally; may be helpful in localizing other independent or comorbid cerebral conditions.

Differential diagnosis

Delirium.
Amnestic disorder.
Vascular dementia.
Dementia due to other general medical conditions (*eg,* Pick's disease, head trauma, HIV, Parkinson's disease, Huntington's disease, Creutzfeldt–Jacob disease).
Pseudodementia secondary to major depression.

Etiology

Risk factors include the following:
Family history: there is no definitively known genetic predisposition, although it is presumed that genetic factors play a role in the disorder.
Advancing age.
History of significant head trauma.

Epidemiology

• Approximately 10% of the population >65 y of age suffer from dementia. Of these, ~60% have dementia of the Alzheimer's type, and 15%–30% suffer from vascular dementia. Mixed dementia (*ie,* patients who suffer from both dementia of the Alzheimer's type and vascular dementia) occurs in 10%–15% of patients who are demented.
• Currently there are ~2.5 million patients in the US who suffer from dementia of the Alzheimer's type. The economic cost to society is currently reported to be $80–100 billion per year.
• Onset occurs most typically in the 7th and 8th decades of life. Duration varies, but most authorities believe the disease course lasts from 8–10 y.

Pathology

Neurofibrillary tangles.
Senile (amyloid) plaques.
Neuronal loss.
Granulovacuolar degeneration of neurons.
Diffuse cortical atrophy.
Degeneration of the nucleus basalis of Meynert.

Treatment

Pharmacologic treatment

Acetylcholinesterase inhibitors

• Two current pharmacologic treatments are commercially available, donepezil (Aricept) and tacrine (Cognex). Both of these drugs are acetylcholinesterase inhibitors and both are efficacious when they are well tolerated. Once these medications have been instituted, they should not be terminated. Both medications slow the progression of the symptoms of dementia of the Alzheimer's type but do not slow down the progression of the underlying disease process. The treatment of the psychiatric manifestations of dementia of the Alzheimer's type is initiated as the symptoms appear.

• It should be emphasized that anticholinergic medications should be avoided whenever possible because one of the major pathologic changes in dementia of the Alzheimer's type is the gradual depletion of central nervous system acetylcholine. Elavil and Benadryl are especially anticholinergic.

Antipsychotic medications

• Typical antipsychotic medications (Haldol, Stelazine, and Navane) are helpful in treating the psychotic symptoms but are given in much lower doses in younger patients. The newer antipsychotic agents (Risperdal and Zyprexa) are also very beneficial in small amounts.

Other medications

• The unpredictable explosive behavior seen in many Alzheimer's patients is frequently improved with valproic acid, carbamazepine, or lithium. These medications should be initiated at low amounts and gradually increased to a low therapeutic range. Some studies have shown that valproic acid may be helpful in a less-than-therapeutic amount. When using valproic acid, it is important to remember that serum ammonia levels may be increased (resulting in hypersomnolence and an encephalopathic picture) in the face of normal liver function tests and a therapeutic level of valproic acid. This condition is rare and reversible if the medication is promptly discontinued.

General references

American Psychiatric Association: *Diagnostic and Statistical Manual of Mental Disorders*, ed 4. Washington, DC: American Psychiatric Association; 1994.

Kaplan HI, Sadock BJ: Synopsis of psychiatry. In *Behavioral Sciences/Clinical Psychiatry*, ed 8. Baltimore: Williams & Wilkins; 1998.

Rogers SL, Friedhoff LT, Donepezil Study Group (Kinney FC): The efficacy and safety of donepezil in patients with Alzheimer's disease: results of a US multicentre, randomized, double-blind, placebo-controlled trial. *Dementia* 1996, 7:293–303.

Diagnosis

Definition
• The patient with dependent personality disorder suffers from an unrealistic belief that he or she is unable to function without help from others and needs to be taken care of. As a result, these individuals subordinate their own needs to elicit and maintain caregiving from others.

Symptoms and signs

General characteristics
Submissive, clinging, passive, suggestible, hypoaggressive; belittles abilities, avoids autonomy, lacks perseverance in tasks for personal fulfillment; may be quite assertive when acting on behalf of dependents; responds feebly to situations requiring action, portrays self as inept to get others to feel responsible for them and take over; may nevertheless complain about "being controlled."

Subjective complaints
Views self as helpless; fears separation or abandonment from close attachments; feels depleted of energy; considers self undeserving; believes others are more capable.

Occupational dysfunction
Avoids positions of responsibility; irritates superiors with excessive guidance-seeking and inability to complete projects without help; demonstrates inadequate performance due to failure to take responsibility for job duties and make vital decisions.

Social dysfunction
Forms strong attachments, usually to one main person; few relationships beyond caregiver–patient relationship; fails to develop independent living skills; lets others make important decisions for them.

Relationships often imbalanced; tolerates exploitation and abuse; may choose partners with extreme narcissism, sociopathy, or substance abuse; fails to express needs or anger when mistreated; often rejected for needy behavior; when relationship ends, desperately seeks new one; makes rapid, indiscriminate choices; rifts in close relationships often the incentive to seek care.

DSM-IV diagnostic criteria
• The disorder is indicated by the presence of five or more of the following:

Dependent behaviors: requires excessive advice from others to make mundane decisions; resists disagreeing with others due to fear of loss of approval (even in situations that easily tolerate debate); does not initiate activities independently due to lack of confidence in own abilities; manipulates others into assuming responsibility for most areas of patient's life; goes to extreme measures to obtain caregiving and support; on the termination of a close relationship, shows urgency in replacing it with another.

Subjective anxieties: discomfort with being alone due to excessive fears of being unable to care for oneself; preoccupation with fear of being left.

• These symptoms cause severe distress or social or occupational impairment.

Investigations
History: assess developmental history; look for mismatch between education versus occupational standing or social status of patient and partner; assess behavior and demeanor during interview; history from significant others can be helpful but may be distorted.

Psychologic testing and questionnaires: Minnesota Multiphasic Personality Inventory and Millon Clinical Multiaxial Inventory administered by a psychologist can suggest clustering of personality traits; physician-rated questionnaires such as Structured Clinical Interview for DSMIII-R Personality Disorders (SCID-II) and the Personality Disorder Examination (PDE) are valid and useful; the patient-rated Personality Diagnostic Questionnaire-Revised (PDQ-R) and the SCID-II self-report questionnaire are also available.

Differential diagnosis
• Some dependency traits are normal at extremes of age, during times of illness, and in certain cultures.
• Dependency is part of many axis I psychiatric conditions, especially chronic major depression, panic disorder with agoraphobia, mental retardation, and schizophrenia.
• Rule out personality change due to a medical condition or substance dependency and other personality disorders (eg, borderline, histrionic, and avoidant).

Etiology
Psychosocial factors: most theories focus on these; overindulgent or controlling parents reward dependency and threaten rejection for independence.
Cultural: women in certain cultures are shaped to take on dependent roles.
Experiential: eg, chronic physical illness.
Biologic: eg, chronic depression.
Constitutional: eg, anxious-inhibited temperament.
Genetic: factors predisposing toward submissive (vs dominant) behaviors.

Epidemiology
• Dependent personality disorder is the most prevalent personality disorder reported in psychiatric settings.
• Prevalence in the general population is 2%–4%; in outpatient psychiatric settings, 23%.
• General prevalence is greater in females; in clinic populations, the proportion of males versus females is equal.

Complications
Comorbid psychiatric conditions: depression, anxiety disorders, adjustment disorders in times of crises, eating disorders, and other personality disorders especially borderline, avoidant, and histrionic.
Repeated disappointed relationships.
Injury, accidental death, suicide.
Misuse of alcohol, drugs, and food: to assuage negative feelings or meet dependency needs with resultant addictions and related health problems.
Bankruptcy: prone to financial exploitation in personal and business relationships.

Treatment

Diet and lifestyle
• Help the patient use healthy and self-nurturing behaviors (*ie*, exercise, writing in journal) for stress management instead of food and drugs.
• Encourage regular sleep habits, reduce potentially dangerous behaviors (*ie*, going to private settings with strangers, frantic late-night car rides).

Pharmacologic treatment
• Medications help only minimally with the underlying condition; an aggressive pharmacologic approach to comorbid psychopathology reduces dependency.
• Antidepressant medications are helpful when depressive symptoms present; can induce nonspecific increased stress tolerance, decreased hypersensitivity to rejection, decreased anxiety, and increased energy (with resultant increased assertiveness).
• Selective serotonin reuptake inhibitors are particularly well tolerated.
• Tricyclic antidepressants have demonstrated efficacy. *Caution: dangerous in overdose; administer sublethal amount to suicidal patients.*

For associated anxiety symptoms
• Buspirone, paroxetine, and sedating antidepressants (*eg*, imipramine, trazodone) are effective and nonaddictive.
• Benzodiazepines (*eg*, clonazepam, alprazolam) can be used on a short-term crisis basis to control anxiety and prevent undesirable behaviors. Avoid long-term use; dependent patients may be a higher risk for habituation.

For insomnia
• Antidepressants (*eg*, trazodone, imipramine) in low doses are helpful and can be given without risk of dependence. For infrequent problems, Ambien or triazolam can be used.

Nonpharmacologic treatment
Psychotherapy
• Insight-oriented psychotherapy is often the treatment of choice; the focus is often on discussing the dependency that develops on the therapist and helping the patient learn to call upon his or her own resources in coping with life situations. Brief therapy helps patients with circumscribed problems. Long-term therapy is necessary for more pervasive problems. Supportive therapy for crisis periods.

Behavioral therapies
Cognitive-behavioral, assertiveness, exposure therapies, anxiety management.

Group therapy
• Patients see how others respond to their behavior, learn to recognize their own feelings, and practice asserting themselves in a safe environment.

Psychiatric hospitalization
• Psychiatric hospitalization relatively contraindicated in dependent personality disorder patients due to the tendency to promote regression, except when patient is suicidal or suffers a serious comorbid psychiatric condition.

Pitfalls
• Dependent personality disorder patients are "experts" in getting others to feel responsible for them. They can become very dependent on and demanding of their treating clinician. Address these behaviors as part of treatment. Resist the urge to reject patient for excessive demands; also avoid becoming yet another caretaker.
• Clinicians become frustrated hearing patient constantly complain about bad relationships without acting to change their situation. Resist aggressively pushing patient to challenge or terminate imbalanced relationships; due to extreme dependency they may be unable to do this and become markedly distressed or terminate treatment.

Treatment aims
To increase self-reliance and self-esteem. To help patient feel independent enough to assert needs within relationships, abandon disturbed relationships, and tolerate loneliness long enough to make discriminating choices in partners.

Prognosis
• In many cases, dependency decreases with maturity.
• Treatment is often successful.

Follow-up and management
For the acute phase
• Establish supportive role, be reliable and consistent, set rules for appropriate availability while allowing for a reasonable degree of dependence (*ie*, available emergently for true crises, with limits set on frequent, trivial phone calls).
• Have patient set personal goals for treatment.

For the continuation phase
• Brief and behavioral therapies typically take 3–5 mo; long-term therapies can take several years.
• Reassess degree to which goals are accomplished at intervals; reframe or set new goals if necessary.
• Help patient work through resistance to changing ways of relating toward eventually becoming independent from therapy.
• Taper sessions toward end of treatment; at termination, allow patient option of as-necessary sessions over the long term.

General references
Diagnostic and Statistical Manual of Mental Disorders, ed 4. Washington, DC: American Psychiatric Association; 1994.

Maier W, Lichtermann D, Klingler T, et al.: Prevalences of personality disorders (DSM-III-R) in the community. *J Pers Disord* 1992, 6:187–196.

Perry JC: Dependent personality disorder. In *Treatments of Psychiatric Disorders*, ed 2. Edited by Gabbard GO. Washington, DC: American Psychiatric Association; 1995:2355–2366.

Perry JC, Vaillant GE: Personality disorders. In *Comprehensive Textbook of Psychiatry*, ed 5. Edited by Kaplan H, Sadock B. Baltimore: Williams & Wilkins; 1989:1352–1387.

Diagnosis

DSM-IV diagnostic criteria

1. Performance in daily activities that require motor coordination is substantially below that expected given the person's age and measured intelligence. This may be manifested by marked delays in achieving motor milestones (eg, walking, crawling, sitting), dropping things, "clumsiness," poor performance in sports, or poor handwriting.

2. The disturbance in criterion 1 significantly interferes with academic achievement or activities of daily living.

3. The disturbance is not due to a general medical condition (eg, cerebral palsy, hemiplegia, or muscular dystrophy) and does not meet criteria for a pervasive developmental disorder.

4. If mental retardation is present, the motor difficulties are in excess of those usually associated with it.

Symptoms and signs

Infancy
Delayed early gross and fine motor milestones well beyond reasonable allowance for individual differences in most cases.

Early childhood
Poor gross motor skills: in running, throwing and kicking a ball, riding a bicycle, and skating and balancing skills.

Poor fine motor skills: in managing tools, crafts and artwork, use of crayons and pencils, tying shoelaces, buttoning clothes, dressing skills, and feeding skills (eg, pouring liquids, holding a knife).

Middle childhood
Delayed development in visual-perceptual-motor skills: writing, printing, assembling puzzles, building models.

Delayed development of sporting skills.

Motor dyspraxia (poor motor planning).

Clumsiness: generalized or restricted to a group of similar tasks.

Persistent patterns of task avoidance.

Newly learned motor tasks performed slowly and inconsistently.

Investigations

History: parents and teachers report of poor performance in self care, recreational tasks, gross and fine motor skills.

Traditional neurologic examination: largely unhelpful, although quantitative neurologic signs (soft signs) can be used to estimate the severity and response to intervention.

Occupational and physical therapy assessment: can provide more detailed information about the child's gross and fine motor development.

Degree of delay or deviation: aids in distinguishing a permanent disorder from a transient clinical problem.

Checklists and rating scales: eg, Test of Motor Impairment, Motor Competence Checklist, Movement Assessment Battery of Children.

Complications

Poor social competence.

Poor motivation: child is often labeled "lazy" or "immature."

Low self-esteem.

Unhappiness.

Reluctance to engage in physical activities.

Poor physical fitness in adolescence.

Differential diagnosis

General medical conditions
Cerebral palsy, muscular dystrophy, congenital hypotonia, neurodegenerative disorders, metabolic disorders, ataxia, progressive lesions of the cerebellum, neurocutaneous diseases, history of closed head injury, arrested hydrocephalus.

Mental disorders
Mental retardation, autistic disorder.

Comorbid disorders
Attention deficit–hyperactivity disorder, reading disorder, mathematics disorder, written expression disorder, phonological disorder, expressive language disorder, mixed receptive-expressive disorder

Etiology
• The central nervous systems responsible for various aspects of motor performance are not yet fully understood. Several theories await experimental confirmation and include the following:
1. Developmental coordination disorder (DCD) is the result of a developmental delay or maturational lag that will correct itself with time.
2. DCD has a physiologic origin that requires treatment to remediate the deficits (eg, the sensory integration theory, which implicates multisensory deficits, and the unisensory deficit theory, in which a specific problem in one of these systems is identified [ie, vestibular, visual, or proprioceptive].
3. DCD is caused by an increased incidence of prenatal and perinatal complications, presumably affecting normal brain development.

Epidemiology
• Prevalence estimates range from 5%–15% for children 5–11 y of age (the 6% quoted in DSM-IV is widely accepted).
• Boys are more commonly affected than girls.
• Diagnosis is difficult in the first year of life but becomes increasingly obvious as expectations increase for the development of complex motor skills.
• There is a strong association with learning disabilities and psychiatric disorders in adolescence.

Treatment

General information
- Developmental coordination disorder is a long lasting but not life-threatening condition that cannot be cured.

Lifestyle management

Education
- The family and the school must be informed about the nature of the condition. The child's problem are not due to lack of effort or intelligence, poor parenting, allergies, or active brain disease. The condition never gets worse, but motor learning continues to be a weakness. Some motor skills are never learned; others are learned but always performed awkwardly. Learning could be painful for the child, and simple repetition is unlikely to benefit.

The better informed the family, the less likely that the child will become involved in alternative treatments or that the parents will become involved in "pathological shopping around."

- Several studies have demonstrated small or nonexisting gains after various intensive therapies (sensory integration, perceptual-motor therapy, task-oriented and process-oriented techniques). Intensive teaching of a specific task or the use of verbal self-guidance has demonstrated some improvement in motor performances.

Changing attitudes
- Modified expectations and increased understanding at home and at school can help with the child's self esteem.
- Specific adaptations include 1) the use of self-gripping fasteners rather than knots and buttons, and 2) not insisting on the use of knives.

Sports
- Deemphasize competitive leisure activities that demand strong motor skills in favor of activities in which children compete against their own prior records.
- Physical education should encourage fitness rather than athletic skills.

School
- Children with DCD are entitled to modifications as other physically disabled students if they face academic failure due to untidy writing
- Teachers can help by granting more time for written assignments, encourage a child's own choice of printing or cursive writing, reducing the length of assignment, providing handouts (rather than requiring the child to copy from the board), helping with note-taking, and encouraging typing for long assignments.

Pharmacologic treatment
- Stimulant medication might help in some cases of properly diagnosed comorbid attention deficit disorder.

Nonpharmacologic treatment

Occupational therapy
- Assessment and follow-up by an occupational therapist is encouraged to 1) quantify the disability; 2) advocate for relevant modifications in the child's environment, including changed expectations; 3) provide information for parents, teachers, and children; 4) assess whether certain children would benefit from specific intervention techniques; and 5) offer children one-on-one mentoring for a range of motor activities related to school work, leisure, and daily living.

Treatment aims
To demystify the disorder.
To provide support for the family.
To provide early intervention.
To prevent school failure.
To reduce the development of secondary emotional disorders.

Prognosis
- Prognosis is good if treatment is implemented.
- For most children, poor motor coordination will be a persistent problem that is likely to be associated with difficulties in mood, behavior, relationship, and academic performance.
- A longitudinal follow-up to 16 y of age showed increased incidence of psychiatric and personality disorder (in 60% of patients), substance abuse (13%), and attempted suicide (5%).

Follow-up and management
- Parents and school should be educated about DCD and implement specific modifications to help the child cope with his or her frustrations.
- Follow-up with an occupational therapist who can decide about the scope and length of the intervention.

General references
Mervyn FA, Lent B: Clumsy children: primer on developmental coordination disorder. Can Fam Physician 1996, 42:1965–1971.

Piek J, Edwards K: The identification of children with developmental disorder by class and physical education teachers. Br J Educ Psychol 1997, 67:55–67.

Willoughby C, Polatajko H: Motor problems in children with developmental coordination disorder: review of the literature. Am J Occup Ther 1995, 49:787–794.

Diagnosis

Symptoms

Genital pain associated with sexual intercourse: usually occurring during intercourse but may precede or follow it.

• The disorder can occur in both males and females.

Signs

Normal genital anatomy.

Chronic vaginal or vulvar irritation: may result from trauma during attempted intercourse.

Spasm of the muscles surrounding the vaginal introitus (vaginismus): may be seen during intercourse and vaginal examination.

• Four categories of pain experience have been identified:

1. Momentary sharp pain of varying intensity.
2. Intermittent painful twinges.
3. Repeated intense discomfort.
4. Aching sensation.

Investigations

History: the diagnosis is usually based on history.

Routine vaginal examination: tender areas often appear normal to the naked eye; using a cotton swab to touch gently in a circular pattern around vaginal entrance will identify very painful areas [1]; rule out causative physical abnormalities (*eg*, vulvar or vaginal inflammation or infection, endometriosis, cystitis, remnant hymenal tissue, lack of lubrication, and Peyrone's disease [in men]).

Psychologic testing and interview: may offer information concerning other psychopathology that exacerbates or contributes to the pain experience.

Complications

Aversion to intercourse due to pain: causes distress or conflict in intimate relationships.

Vaginal or penile irritation and inflammation: with repeated, unsuccessful attempts at intercourse; in some cases can be perceived as abusive by the female.

Vaginismus, hypoactive sexual arousal, inhibited orgasm, and sometimes sexual aversion disorder: may be primary or secondary to the dyspareunia.

Self-medication with alcohol or other intoxicating substances: drug effects may cause increased sensitivity and irritation of the painful area.

Differential diagnosis

Dyspareunia due to a general medical condition (pain caused solely by anatomic or physical or medical problems). Substance-induced dyspareunia (some substances can be associated with painful intercourse, depending upon the type of drug and frequency of use). Lack of vaginal lubrication (may result from inadequate mental or physical erotic stimulation or a variety of other reasons, creating the experience of pain).

Etiology

• A history of sexual abuse and resultant fear of sexual contact occurs in many cases. Other learning factors that associate anxiety, fear, pain, danger, threat, or emotional upset with sexual intercourse may also occur. Lack of sexual knowledge or patience by one or both partners may contribute.

• Physical difficulties (eg, vulvar or vaginal inflammation or infection, endometriosis, cystitis, remnant hymenal tissue, lack of lubrication, and Peyrone's disease) may result in painful intercourse. If the pain is attributed completely to a physical problem, the diagnosis of dyspareunia due to that particular medical condition is made rather than general dyspareunia.

• In some cases, the disorder has the characteristics of a local neuralgia.

Epidemiology

• Dyspareunia occurs in ~10%–20% of females aged 20–40 y.

• Most have a fair complexion or sensitive skin [1].

• Comorbid sexual aversion disorder is common.

Treatment [1,2,3]

Nonpharmacologic treatment

• A comprehensive program designed to address both medical and psychologic factors is often necessary. Individuals are often averse to being told it is purely psychologic. Treatment should most likely include the following facets:

1. Addressing history of sexual abuse or trauma if present.

2. Addressing relationship problems and conflicts over intimacy and sexuality.

3. Education regarding sexual anatomy and normal sexual function.

4. Enlistment of the partner's cooperation, understanding, and patience.

5. Sex therapy: may include exercises to relieve pelvic floor muscle tension, use of lubricants and anesthetic gels, sensate focus exercises, relaxation therapy, and therapeutic insertion of graduated sizes of vaginal dilators; individuals opposed to the use of dilators have successfully utilized fingers or penile insertion in a graduated manner.

• If a medical condition is contributing or responsible for the experience of pain, the medical condition should be properly treated. It is likely, however, that psychologic treatment will be beneficial regardless of the etiology of the dyspareunia. This is especially true in situations in which the individual or couple has begun experiencing anticipatory or performance anxiety.

• Rare cases may require surgical intervention (eg, perineoplasty).

Prognosis

• Prognosis varies widely, and there have been few factors that consistently indicate treatment success or failure. Without treatment, it is likely that the disorder will persist.

Key references

1. Heiman, Julia R: Genital pain in the context of chronic pain and an incest history. In *Case Studies in Sex Therapy*. Edited by Rosen R, Leiblum S. New York: The Guilford Press; 1995.

2. Lazarus AA: Dyspareunia: a multimodal psychotherapeutic perspective. In *Principles and Practice of Sex Therapy*. Edited by Leiblum SR, Rosen RC. New York: The Guilford Press; 1989.

3. Wincze J: *Sexual Dysfunction* New York: Guilford Press; 1991.

General reference

Levine SB: *Sexual Life*. New York: Plenum Press; 1992.

Diagnosis

Symptoms and signs

• Persons with dysthymic disorder experience a depressed mood for most of the day (on more days than not) for a period of at least 2 years (as indicated either by subjective account or observation by others). It is further indicated by the presence of two or more of the following:

1. Decreased or increased appetite.
2. Decrease or increase in sleep.
3. Fatigue.
4. Decreased self-esteem.
5. Hopelessness.

• Mood in children and adolescents can be irritable, with duration of at least 1 year.

• Person has never been without above symptoms for >2 months sequentially during the 2-year period (1-y period for child or adolescent).

• If major depression is not present during first 2 years of episode, patient should be excluded from this diagnosis.

Investigations

History: diagnosis can generally be made on this basis.

Sleep studies: may show decreased latency or increased density of rapid eye movement.

Physical examination and indicated laboratory studies: to rule out medical contributors (eg, hypothyroidism, urine, drug and alcohol screening).

Biochemical and neuroendocrine findings: less robust than in cases of major depressive disorder.

Complications

Impairment in social and occupational functioning.

Higher risk of suicide.

Increased risk of major depressive disorder and bipolar disease: in cases of early-onset dysthymic disorder.

Differential diagnosis

Major depressive disorder.
Substance-induced mood disorder (especially in cases of chronic use).
Personally disorder.

Etiology

• Psychosocial factors include faulty personality/ego development as well as factors relating to difficulty in adapting to adolescence and young adulthood.
• Family history is frequently positive for mood disorder, which may represent chronic, mild, or major depressive disorder.

Epidemiology

• Incidence is 3%–5% of the general population; 8% of adolescent boys, 5% of adolescent girls; however, more frequent in women than in men overall.
• Other factors include young age, single, low socioeconomic status.

Treatment

Diet and lifestyle

• No specific precautions are noted; increasing exercise is often helpful.

Pharmacologic treatment

• Antidepressants (eg, selective serotonin-reuptake inhibitors [SSRIs], bupropion, tricyclics [TCAs]) are often helpful. Monoamine oxidase inhibitors (MAOIs) may be helpful for treatment of refractory cases. Occasional patients may benefit from stimulants.

• Concurrent use of SSRIs and MAOIs are contraindicated; 6 weeks should elapse after discontinuance of fluoxetine before an MAOI is initiated.

• Side effects include nausea, gastrointestinal upset, agitation, and sexual dysfunction (with SSRIs); hypotension, weight gain, and food and drug interactions (with MAOIs); and cardiac dysrhythmias, lowering of seizure threshold, and anticholinergic side effects (with TCAs).

• Generally, continue maximally tolerated dose for period of 4–8 weeks before determination of medication trial as a failure. Be prepared to reconsider diagnosis and/or possible comorbidity. Dysthymic disorder patients may experience less robust response to pharmacotherapy than those with major depression.

Nonpharmacologic treatments

• Insight-oriented psychotherapy, cognitive-behavioral therapy, and family therapies may all be helpful.

• Hospitalization should be considered in cases with severe suicidal ideation or in which the individual shows severe social or occupational dysfunction.

Treatment aims

To alleviate symptoms.
To obtain remission.
To prevent relapse and complications.

Prognosis and course

• Insidious onset in young adulthood or earlier occurs in 50% of patients.
• Patients with early-onset (<21 y of age) dysthymic disorder are at increased risk for development of major depressive disorder or bipolar affective disease.
• Late-onset (>21 y of age) dysthymic disorder generally follows a unipolar course.
• Major depressive disorder (and/or "double depression" [ie, dysthymia plus major depressive disorder]) develops in 20% of patients.
• Bipolar affective disease, type II (no florid or psychotic manic episodes), may develop in 15% of patients.
• Full remission is never attained in 25% of patients.

Follow-up and management

• Provide limited amount of medications for patients who have suicidal ideation.
• Provide emergency number in case of crisis situation.
• Provide psychotherapy or supportive follow-up on a weekly basis initially.
• Provide psychopharmacologic management on frequent basis initially; however, once stabilized, patient may be monitored on a 3–6-mo check-in basis.

General references

Janicak PC, et al.: Indications for antidepressant therapy. In Principle and Practice of Pharmacotherapy. Baltimore: Williams & Wilkins; 1995:227–230.

Kaplan HI, Saddick BJ, Grebb JA: Mood disorders. In Synopsis of Psychiatry. William & Wilkins; 556–559.

Diagnosis

General information

• There are two types of encopresis—encopresis with constipation and overflow incontinence (or retention encopresis, in which feces are poorly formed, leakage is continuous, and small amounts are passed in toilet; resolves with treatment of constipation) and encopresis without constipation and overflow incontinence (or nonretention encopresis, in which feces are of normal form and consistency, soiling is intermittent, and depositing is in prominent places).

Symptoms and signs (of both types)

Passage of feces in inappropriate places: whether intentional or involuntary at least once per month for 3 months

Mental or chronologic age of at least 4 years.

Nonmedical cause.

Investigations

• Rule out Hirschsprung's disease.

Detailed history: including time, frequency, and circumstances.

Assessment of child's and family's overall functioning and dynamics.

Psychologic testing: may be helpful.

Complications

Social, familial, and personal issues; shame.

Avoidance of school, camp overnights, etc.

Diminished esteem.

Conflict with parents.

Isolation from peers, ostracization.

Differential diagnosis

Rectal or anal stenosis.
Endocrine abnormalities.
Smooth muscle disorder.
Hirschsprung's disease.
Developmental delay.
2° to overall impulsivity and overactivity, lending to poor attention to stimuli.

Etiology

Chronic, significant constipation.
"Chronic neurotic encopresis": has been associated with distant father and neurotic mother; early, harsh bowel training; neurologic delay; abnormal anal and rectal expulsion; abnormal sphincter control; no correlation shown between social class and encopresis.

Epidemiology

• Incidence among 10–12-year-olds is 1.35% of boys, 0.3% of girls; among 7–8-year-olds, 1.5% of boys.
• Correlation exists between encopresis and enuresis.

Treatment

Diet and lifestyle

Well-rounded nutritious diet with fiber and vitamins.

Exercise.

Regular time periods on toilet without emphasis on production.

Pharmacologic treatment

Stool softeners, laxatives.

Careful administration of mineral oil: if constipation is severe.

Imipramine: there have been case reports of some children responding to imipramine in doses appropriate for age and size of child; cardiac is monitoring necessary.

Nonpharmacologic treatment

Behavioral.

Parental guidance: essential to diminish struggles and implement programs in nonpunitive fashion.

Family therapy.

Behavioral programs: to reinforce success.

More intensive psychotherapy: for children and families with more disturbed profile.

Treatment aims

To educate about regular time periods on the toilet, diet, medications, and undue stress.

To address disturbances in parent–child relationship that may contribute to the disorder.

Prognosis

• Maturation improves prognosis.

• There is a 78% improvement when educational, behavioral, and psychologic components are addressed.

General references

Comprehensive Textbook of Psychiatry, ed 6. Kaplan H, Saddock B. Williams & Wilkins; 1995.

Levine MD: Encopresis: it's potentiation, evaluation, and alleviation. Pediatr Clin North Am 1982, 29:315–330.

Loening-Bauke V, Cruikshank, BM: Factors responsible for persistence of childhood constipation. J Pediatr Gastroenterol Nutr 1987, 6:915–922.

Sprague-McRae JM, Lamb W, Homer D: Encopresis: a study of treatment alternatives and historical and behavioral characteristics. Nurse Pract 1993, 18:52–56.

Diagnosis

General information
• There are two types of enuresis—primary enuresis (in which an individual has never established urinary continence; begins at 5 y of age) and secondary enuresis (in which enurectic episodes develop after urinary continence has been established). Additional qualifiers include nocturnal only, diurnal (waking) only, and both nocturnal and diurnal.

Symptoms and signs
Repeated voiding of urine into bed or clothes: either intentionally or unintentionally; frequency of episodes occur at least twice per week for 3 consecutive months or creates significant distress or impairment.

Mental or chronologic age of at least 5 years.

Nonmedical cause.

Investigations
History.

Physical examination.

Urinalysis: to rule out urinary tract infection.

Contrast studies: are indicated *only* if there is significant evidence for functional or anatomical abnormalities based on the history or physical examination.

Complications
Increased psychologic distress, lowered self-esteem.

Increase in family conflicts.

Impairment in social, academic functioning; ostracization by peers.

Differential Diagnosis
Urinary tract infection.
Neurologic disease.
Anatomical malformations (uncommon).
Obstructive lesions (uncommon).
• When enuresis is intentional, coexisting behavioral and psychologic issues should be identified and treated.

Etiology

For intentional enuresis
Oppositional defiant disorder.
Psychotic disorder.

For involuntary enuresis
Developmental delay.
Psychosocial stress.
• A genetic link has been implicated, although no specific genetic pattern has been found.
• A decreased ability to concentrate urine due to nocturnal decreases of plasma atrial natriuretic peptide has been implicated but not consistently demonstrated in clinical studies.

Epidemiology
• At 5 years of age, prevalence is 7% of boys and 3% of girls.
• At 10 years of age, prevalence is 3 % of boys and 2% of girls.
• At 18 years of age, prevalence is 1% of boys and <1% of girls.
• Secondary enuresis may begin at any age but most commonly occurs between 5–8 y of age.

Treatment

General information
• For mild cases, often no treatment is necessary given the high rate of spontaneous remission with reassurance and time.

Diet and lifestyle
• Limit fluid intake in evening (although, the merits of this have been debated).

Pharmacologic treatment
• *Note*: medicine-free trials should be given every 4–6 months to monitor for spontaneous remission.

Imiprimine
Standard dosage	Start at 25 mg at bedtime. Titrate up by 25 mg every 4 days until therapeutic level is reached (maximum 5 mg/kg body weight).
Special points	Baseline electrocardiogram and monitoring >3.5 mg/kg are recommended.

Antivassopressors
Standard dosage	Start at 5–10 µg at bedtime. Titrate up by 5–10 µg every few nights to a minimum of 40 µg.
Special points	May be used as needed only for overnight trips, etc.

Nonpharmacologic treatment
• Behavioral interventions are effective in >75% of cases. Common types of behavioral interventions included:

Bell and pad utilization.

Reward contingencies.

Combination approach.

Psychotherapy: has limited use in some cases of secondary enuresis.

General references

Child and Adolescent Psychiatry, ed 2. Edited by Lewis M. Baltimore: Williams & Wilkins; 1996.

Comprehensive Textbook of Psychiatry, ed 6. Edited by Kaplan H, Saddock B. Baltimore: Williams & Wilkins, 1995.

ERECTILE DISORDER, MALE

Diagnosis

Symptoms and signs

Persistent or recurrent inability to attain or maintain an erection for sexual activity: erection may fail to occur for any sexual function, be inadequate for penetration, or fail during intercourse itself; masturbatory and rapid eye movement (REM)–associated erections usually occur without problem.

Preoccupied with erectile function: to the point where the preoccupation or associated (performance) anxiety causes or contributes to erectile failure.

Significant distress or interpersonal difficulties.

Investigations

History: the diagnosis is made from history; need to inquire regarding associated psychiatric disorders (especially depression and chronic anxiety), relationship problems, and lack of education or understanding by patient or partner regarding normal sexual function; inability to achieve an erection during masturbation or REM sleep suggests an underlying physical cause (*eg,* vascular disease [most common], endocrinopathy, and diabetes); screen also for alcohol and drug abuse, which are common contributors to this disorder.

Psychologic assessment and testing: may reveal characteristics, behaviors, or disorders that may be contributing to the intensity, duration, or frequency of erectile disorder.

Complications

Relationship problems: disorder may interfere with development of normal intimacy and romantic relationships; this disorder has been associated with marital affairs; some men may have "experimented" to determine if the erectile difficulties exist with another partner.

Impaired procreation.

Sexual inadequacy: in those afflicted; partners may feel rejected or undesirable.

Physical injury or damage: from homemade remedies or usage of poorly constructed devices (*eg,* misused vacuum device).

Differential diagnosis

• Medical and physical factors must be ruled out before labeling the problem as psychogenic.
• There will usually be an overlay of psychogenic factors with any medical cause.

Etiology [1]

• The majority of cases of impotence (erectile failure) seen in the primary care setting have physical or medical abnormalities that contribute or cause the dysfunction.
• Generally, psychologic factors (eg, anxiety, relationship concerns, fear of erectile failure, and fear of pregnancy) are also present and can contribute and occasionally cause the dysfunction.
• The primary cause is less likely to be psychogenic if the patient is >50 y of age or if the occurrence of erectile dysfunction was gradual [2].
• Many medications, especially most antidepressants and some antihypertensives, can cause erectile failure.
• Organic impotence is more commonly seen in chronic cigarette smokers and in those with arteriovascular disease.
• There has been an association between alcoholism and erectile disorder. This association has been demonstrated during the time of alcohol abuse as well as when the individual becomes sober.

Epidemiology

• It is estimated that this problem affects at least 2% of men. This may be an low estimate because there are many males who are reluctant to acknowledge the problem.

Treatment

Diet and lifestyle
• Tobacco, alcohol, and drug use can all contribute and must be minimized or eliminated.

• Obesity can make sustained intromission more difficult and requires greater energy expenditure for sexual activity.

Pharmacological treatment [2,3]

Standard dosage	Yohimbine 5.4 mg as necessary or up to three times daily.
	Trazodone, 50–150 mg/d
	Wellbutrin, 200–450 mg/d.
	Alprostadil (MUSE) suppository, insert into urethra 5–10 minutes before sex; erection can last 1 hour.
Main side effects	*Yohimbine*: may cause anxiety, sweating, increased blood pressure.
	Trazodone: sleepiness, dizziness, increase in frequency and duration of REM-associated erections, priapism (rare).
	Wellbutrin: enhancement of sexual function, increase ability to obtain and maintain erection.
	Alprostadil (MUSE) suppository: local pain and discomfort are common.
Special points	*Trazodone*: may be helpful in some men, although the benefit may be largely a placebo effect given the drug's reputation for causing priapism.

Other drugs
• Sildenafil (Viagra) is a phosphodiesterase inhibitor that increases penile blood flow and retention. It is expected to be released in 1998 and holds considerable promise for treatment of erectile failure.

• Topical creams for delivery of vasoactive drugs are under development for impotence. It appears that creams may result in erections that are less firm and reliable than erections produced from injection.

• Testosterone replacement may be helpful if serum testosterone levels are low.

Nonpharmacologic treatment
Vacuum erection devices: may be useful in otherwise treatment-refractory cases; these devices have specific instructions and should be used with caution; permanent damage could result from misuse.

Intracorporal injections and implanted penile prostheses: not generally recommended for psychogenic male erectile disorder but are certainly useful in treatment-refractory cases of permanent impotence; possible short-term adverse effects include pain and priapism; possible long-term adverse effects include build-up of scar tissue, penile curvature, and permanent damage in ability to obtain a spontaneous erection.

Sex therapy: although medical treatments positive but not perfect solutions, it is suggested that all affected individuals (preferably couples) should receive some counseling regarding sexual function and the enjoyment of the induced erection; in general, sex therapy would include 1) education regarding normal sexual function (including adequate foreplay), 2) altering sexual expectations and reducing performance anxiety, 3) improving mutual understanding and cooperation to identify alternate expressions of sexual intimacy (other than penetration), 4) sensate focus exercises with gradual increase in sexual activity progressing from penetration only to thrusting, and 5) exploration and treatment of psychologic and relationship problems (when present).

Prognosis
• Prognosis is generally good regardless of the causative factors. Whatever the treatment choice, couples are encouraged to express their sexuality in multiple ways, which will enhance enjoyment and increase acceptance of their level of function.

Key references
1. Zilbergeld B: *The New Male Sexuality.* New York: Bantam Books; 1992.
2. Tiefer L, Melman A: Comprehensive evaluation of erectile dysfunction and medical treatments. In *Principles and Practice of Sex Therapy.* Edited by Leiblum SR, Rosen RC. New York: The Guilford Press; 1989.
3. Levine S: *Sexual Life.* New York: Plenum Press; 1992.

General reference
Crenshaw TL, Goldberh JP: *Sexual Pharmacology.* New York: WW Norton & Co., Inc.; 1996.

Diagnosis

Symptoms and signs

• This paraphilia involves sexual excitement from exposing genitals to an unsuspecting stranger with no attempt at further sexual activity with the stranger. Individuals are only diagnosed if the following criteria are met:

Significant distress or impairment in functioning due to fantasies, urges, or actual exhibitionistic behaviors.

Symptoms present for at least 6 months.

• Exhibitionism is usually evident by the following signs:

Hobbies or occupations that allow for or facilitate exhibitionistic behavior.

Arousal directly prior to the exposure (as it is imagined) and masturbation and/or ejaculation immediately upon exposure.

Unhappy marriages and dissatisfying sexual relationships with their partners: reported by more than half of exhibitionists who are married.

• Previous information suggesting that exhibitionists are harmless has been strongly questioned. Exhibitionism has been linked to more serious sex crimes such as rape and child molestation.

• In comparison with other sex offenders, exhibitionists are more likely to underreport the frequency of their behavior, more likely to deny other paraphilias, more likely to have committed other sex crimes, and less likely to believe that exposing has harmed the victim.

Investigations

Laboratory investigations: none are indicated.

Psychologic testing: may indicate additional psychologic features that may contribute to the frequency and severity of exhibitionistic behavior; the Minnesota Multiphasic Inventory-2 results for individuals with exhibitionism indicate elevations on antisocial and impulsive behavior subscales; however, these data are descriptive, not diagnostic.

Penile plethysmography: may offer additional information to establish arousal associated with exhibitionism and to assess for arousal associated with other paraphilias; the reliability of this measure is questionable, however, and may result in false-negative information.

• For additional testing information, *see* Fetishism.

Complications

Legal implications of behavior: exhibitionism itself is illegal. Other charges may include loitering, trespassing, disorderly conduct, or illegal entry; individuals are more likely to be brought to treatment through the court system than on their own accord.

Impaired social functioning: the exhibitionist withdraws from social situations and networks in order to engage in exposure behavior; this tendency may be associated with loneliness and social impairment.

Impaired occupational functioning: the exhibitionist may neglect job requirements (especially if job facilitates exposure behavior) in order to expose.

Impairment in sexual functioning: the individual may only be able to achieve sexual arousal through exhibitionistic behaviors.

Differential diagnosis

Public urination: in public urination, the individual exposes self to urinate (often an excuse offered by exhibitionists who are "caught in the act").

Psychosis: individuals with psychotic disorders such as schizophrenia and bipolar disorder may engage in exhibitionistic behavior; however, this behavior is related to the symptomatology associated with these disorders.

Mental retardation or dementia: for many of these individuals, this behavior is associated with poor judgment and disinhibition rather than with sexual arousal.

Substance intoxication: individuals may engage in exposure behavior that is limited to the time while the individual is intoxicated.

Etiology

Biologic theory: serotonergic dysregulation has been suggested, but is uncertain; also suggested is a predisposition toward this behavior.

Behavioral theory: exposure of genitals is associated with sexual arousal (classic conditioning) and is reinforcing; the behavior is further reinforced by masturbatory practices.

Courtship disorder theory: suggests that exhibitionism is a disturbance in pretactile courtship interactions and is related to voyeurism, frotteurism, and rape, which are also seen as courtship disorders.

Epidemiology

• Exhibitionism is one of the more common paraphilias.
• Patients are typically male.
• Victims are predominately female.
• Onset occurs during adolescence or early adulthood.

Treatment

Pharmacologic treatment

• Psychopharmacologic treatment has varying results. Most research is based on case studies. Combination of drug treatment and psychotherapy may prove most effective.

Psychotropic medication

• Most medications given for paraphilias are thought to work by treating the "obsessional" nature of the disorder, and by taking advantage of the sexual side-effect profile of these medications. Other medications have been reported in case studies and are potentially beneficial for unspecified reasons.

• Appropriate dosage has not been determined. It is generally accepted that medications will be prescribed similarly to treatment of obsessive-compulsive disorder or depression and adjusted until symptoms are controlled or side-effects intolerable.

Standard dosage	Fluoxetine, 20–80 mg/d; paroxetine, 20–60 mg/d; clomipramine, 150–300 mg/d; fluvoxamine, 50–300 mg/d; sertraline, 50–200 mg/d; desipramine, 150–300 mg/d; imipramine, 150–300 mg/d.

Hormonal agents

• Antiandrogens have been shown to be effective in suppressing sexual urges, but they also may truncate an individual's sexual life; sooner or later the individual may wish to stop them.

• Medroxyprogesterone acetate lowers testosterone levels and has demonstrated efficacy for decreasing sexual urges, fantasies, and behaviors for most paraphilias.

• Cyproterone acetate (in Canada) blocks the action of testosterone and has demonstrated efficacy in treatment of paraphilias.

• Long-acting gonadotropic hormone-releasing hormone agonists have recently shown efficacy in paraphilic populations. These agents result in decreased secretion of luteinizing hormone and follicle-stimulating hormone, which results in lowered testosterone secretion.

• Usually symptoms of the paraphilia rapidly recur on discontinuation of psychotropic medications or hormonal agents.

Standard dosage	Luteinizing hormone–releasing hormone (LHRH) agonist in combination with flutamide, 500 µg; LHRH agonist plus 250 mg flutamide every 8 hours.
Special points	Permanent reduction in sperm motility and density.

Selective serotonin reuptake inhibitors

• Selective serotonin reuptake inhibitors generally have fewer side effects and may be considered first-line agents, especially for patients on few or no other medications.

• Dosage has not been well established. Dosing may be similar to that for obsessive-compulsive disorder. Titrate dose until symptoms are lessened or until side-effects become too severe.

Standard dosage	Fluoxetine, 20–60 mg.
	Fluvoxamine, 300 mg.
Main drug interactions	Potentially fatal interaction with monoamine oxidase inhibitors, potentially fatal interaction with antiar-rythmic medications; serotonergic crisis (hypertension, hyperpyrexia, and seizure) is possible in patients on other serotonergic medications.
Main side effects	Agitation, anxiety, sleep disturbance, tremor, sexual dysfunction (primarily anorgasmia), headache.

Antianxiety agents

Standard dosage	Buspirone, 30–60 mg.
Side effects	Dizziness, headache, nausea, nervousness, lighthead-edness, and agitation.

Treatment aims

• Abstain from exposure behavior.
• Decrease arousal to exposure fantasies, urges, and behavior.

Prognosis

• Without treatment, there appears to be a general decline in exhibitionism after 40 y of age, although the individual may continue to have fantasies of the deviant behavior.
• High relapse rates follow discontinuation of hormonal or psychotropic medications.
• Psychologic treatment outcome is dependent on individual's motivation to change and willingness to comply with treatment requests.

Follow-up and management

• Some individuals benefit from support groups for sexual addictions or paraphilias.
• Sexual therapy may be warranted for individuals with dissatisfying sexual relationships outside their exhibitionistic behavior.
• Individual therapy may be indicated for related psychopathology.

Nonpharmacologic treatment

• Behavior therapy aims to reduce inappropriate sexual arousal and increase appropriate sexual arousal. This is done in the following ways:
Covert sensitization.
Orgasmic reconditioning.
Plethysmographic biofeedback.
Satiation.
Challenging of distorted thinking and beliefs that contribute and maintain the behavior.
Social skills training, assertiveness training, communication skills training, and anger management.
Relapse prevention.
Aversion therapy.

General references

Travin S, Protter B: *Sexual Perversion: Integrative Treatment Approaches for the Clinician.* New York: Plenum Press; 1993.

Zohar J, Kalan Z, Benjamin J: Compulsive exhibitionism successfully treated with fluvoxamine: a controlled case study. *J Clin Psychiatry* 1994, 55:86–88.

Diagnosis

Definition

• Factitious disorders are defined as the intentional production or feigning of physical or psychologic signs or symptoms. The motivation for the behavior is to assume the sick role. External incentives for the behavior (eg, economic gain, avoiding legal responsibility, or improving well-being [as in malingering]) are absent.

• Research criteria for the designation factitious disorder by proxy (FDP) apply when a caregiver produces or feigns physical or psychologic signs or symptoms in another person. The motivation for the perpetrator's behavior is to assume the sick role by proxy.

Symptoms and signs [1]

• Individuals may engage in the following:

Total fabrications: (eg, asserting falsely that one is HIV-positive).

Simulations: (eg, mimicking a grand mal seizure).

Exaggerations: (eg, claiming that mild pain is incapacitating).

Aggravations: (eg, manipulating a pre-existing wound to impede healing).

Self-inductions: (eg, injecting oneself with fecal bacteria to cause sepsis).

• Factitious psychologic symptoms are most frequently seen in conjunction with factitious physical disorders. The most common manifestation is feigned depression, often linked to false claims of bereavement or posttraumatic stress disorder.

• In severe and chronic cases (sometimes termed Munchausen syndrome), patients have a history of repeated hospitalization, peregrination, and gratuitous lying (pseudologia fantastica).

Investigations [2]

• Common findings include the following:

1. Signs and symptoms are not controllable: there is continual escalation, or improvement is reliably followed by relapse.

2. The magnitude of symptoms consistently exceeds objective pathology.

3. There has been a remarkable number of tests, consultation, and treatment efforts to little or no avail.

4. The patient predicts deteriorations, or there are exacerbations shortly before discharge is to occur.

5. The patient has sought treatment at numerous facilities.

6. The patient emerges as an inconsistent, selective, or misleading informant.

7. The patient restricts access to outside informants.

8. Evidence from laboratory or other tests disputes information provided by the patient.

9. The patient engages in gratuitous lying.

10. Symptoms are present only when observation by others is evident to the patient.

• Standardized psychologic instruments most often show an average or above-average IQ, absence of a formal thought disorder, a poor sense of identity, strong dependency needs, poor frustration tolerance, and narcissism.

• In certain cases, covert video surveillance during hospitalization may be used to establish or disconfirm FDP.

Complications

Morbidity or mortality associated with self-induced illnesses.

Drug abuse: eg, opioids or benzodiazepines originally prescribed for factitious ailments.

Other iatrogenic complications.

Differential diagnosis

Authentic illness.

Somatoform disorders: somatoform disorder patients do not intentionally mislead others or produce their symptoms.

Personality disorders: comorbid personality disorders (especially borderline) are almost invariable.

Malingering: involves pursuit of external incentives rather than the sick role.

• In FDP, the differential includes the parent who is overanxious; illness that is authentic but variable or undiagnosed; and malingering or factitious disorder in an older child.

Etiology [3]

• Potential psychosocial etiologies include desire for attention and nurturance, gratification of dependency needs, defense against psychosis, need for identity, need for role mastery through imposture, and internalized anger or masochism.

• Emotionally-deprived childhoods are common, sometimes involving physical or sexual abuse.

• Potential biologic factors (eg, anatomic brain abnormalities in some patients) are of uncertain significance.

• No genetic pattern has been established.

Epidemiology

• Because factitious disorders involve willful deception and sometimes involve itinerancy as well, population-based epidemiologic techniques are not applicable. Data from case series and referral patterns suggest that ~1% of medical and surgical inpatients on whom psychiatrists consult are diagnosed with factitious disorder.

• Factitious psychologic disorders occur in 0.1%–0.5% of inpatient psychiatric admissions. Such patients are commonly employed in or intimately familiar with health care occupations.

• FDP appears to occur in 1.0%–1.5% of children seen in subspecialty pediatric settings. In 95%–98% of reported cases, the abusive individual is the mother and the victim is her own child.

Treatment [2]

Diet and lifestyle management

• Patients with factitious disorders often lack stable employment and consistent sources of support. Efforts should be made to change the lifestyle of these patients through psychosocial interventions.

Pharmacologic treatment

• Pharmacotherapy of factitious disorders is largely limited to treatment of any comorbid Axis I disorders. Medications should be carefully monitored because of patients propensity to act in self-destructive ways.

Nonpharmacologic treatment

• There is no specific treatment that has proved to be the gold standard.

Psychiatric consultation: should be initiated when the diagnosis is first seriously considered, and a multidisciplinary management team should be established.

Confronting the patient in a supportive manner: authorities generally advocate doing this in a way that redefines the patient's illness from physical disease to psychologic distress; angry rejection by caregivers should be avoided.

Psychotherapy: directed to the underlying personality disorder; supportive therapies may facilitate containment of symptoms.

Face-saving or strategic interventions: have been used with success.

Family and behavior therapy: can be useful in diminishing the reinforcement of sick-role behaviors.

Treatment aims

To reduce the patient's dissimulation and medical or surgical overutilization.
To ensure the ongoing protection of actual or potential victims (in FDP).

Prognosis

• Favorable prognostic indicators include the following:
Underlying psychiatric diagnosis (eg, mood or anxiety disorders).
Personality traits lacking borderline or antisocial elements.
Psychosocial supports (eg, ongoing relationships with others).
Ability to establish a therapeutic alliance.
• FDP has a mortality rate of 5%–10%. Long-term psychologic and physical morbidity are common.

Follow-up and management

• Treating clinicians must have modest expectations, anticipating relapse and accepting periods of symptomatic relief rather than cure. Clinicians should also be aware of their countertransference toward these patients (eg, therapeutic nihilism or anger).
• In FDP, suspicions must be reported to child abuse authorities. Categorical denial by perpetrators is extremely common. Legal mechanisms should be in place to prevent the perpetrator's removal of the child. The child's safety generally can be assured only by removing him or her from the home. Reunification should be undertaken only if a plan is in place to help ensure the child's continued safety.

Key references

1. Feldman MD, Ford CV: *Patient or Pretender: Inside the Strange World of Factitious Disorders.* New York: Wiley; 1995.
2. Feldman MD, Eisendrath SJ (eds): *The Spectrum of Factitious Disorders.* Washington, DC: American Psychiatric Press; 1996.
3. Ford CV: *Lies! Lies!! Lies!!!: The Psychology of Deceit.* Washington, DC: American Psychiatric Press, 1996:159–171.

General reference

American Psychiatric Association: *Diagnostic and Statistical Manual of Mental Disorders* ed 4. Washington, DC: American Psychiatric Press; 1994.

Diagnosis

Symptoms and signs

Persistent inadequate caloric intake.

Deceleration of weight gain or significant weight loss over at least 1 month.

Deceleration of linear growth and head circumference.

Delayed emotional and developmental milestones.

Age of onset <6 years.

• Associated factors include 1) emotional deprivation and inadequate caloric intake, leading to developmental delays and malnutrition; 2) persistent disturbance in the attunement between infant and caregiver; and 3) parental mental illness.

Investigations

Thorough physical and neurologic examination.

Laboratory tests: including complete blood count, lead level, free erythrocyte protoporphryn, tuberculin, urinalysis, urine culture, sweat test to rule out cystic fibrosis.

Thorough family assessment: including assessment of feeding routine, style, interaction.

Complications

Recurring infections: secondary to malnutrition-induced immunosuppression.

Other complications of malnutrition: *eg,* elevated blood levels of heavy metals, mineral deficiencies, and apathetic withdrawal similar to that seen in depression.

Developmental, emotional, and cognitive delays.

Differential diagnosis

Esophageal reflux.
Psychosocial dwarfism.
Malabsorption syndromes.
Depression.
Anorexia nervosa.
Rumination disorder.

Epidemiology

In pediatric hospital admissions, 1%–3%.
In lower socioeconomic outpatient populations, 10%–15%.
Sex ratio, ~1:1; with a slightly higher preponderance of boys in older infants.

Treatment

Diet and lifestyle
• Compensate for the degree of malnutrition with correct nutritional treatment.
• Focus family assessment particularly upon the relationship between the child and primary care giver.

Pharmacologic treatment
• Antidepressants may be helpful to treat depressive symptoms.

Nonpharmacologic treatment
Parental guidance, education.

Family therapy.

Referral to social services or child protective services: if necessary.

Treatment aims
To restore nutritional status to normal.
To treat comorbid depression if present.
To improve child–care giver interaction.
To ensure child has as nurturing an environment as possible, minimizing risk for future understimulation.

Prognosis
• Frequently, young infants respond rapidly to refeeding with interested caretaker. Infants with recurrent episodes resist adequate caloric intake, resulting in stunted linear growth and head circumference. Outcome is influenced by socioeconomic status, maternal education, parental mental illness, family social functioning, and extent of follow-up support and monitoring.

Follow-up and management
• Regular appointments should be made to assess the nutritional status, linear growth, and head circumference and emotional development.
• Social services support and visiting nurse care may be helpful for maintenance of recovery and minimization of long-term risk.

General references
Benoit D: Failure to thrive and feeding disorders. In *Handbook of Infant Mental Health* Edited by Zeanah CH Jr. New York: Guilford Press; 1993:317–331.

Livingston R: Anxiety disorders. In *Child and Adolescent Psychiatry: A Comprehensive Textbook.* Edited by Lewis M. Baltimore: William & Wilkins; 1996:674–678.

Woolston JL: Eating and growth disorders in infants and children. In *Child and Adolescent Psychiatry: A Comprehensive Textbook.* Edited by Lewis M. Baltimore: William & Wilkins; 1996:577–582.

Diagnosis

Symptoms and signs [1–3]

• Fetishism is a type of paraphilia (pathologic erotic preference) in which the individual has recurrent, intense sexually arousing fantasies, sexual urges, or behaviors involving the use of nonliving objects (the "fetish"). Individuals are diagnosed only if 1) there is significant distress or impairment in functioning due to their fantasies, urges, or actual behaviors utilizing the fetish, and 2) symptoms present for over 6 months.

• Fetishism is not diagnosed if the nonliving objects are limited to those specifically designed for the purpose of tactile genital stimulation, such as a vibrator, or articles of female clothing for use in cross-dressing as in transvestic fetishism.

• Articles of clothing are the most common fetish objects.

• Fetish objects frequently reported include underwear (eg, panties, bras, diapers), outer clothing (eg, scarves, blouses), rubber objects (eg, raincoats, enemas, galoshes), body parts (eg, foot, toes, leg, hair), leather objects (eg, boots, pants, jackets), and other specific items (eg, feathers, baby cribs).

• Most individuals have more than one fetish.

• The fetish may be used during masturbating or during sexual intercourse.

• Some individuals are reliant on the fetish to obtain sexual satisfaction. Most fetishists engage in more than one type of behavior, including wearing it, stealing it, adorning someone else with it, gazing at it, placing it in the rectum, hoarding it, fondling it, and sucking it.

Investigations

Laboratory investigations: no routine labwork is indicated.

Collateral sources of information and more objective measures of pathology: are vital; patients reveal substantially more acts when confronted with other evidence.

Penile plethysmography: may offer additional information to establish arousal associated with this behavior and assess for arousal associated with other paraphilias; the reliability of this measure is questionable and may result in false-negative information.

Abel Assessment for Sexual Interest: is an objective measure based on patient's reaction time responses to various slides; may be a less intrusive alternative to plethysmography.

Psychologic testing: may suggest additional psychiatric disorders and paraphilias contributing to the severity of the paraphilic behavior.

Complications

Legal implications of behavior: depending on the nature of the fetish, the individual may engage in illegal activities to increase arousal or obtain the fetish object.

Impaired social or sexual functioning: may include impaired procreation (males may have erectile dysfunction in the absence of the fetish).

Medical concerns: depending on the fetish object and the activities performed with the object, the individual may be at risk for infection or injury.

Differential diagnosis [3]

Normal sexual arousal: fetish object is used only during the arousal phase and is not used throughout the entire sexual response cycle.

Other conditions: may cause impaired judgment, social skills, or impulse control that result in fetishistic activity; behavior is not preferred or usual pattern, occurs exclusively during the course of illness, is usually isolated rather than recurrent, and usually has a later age at onset.

Etiology [1,3,4]

Biologic theory: biological predisposition; neurochemical and hormonal abnormalities that establish and maintain the fetish; possible association with temporal lobe epilepsy or neurologic damage.

Behavioral theory: fetish object is paired with sexual arousal (classic conditioning), which is generally reinforcing; further reinforced by masturbatory fantasies involving the fetish object; person likely to use fetish objects if they have poor learning histories for interpersonal skills, sexual trauma, or other learning factors.

Psychodynamic theory: fetish unconsciously linked with important people of childhood and has qualities associated with those loved, needed, and traumatizing persons; serves as a magical (hence, "fetish") bridge to relatedness, a binder of aggression, a representation of the female phallus, and a general process of "dehumanization."

Epidemiology [1,2]

• Incidence in psychiatric populations is 0.8%.

• Patients are typically male.

• Onset during adolescence with chronic course.

Treatment

General information

• Because of the scant literature on fetishism alone and the high rate of multiple paraphilias in one individual, treatment plans for fetishism are based on those developed for paraphilias in general.

Pharmacologic treatment [4]

Psychotropic medication

• Most medications given for paraphilias are thought to work by treating the obsessional nature of the disorder and by taking advantage of the sexual side-effect profile of these medications. Other medications have been reported in case studies and are potentially beneficial for unspecified reasons.

• Appropriate dosage has not been determined. It is generally accepted that medications will be prescribed similarly to treatment of obsessive-compulsive disorder and adjusted until symptoms are controlled or side effects intolerable.

• Selective serotonin reuptake inhibitors generally have fewer side-effects and may be considered first-line agents, especially for patients on few or no other medications.

Standard dosage	Fluoxetine, 20–80 mg/d; paroxetine, 20–60 mg/d; clomipramine, 150–300 mg/d; fluvoxamine, 50–300 mg/d; sertraline, 50–200 mg/d.

Hormonal agents

• Hormonal agents have been shown to be effective in suppressing sexual urges, but they also may truncate an individual's sexual life; sooner or later an individual may wish to stop them.

Standard dosage	Medroxyprogesterone acetate, 500 mg/wk i.m. or 80 mg/d orally.
	Leuprolide acetate, 7.5 mg/mo i.m. or 1 mg/d s.c.
Contraindications	*Medroxyprogesterone acetate*: should be used cautiously in patients with hyperlipidemia. Serum lipoproteins (high- and low-density lipoproteins) should be monitored during therapy with medroxyprogesterone. Medroxyprogesterone can cause fluid retention.
	Leuprolide acetate: patients with urinary tract obstruction may have worsening of symptoms during the first weeks of leuprolide therapy.
Main side effects	*Medroxyprogesterone acetate*: weight gain, hypertension, lethargy, hot flashes, mood lability (during early treatment), phlebitis (rare), gynecomastia (rare).
	Leuprolide acetate: weight gain, hypertension, headaches, mood lability (during early treatment), phlebitis (rare), gynecomastia (rare).
Main drug interactions	*Medroxyprogesterone acetate*: should not be used with bromocriptine because the combination would be counterproductive.
	Leuprolide acetate: although no drug interactions have been reported with leuprolide, therapy with androgens or estrogens are relatively contraindicated and would defeat the purpose of leuprolide therapy.
Special points	*Medroxyprogesteron acetate*: may exacerbate major depression, migraine, or seizure disorder.
	Leuprolide acetate: flutamide (250 mg orally 3 times daily) should be given concurrently during first 2 weeks of therapy to prevent a possible transient increase in sex drive.

Treatment aims

To reduce the target behavior of fetishism and any other paraphilic behaviors present so that the patient can live in society without violating the rights of others. To modify the patient's sexual interests such that they may enjoy healthy sexual functioning.

Prognosis [1]

• The earlier the age of onset, the worse the prognosis.
• Better prognosis is indicated if there is some evidence for guilt.
• Higher frequencies of the behavior lead to a higher recidivism rate.
• Behavior tends to decrease with age.

Follow up and management [1]

• Involvement of the legal system or significant others to assist in the treatment is important.
• Family members should be educated about the disorder so that they can help monitor the patient and report any worrisome activity to the patient's therapist.

Nonpharmacologic treatment

• Behavior therapy aims to reduce inappropriate sexual arousal and increase appropriate sexual arousal. This is done in the following ways:
Covert sensitization.
Orgasmic reconditioning.
Plethysmographic biofeedback.
Satiation.
Challenging of distorted thinking and beliefs that contribute and maintain the behavior.
Social skills training, assertiveness training, communication skills training, and anger management.
Relapse prevention
Aversion therapy.

Key references

1. Laws DR, O'Donohue W: *Sexual Deviance.* New York: The Guilford Press; 1997.
2. *Diagnostic and Statistical Manual of Mental Disorders,* ed 4. Washington, DC: American Psychiatric Association; 1995.
3. *Comprehensive Textbook of Psychiatry.* Edited by Kaplan HI, Sadock BJ. Baltimore: Williams & Wilkins; 1995.
4. Gabbard GO: *Treatments of Psychiatric Disorders.* Washington, DC: American Psychiatric Association; 1995.

Diagnosis

Symptoms

Mental retardation: mild to profound in males, most with IQ of 30–55; 50% of females with the full mutation are mentally retarded or have education difficulties.

Attentional deficits, hyperactivity, autism or autistic-like behaviors.

"Cluttered" speech or short bursts of repetitive speech.

Anxiety or unstable mood.

• Males are typically more severely affected than females.

Epidemiology

• Fragile X syndrome is the most common cause of inherited mental retardation. It affects ~1:1200 boys patients and ~1:2500 girls worldwide. The prevalence of carriers in the population is estimated at ~1:300–600.

Signs

Facies.

Macrocephaly.

Large ears.

Long face.

Prognathism.

Dental crowding.

Mild connective tissue dysplasia.

Hyperextensible joints.

Mild cutis laxa.

Pectus scoliosis, flat feet.

Mitral valve prolapse, aortic dilatation.

Enlarged testes (macro-orchidism).

Occasional ocular anomalies.

Pale blue irises.

Myopia.

Nystagmus.

Strabismus.

Investigations

Chromosomal analysis: should be considered for 1) persons of either sex with mental retardation or autism (especially if they have physical or behavioral characteristics of Fragile X, 2) those with a family history of Fragile X or undiagnosed mental retardation or autism, 3) patients seeking reproductive counseling due to a family history of Fragile X, and 4) those with undiagnosed mental retardation or autism.

Prenatal testing: can be done on fetuses of known carriers via chorionic villus sampling or amniocentesis.

DNA base molecular analysis

• DNA base molecular analysis for mutations and methylation within the Fragile X gene locus is the preferred adjunct to diagnosis.

• The Fragile X gene locus is on the X chromosome and contains a variable number of "repeats" of the trinucleotide CGG. Normal individuals have six to ~50 CGG repeats.

• There are two main categories of mutations:

1. Premutations of ~50–200 CGG repeats: these individuals are phenotypically normal; further expansion of a premutation can occur during female meiosis, leading to full mutations.

2. Full mutations of >200 CGG repeats within the locus: this large expansion allows for excess methylation and inactivation of the promoter region of the gene; all male patients and 30%–50% of female patients with the full mutation are phenotypically affected.

Treatment

General information

- There is no cure for the Fragile X syndrome at this time.
- Treatment consists of special education, speech, and physical and occupational therapy.
- Behavioral problems may be addressed by behavior modification programs.
- Neducatui can be helpful with some of the more common behavior problems, including hyperactivity, impulsive behavior, attentional difficulties, mood fluctuations, aggressive outbursts, anxiety, and obsessive-compulsive behavior.

Treatment aims

To optimize learning and development.
To provide symptomatic relief.
To provide genetic counseling.
To provide family and caretakers with information and support.

Prognosis

- Lifespan is normal.
- Early somatic growth is often accelerated.
- Developmental milestones are delayed but with no evidence of regression.

General reference

Turner G, Eastman G, Casey J, et al.: X-linked mental retardation associated with macro. *J Med Genetics* 1975, 12:367.

Diagnosis

Symptoms and signs [1–3]

• Frotteurism is a type of paraphilia (pathologic erotic preference) in which the individual has recurrent, intense sexually arousing fantasies, sexual urges, or behaviors involving touching and rubbing against a nonconsenting person. Individuals are diagnosed only if the following criteria are met:

Significant distress or impairment in functioning due to their fantasies, urges, or actual behaviors utilizing the fetish.

Symptoms present for over 6 months.

• Frotteurs usually choose crowded places where escape is easy (busy sidewalks, public transportation, sporting events, malls, city fairs).

• Frotteurs may rub their genitals or hands against the victim or may fondle the victim.

• Primary target areas include the thighs, buttocks, genitals, and breasts.

• Because of the crowded conditions, the victim is frequently unsure of what has occurred.

• Upon discovery, the frotteur usually flees and completes the sexual act by masturbation if the excitement was not intense enough to lead to instant ejaculation.

• Frotteurs are rarely self-referred because most have little insight into their pathologic behavior. Legal charges are often necessary.

• Some, but few, frotteurs report extreme guilt, shame, and depression secondary to their compulsion that they may regard as immoral.

• The average frotteur has approximately four additional paraphilias.

• Frotteurs often have numerous victims, are rarely caught, and serve short sentences.

• There are two subtypes of frotteurs [1]:

1. Exclusive type: paraphilic fantasies or stimuli are obligatory for erotic arousal and are always included in sexual activity.

2. Nonexclusive: paraphilic preferences occur only episodically (eg, perhaps during periods of stress), whereas at other times the person is able to function sexually without paraphilic fantasies or stimuli.

Investigations [1]

Laboratory investigations: no routine labwork is indicated.

Collateral sources of information and more objective measures of pathology: are vital; patients reveal substantially more acts when confronted with other evidence.

Penile plethysmography: may offer additional information to establish arousal associated with this behavior and assess for arousal associated with other paraphilias; the reliability of this measure is questionable and may result in false-negative information.

The Abel Assessment for Sexual Interest: examines reaction time responses to various slides; may be a less intrusive alternative to plethysmography.

Psychologic tests: Clarke Sexual History Questionnaire for Males (probes for multiple paraphilias), Derogatis Sexual Functioning Inventory (surveys the individual's sexual functioning), assessment for comorbid psychiatric illness (eg, increased rates of depressive disorders, personality disorders, substance abuse, attention-deficit hyperactivity disorder, conduct disorders, sexual disorders, and other paraphilias).

Complications

Legal implications of behavior: frotteurism is an illegal activity. In addition, the individual may engage in illegal activities to increase arousal or place himself into position to locate a victim.

Impaired social or sexual functioning: these individuals tend to have very poor social and sexual relationships, which may be further impaired due to their need for the deviant behavior.

Differential diagnosis [3]

Normal sexual arousal: in normal sexual behavior, the target individual consents to being touched.

Other conditions: may cause impaired judgment, social skills, or impulse control that result in fetishistic activity; behavior is not preferred or usual pattern, occurs exclusively during the course of illness, is usually isolated rather than recurrent, and usually has a later age at onset.

Etiology

Biologic theory: biologic predisposition; neurochemical or hormonal abnormalities that establish and maintain the fetish; possible association with temporal lobe epilepsy or neurologic damage.

Behavioral theory: frotteurism is paired with sexual arousal (classic conditioning), which is generally reinforcing; further reinforced by masturbatory fantasies involving behavior; history of sexual or physical abuse is common.

Psychodynamic theory: contact and fondling represent eroticized maternal contact; this elicits merger and castration fears, and thus contact is brief and orgasm is necessary to reassert bodily integrity.

Courtship disorders: suggests that frotteurism is a disturbance in tactile courtship interactions and is related to voyeurism, exhibitionism, and rape, which are also courtship disorders.

Epidemiology

• Frottage usually begins by adolescence and occurs between ages 15–25, frequency gradually declining with age.

• Female frotteurs are considered extremely rare.

• The mean number of acts per frotteur has been found to be as high as 850.

Treatment

General information
• Because of the scant literature on frotteurism alone and the high rate of multiple paraphilias in one individual, treatment plans for frotteurism are based on those developed for paraphilias in general.

Pharmacologic treatment [4]
Psychotropic medication
• Most medications given for paraphilias are thought to work by treating the obsessional nature of the disorder and by taking advantage of the sexual side effect profile of these medications. Other medications have been reported in case studies and are potentially beneficial for unspecified reasons.

• Appropriate dosage has not been determined. It is generally accepted that medications will be prescribed similarly to treatment of obsessive-compulsive disorder or depression and adjusted until symptoms are controlled or side effects intolerable.

• Selective serotonin reuptake inhibitors generally have fewer side effects and may be considered first-line agents, especially for patients on few or no other medications.

• Usually symptoms of the paraphilia rapidly recur on discontinuation of psychotropic medications or hormonal agents.

Standard dosage	Fluoxetine, 20–80 mg/d.
	Paroxetine, 20–60 mg/d.
	Clomipramine, 150–300 mg/d.
	Fluvoxamine, 50–300 mg/d.
	Sertraline, 50–200 mg/d.
	Desipramine, 150–300 mg/d.
	Imipramine, 150–300 mg/d.

Hormonal agents
• Antiandrogens have been shown to be effective in suppressing sexual urges, but they also may truncate an individual's sexual life; sooner or later the individual may wish to stop them.

• Medroxyprogesterone acetate lowers testosterone levels and has demonstrated efficacy for decreasing sexual urges, fantasies, and behaviors for most paraphilias.

• Cyproterone acetate (in Canada) blocks the action of testosterone and has demonstrated efficacy in treatment of paraphilias.

• Long-acting gonadotropic hormone-releasing hormone agonists have recently shown efficacy in paraphilic populations. These agents decrease secretion of luteinizing hormone and follicle-stimulating hormone, which results in lowered testosterone secretion.

Nonpharmacologic treatment
• Behavior therapy aims to reduce inappropriate sexual arousal and increase appropriate sexual arousal. This is done in the following ways:

Covert sensitization.

Orgasmic reconditioning.

Plethysmographic biofeedback.

Satiation.

Challenging of distorted thinking and beliefs that contribute and maintain the behavior.

Social skills training, assertiveness training, communication skills training, and anger management.

Relapse prevention.

Aversion therapy.

Treatment aims
To reduce the target behavior of frotteurism and any other paraphilic behaviors present so that the patient can live in society without violating the rights of others.
To modify the patient's sexual interests such that they may enjoy healthier sexual functioning.

Prognosis
• The earlier the age of onset, the worse the prognosis.
• Better prognosis is indicated if there is some evidence for guilt.
• The higher the frequency of the behavior, the higher the recidivism rate.
• Behavior tends to decrease with age.

Follow-up and management
• Involvement of the legal system or significant others to assist in the treatment is important.
• Family members should be educated about the disorder and can then help monitor the patient and report any worrisome activity to the patient's therapist.

Key references
1. Laws DR, O'Donohue W: *Sexual Deviance.* New York: Guilford Press; 1997.
2. *Diagnostic and Statistical Manual of Mental Disorders*, ed 4. Washington, DC: American Psychiatric Assocation; 1995.
3. Kaplan HI, Sadock BJ: *Comprehensive Textbook of Psychiatry.* Baltimore: Williams & Wilkins; 1995.
4. Gabbard GO: *Treatments of Psychiatric Disorders.* Washington, DC: American Psychiatric Association; 1995.

Diagnosis

Symptoms and signs

• Strong, persistent cross-gender identification (desire to be or feeling like one is of the opposite sex).

• Persistent discomfort about one's sex (or sense of inappropriateness in the gender role of that sex).

• Clinically significant distress or impairment in function.

Common behavior in male children

• Preoccupation with traditionally feminine activities wearing girls' clothes, playing with dolls.

• Avoidance of stereotypical male activities (rough play and competitive sports).

• Sitting to urinate or pretending not to have a penis.

• Expressing wish to be a girl or belief about growing up to be a woman.

Common behavior in female children

• Preference for boys' clothing and short hair, aversion to feminine attire.

• Stereotypical male activities and identification with powerful male figures.

• Standing to urinate or claiming to have a penis.

• Expressing wish to be a boy or belief about growing up to be a man.

Common behavior in adults

• Preoccupation with desire to live as member of opposite sex.

• Adoption of behavior, dress, and mannerisms of other sex (to various extents).

• Sexual attraction may be to same sex, opposite sex, both, or neither.

• Males may display breast enlargement, hair denuding, and other physical changes from hormone ingestion, depilation, and so on.

• Females may have distorted breasts or breast rashes from wearing breast binders.

• Extreme form of the disorder is known as transsexualism.

Course in children

• Onset occurs typically between 2 to 4 years of age.

• Homosexual or bisexual orientation by late adolescence in three-quarters of boys with childhood gender identity disorder.

• Small percentage still diagnosed with gender identity disorder in adulthood.

Course in adults

• There are two distinct courses in adults: 1) continuation from childhood or adolescence, and 2) onset in early to mid-adulthood, usually following or concurrent with transvestic fetishism.

• Males who are sexually attracted to males tend to present for treatment earlier than others.

Investigations [1]

Physical diagnostic tests: none are available.

Psychological testing: can provide evidence of opposite-gender identification and behavior.

Karyotyping for sex chromosomes, sex hormone assays: usually not indicated if the physical examination is normal (unless hormonal or surgical gender reassignment is to be done).

Routine electroencephalogram: should be performed at least once in transsexual patients to rule out temporal lobe epilepsy.

Differential diagnosis

Transvestic fetishism: cross-dressing for sexual excitement, rather than feeling like a member of opposite sex.

Psychosis: may have delusions that one is a member of the opposite sex, rather than just feeling like the opposite sex.

"Tomboyishness" in girls or "sissy" behavior in boys: nonconformity to stereotypical sex role behavior without profound disturbance in gender identity.

Physical intersex problem (eg, androgen insensitivity syndrome or congenital adrenal hyperplasia) plus gender dysphoria: diagnose as a gender identity disorder not otherwise specified.

Etiology

• Etiology remains undetermined.

• Fundamental disturbance is possibly neurobiologic, involving sex differences in hypothalamic and adjacent brain regions.

Epidemiology

• The prevalence is estimated at 3% for boys in childhood and less than 1% for girls; there is no comparable estimate for adults, although the prevalence estimate for transsexualism is ~1:50,000.

• In child clinics, the gender ratio is five males per female; in adult clinics, two to three males per female.

• Onset may be in childhood, adolescence, or adulthood.

Complications

Social isolation, ostracism, or ridicule: may result in low self-esteem or dropping out of school; more common for males than females.

Impaired social relationships: poor same-sex peer relationships, difficulty relating to parents, marital problems.

Substance-related and axis II disorders: high comorbidity.

Sexually transmitted diseases: prostitution is common in males, resulting in high HIV risk.

Anxiety, depression, suicidality: common in children, adolescents, and adults with the disorder.

Legal issues: increased criminality, difficulties with legal definitions of male and female.

Medical concerns: possible risk of infection, injury, and death from self-inflicted body changes and self-prescribed hormones.

Treatment [1–3]

General information

• For hormonal and surgical sex reassignment, standards of care have been developed and should be followed.

• Wearing cross-gender clothing in daily life under psychiatric supervision for at least 1 year is advised before beginning hormone or surgical treatment.

Pharmacologic treatment

• No pharmacologic treatments have been identified for children.

• Pharmacologic treatment has not been effective in reducing cross-gender desires in adults.

Hormonal treatment

• Hormonal treatment for adults modifies physical sex characteristics to agree with gender identity, ie, gender reassignment.

Standard dosage	Estrogens for men (may take ≥2 y to achieve maximal breast growth).
	Androgens (testosterone) for women.
Contraindications	*Estrogens*: active or past thrombophlebitis, thrombosis, or thromboembolic disorders, known or suspected estrogen-dependent neoplasia; use with caution with asthma, epilepsy, migraine, cardiac or renal dysfunction, hypercalcemia, glucose intolerance, and depression.
	Testosterone: patients with high risk of coronary heart disease or severe liver damage.
Main side effects	*Estrogens*: elevated liver enzymes, loss of libido, mood disturbance, hyperprolactinaemia, nausea and vomiting, fluid retention, high blood pressure, possible increased risk of thromboembolic events, coronary heart disease, and malignant tumors.
	Testosterone: acne, elevation of cholesterol and triglyceride levels, libido change, nausea, jaundice, alterations in liver function, suppression of clotting factors, sodium and fluid retention, headache, anxiety, depression.
Main drug interactions	*Testosterone*: anticoagulants, oxyphenbutazone, insulin.
Special points	Hormonal treatment ideally recommended to be accompanied by ongoing psychotherapeutic relationship with patient for a minimum of 3–12 months. Hormonal treatment is not recommended for use with children. Many effects, such as deepening voice in females, may be irreversible. Blood chemistry monitoring is required, including liver function, prolactin levels, hormone status, and serum lipids.

Nonpharmacologic treatment

Psychotherapy: may be helpful if aimed at helping patients accept and function within their biologic sex.

Behavioral treatment: ie, token economy or differential social reinforcement, can reduce cross-gender behavior in children.

Therapies with aim to change disturbed gender identity structure: generally fail.

Supportive and skills-development psychotherapy: vital for candidates of hormonal or surgical sex reassignment.

Sex reassignment surgery.

Treatment aims

In children: to develop social skills and comfort in biologic sex role. Psychotherapy for non–sex-reassignment candidates: to accept biologic sex and increased ability to function within it. Hormonal (males): to increase physical resemblance to female (eg, breast enlargement, feminization of body contour and skin texture, decrease in body and facial hair). Hormonal (females): to increase physical resemblance to male (eg, cessation of menses, increase in hair and muscle mass, clitoral growth, voice deepening). Multistep treatment for transsexuals: to achieve effective functioning in society as member of opposite sex.

Prognosis

• Course tends to be chronic, with cyclical variation in many cases.

• Psychiatric or psychosocial treatment of children may prevent transsexualism, but is unlikely to affect direction of adult sexual orientation.

• The majority of well-screened transsexuals who have sex reassignment treatment report positive outcome in terms of well being, happiness, and psychosocial adjustment. Better surgical results predict better postoperative adjustment.

• Adult onset is associated with lower satisfaction with sex-reassignment surgery.

Follow-up and management

• After hormone or surgical sex reassignment, monitoring and optimizing hormone levels are recommended. Psychotherapy should be focused on development and adaptation to new lifestyle.

Key references

1. Schlatterer K, et al.: Multistep treatment concept of transsexual patients. *Exp Clin Endocrinol Diabetes* 1996, 413–419.
2. Walker P, et al.: Standards of care: the hormonal and surgical sex reassignment of GD persons. *Arch Sex Behav* 1985, 14:79–90.
3. Brown G: A review of clinical approaches to gender dysphoria. *J Clin Psychiatry* 1990, 51:57–64.

Diagnosis

Symptoms

• Generalized anxiety disorder (GAD) is characterized by excessive anxiety and worry for 6 months that is difficult to control and concerns a number of activities or events. The anxiety will be associated with at least three of the following:

1. Restless feelings, being keyed up or on edge.
2. Being easily fatigued.
3. Difficulty in concentrating or mind going blank.
4. Irritability.
5. Muscle tension.
6. Sleep disturbance (falling or staying asleep, restless sleep).

• Patients usually present to their primary care physician and often complain of medically unexplained somatic symptoms (eg, chest pain, irritable bowel symptoms, and hyperventilation) and either ignore or deny symptoms of nervousness. GAD is not diagnosed in 50% of these patients.

Investigations

• Before diagnosing and treating GAD, it is essential to exclude physical disorders. However, most patients with GAD will have a comorbid psychiatric disorder.

Complications

Overall reduction in emotional health.

Impairment in functioning at work.

Impairment in social and family relations.

Low satisfaction with life.

Differential diagnosis

Anticipatory anxiety.
Depression.
Panic disorder.
Delirium and dementia.
Anxiety disorders due to a general medical condition.
Substance abuse.
Personality disorders.
Hypochondriasis.

Etiology

Biologic factors: patients with GAD have prolonged, abnormal responses to stress that appear to be modulated by noradrenergic and serotonergic systems, γ-aminobutyric acid receptors, and the hypothalamic–pituitary–adrenocortical axis.

Psychosocial: a high level of stressful life events is associated with the onset of GAD.

Epidemiology

• GAD is the most common anxiety disorder, with rates of 1.6% current, 3.1% 1-year, and 5.1% lifetime.
• Prevalence in primary care settings is 2.9%
• GAD is more common in women, African-Americans, and young persons.
• Average age of onset varies from mid-teens to mid-20s, and the average age of presentation is 39 y.
• A comorbid psychiatric disorder (most commonly depression) occurs in 66%–90% of patients.

Treatment

Diet and lifestyle
- Minimize stress, alcohol, tobacco, drug use.
- Increase physical exercise.

Pharmacologic treatment

Standard dosage   Benzodiazepines, *eg*, alprazolam (1.5–2.5 mg/d), diazepam (15–25 mg/d), lorazepam (3–5 mg/d), or clonazepam (1.5–2.5 mg/d).

Buspirone, 20–60 mg/d

Cyclic antidepressants, *eg*, imipramine or desipramine (75–300 mg/d).

Beta-blockers, *eg*, propranolol, start at 20 mg/d and titrate up as tolerated.

Contraindications   *Benzodiazepines*: substance abuse, narrow-angle glaucoma, hazardous activities.

Buspirone: patients on a monoamine oxidase inhibitor (MAOI).

Cyclic antidepressants: patients on a MAOI or those recovering from a myocardial infarction.

Propranolol: cardiogenic shock, sinus bradycardia, heart block (greater than first degree), bronchial asthma, congestive heart failure.

Main side effects   *Benzodiazepines*: sedation, fatigue, impaired performance, cognitive impairment, dizziness, and ataxia. A discontinuation syndrome (depending on dose, half-life, and duration of treatment) is common and consists of autonomic symptoms, anxiety, irritability, loss of appetite, insomnia, sweating, diarrhea, vomiting, and dysphoria.

Buspirone: nausea, dizziness, headaches, excitement.

Cyclic antidepressants: cardiac dysrhythmias (usually with underlying cardiac disease), anticholinergic effects (*eg*, dry mouth, orthostasis, constipation, urinary retention), lower seizure threshold.

Main drug interactions   *Benzodiazepines*: central nervous system depression in conjunction with alcohol or barbiturates.

Buspirone: potentially fatal interaction with MAOIs.

Cyclic antidepressants: potentially fatal interaction with MAOIs or antiarrhythmic agents.

Propranolol: possible adverse cardiac effects in combination with calcium-channel blockers, catecholamine-depleting drugs, clonidine, haloperidol, and prazosin.

Special points   *Benzodiazepines*: consider their use with a predominance of psychic symptoms, low level of depression, and acute onset of symptoms.

Buspirone: consider its use with a predominance of somatic symptoms, chronic anxiety, history of substance abuse, and absence of panic attacks.

Treatment aims
To obtain remission and prevent relapse of GAD.

Nonpharmacologic treatment
Psychotherapy: cognitive-behavioral therapy is a short-term treatment that yields long-term improvement; it may shorten the length of time that the patient needs medication.

Other therapies: dynamic and supportive therapies are helpful.

Prognosis
- GAD is a chronic illness requiring long-term treatment. Relapse is typical and should not be considered treatment failure. There are periods of symptom quiescence.

Follow-up and management
- Make sure the diagnosis is correct and that the patient does not have a comorbid disorder (especially depression) that also needs treatment.
- The medication maintenance period should last for several months. Thereafter, the medication should be slowly tapered. If symptoms reappear, consider longer treatment. Short-term, symptom-specific treatment is often helpful.

General references
Brawman-Mintzer O, Lydiard RB: Generalized anxiety disorder: issues in epidemiology. *J Clin Psychiatry* 1996, 57(suppl 7):3–8.

Dubovsky SL: Generalized anxiety disorder: new concepts and psychopharmacologic therapies. *J Clin Psychiatry* 1990, 51:3–9.

Gorman JM, Papp LA: Chronic anxiety: deciding the length of treatment. *J Clin Psychiatry* 1990, 51(suppl 1):11–13.

Roy-Byrne PP: Generalized anxiety and mixed anxiety-depression: association with disability and health care utilization. *J Clin Psychiatry* 1996, 57(suppl 7):86–91.

Schweizer E: Generalized anxiety disorder: longitudinal course and pharmacologic treatment. *Psychiatr Clin North Am* 1995, 18:843–857.

Schweizer E, Rickels K: The long-term management of generalized anxiety disorder: issues and dilemmas. *J Clin Psychiatry* 1996, 57:9–12.

Diagnosis

Definition
• The person with a histrionic personality disorder is typified by attention-seeking behaviors and over-emotionality.

Symptoms and signs
• Persons with histrionic personality have a need to be the center of attention and dress and behave in ways to attract attention. Their emotionality is often excessive and dramatic but lacks depth of feeling. These persons are frequently stylish and use language in a colorful manner, sprinkled with the latest faddish colloquialisms (slang). They may be dramatic, flirtatious, and openly seductive. Their apparent concern for others, including flattery and gifts, may be more to create attention for themselves than out of genuine feelings for others.

• The histrionic person is often naively suggestible and may be a victim of sexual predators or con men. The histrionic often has many briefly intense but basically shallow romantic or sexual relationships. Promiscuity is common, as are multiple marriages.

• Speech and thinking are driven by emotionality rather than logic and detail, and decisions are often made impulsively by "intuition" or hunches. The histrionic is prone to exaggeration, fantasy, and outright deceit.

DSM-IV diagnostic criteria
• Histrionic personality disorder is indicated by the presence of five (or more) of the following:

1. Is uncomfortable in situations in which he or she is not the center of attention.

2. Interaction with others is often characterized by inappropriate sexually seductive or provocative behavior.

3. Displays rapidly shifting and shallow expression of emotions.

4. Consistently uses physical appearance to draw attention to self. Has a style of speech that is excessively impressionistic and lacking in detail. Shows self-dramatization, theatricality, and exaggerated expression of emotion.

5. Is suggestible, ie, easily influenced by others or circumstances.

6. Considers relationships to be more intimate than they actually are.

Investigations
• The diagnosis of histrionic personality disorder is best made by a careful review of life history supplemented by the reports of others, such as family members.

Psychologic testing: standardized valid and reliable self-report instruments include the Minnesota Multiphasic Personality Inventory-2 and Millon Clinical Multiaxial Inventory-II; structured interview instruments include the Structured Clinical Interview for DSM-IIIR Personality Disorders-II.

Laboratory studies: there are no specific laboratory examinations.

Complications
Comorbidity
Many associated personality features of other cluster B personality disorders and dependent personality disorder; alcohol and substance abuse; impulse control disorders: *eg*, compulsive buying or kleptomani; panic disorder; somatization disorder; major depression; rejection sensitivity: excessive response to loss of a relationship.

Behavioral outcomes
Promiscuity and sexually transmitted diseases, divorce, financial irresponsi-bility, substance abuse, unstable work record.

Differential diagnosis
Other cluster B personality disorders. Substance abuse (eg, cocaine). Cyclothymia.

Etiology
• Concepts of histrionic traits as compared with "hysterical traits" have been muddied by the confusing terminology used to describe these persons. Early psychoanalytic theories of fixation at an oedipal level of psychosexual development have largely been discarded.
• Current explanations of etiology include the following:
Cultural and subcultural differences in the degree of emotional demonstrativeness. Constitutional temperamental differences in traits such as novelty seeking. Genetic influences: there is evidence of an increased frequency of histrionic personality disorder and somatization disorder in female relatives and of antisocial personality disorder in male relatives.

Epidemiology
• The prevalence in the general population is 2%–3%; in psychiatric patients (when structured assessment instruments are used), 10%–15%.
• The prevalence is greater in females than in males, although there may be a gender bias for females in favor of histrionic personality over antisocial personality.

Treatment

Diet and lifestyle
• Regular life habits should be encouraged, including meals and sleep. The histrionic patient often needs increased organization of personal finances and work habits.

Pharmacologic treatment
• There is no specific pharmacologic treatment for histrionic personality disorder.
• Target symptoms of comorbid axis I disorders should be treated (eg, major depression, panic disorder, substance abuse).
• The person with histrionic personality disorder is at risk for substance abuse, including habituation to prescribed medication. Those medications with habituation potential (eg, benzodiazepines and opiate analgesics) are relatively contraindicated.

Nonpharmacologic treatment
• Individual psychodynamic psychotherapy remains the cornerstone of treatment, although alternative treatments may be useful adjuncts to therapy.

Psychotherapy
• Individual psychotherapy needs to provide support at times of crisis (eg, the break-up of a relationship) while simultaneously confronting the patient's expectations of a rescuer. The therapist models a well-modulated affective response, and through questions and interpretations emphasizes the need for problem solving and coping strategies rather than the use of emotional displays or somatization to manipulate others into care-taking behaviors. The therapist must also carefully redirect the patient to resolve those emotional conflictual issues that are characteristically avoided or repressed.
• Group therapy may be an useful adjunct to individual therapy in that the group in a supportive manner may confront the patient concerning issues of emotionality and manipulativeness.
• Marital therapy may be needed in order to resolve conflictual issues in the marriage that are related to patient's emotionality. Perhaps most importantly, marital therapy can address problems related to the sabotage of individual therapy that may be motivated by the spouse's need to keep the patient in a more infantile dependent state.
• Behavioral therapy plays an important role in treatment of acute symptomology (eg, somatic symptoms, suicide gestures), particularly during inpatient treatment. Such treatment consists of failing to respond to the patient's dramatic attention-seeking symptoms while providing positive reinforcement of mature means of communication.

Treatment aims
To promote greater organization in life style, increased stability and genuine intimacy in interpersonal relationships, and the capacity to modulate emotions.

Prognosis
• Mild forms of histrionic personality disorder benefit from therapy in terms of increased quality of interpersonal relationships and decreased somatization. Some improvement may occur as the result of aging and increased maturity.
• Severe forms of histrionic personality disorder, those associated with borderline or antisocial features, are prone to continued marital or occupational instability, the effects of substance abuse, acting out behaviors, and even imprisonment.

Follow-up and management

For the acute phase
• The person with histrionic personality disorder frequently presents at times of severe emotional distress, often due to disrupted interpersonal relationships. Supportive care, at times inpatient psychiatric treatment, is required for stabilization.

For the continuation phase
• Long-term psychotherapy (months to years) to address characterologic issues is needed after stabilization of acute episodes of emotional dyscontrol or somatization. Even following successful moderation of histrionic defenses, some brief psychotherapeutic interventions may be required at times of severe stress or loss.

Pitfalls
The histrionic patient will attempt to subvert therapy to a social event. Seductive behavior can not only circumvent the therapeutic process but, if the therapist succumbs, can lead to disaster for both patient and therapist.

General references
Halleck SL: Hysterical personality traits: psychological, social, and iatrogenic determinants. *Arch Gen Psychiatry* 1967, 16:750–757.

Horowitz MJ: Histrionic personality disorder. In *Treatments of Psychiatric Disorders*, ed 2. edited by Gabbard GO. Washington, DC: American Psychiatric Press; 1995:2311–2326.

Horowitz MJ: *Hysterical Personality Style and the Histrionic Personality Disorders*. Northvale, NJ: Jason Aronson; 1991.

Diagnosis

Symptoms

Motor disorders

• Onset is typically insidious, and symptoms have usually been present for some time by the time of diagnosis.

Involuntary movements: chorea primarily but also athetosis, dystonia, myoclonus, and parkinsonism.

Impaired fine motor activities.

Gait changes and problems with balance.

Dysarthria.

Dysphagia.

Behavioral and cognitive abnormalities

• Frank dementia is usually a late finding, but the patient and family may describe a history of depression, anxiety, or other less specific behavior change concurrent with or prior to the onset of motor symptoms. Affective disorders occur in 30%–50% of patients.

Signs

Slowed or incomplete saccadic eye movements.

Chorea: often exacerbated by stress or mental effort.

Motor impersistence: typically with tongue protrusion or forced eye closure.

Poor tandem gait: with difficult maintenance of station.

Investigations

• In a patient with typical clinical signs and a positive family history for Huntington's disease (HD), an experienced clinician may not investigate further. If the family history is incomplete, or other conditions are suspected, the following studies may be informative.

Complete blood count: a thick smear should be done to rule out neuroacanthocytosis.

Thyroid functions: to rule out hyperthyroidism.

Rheumatologic studies: eg, erythrocyte sedimentation rate, rheumatoid factor, antinuclear antibodies; to determine the likelihood of systemic lupus erythematosus (SLE).

Neuroradiologic studies: magnetic resonance imaging and computed tomography scans of the brain may demonstrate atrophy of the caudate nucleus.

Special studies

• There is a direct test for the HD mutation that can be performed on a single specimen of whole blood; however, because the specificity and sensitivity for this test are so high, significant care must be taken in it use. All patients should be counseled thoroughly regarding the consequences of obtaining this test, especially with regard to issues of insurability, long-term care, and employability. Due to the need for a thorough understanding of the ramifications of the test to the patient and his or her family, mutational analysis should not be performed outside of the auspices of a qualified testing center. Testing centers are equipped to deal with presymptomatic and prenatal HD testing. Currently, testing of minors and preadoption screening are considered controversial due to the issue of informed consent.

Complications

• Huntington's disease is a progressive neurodegenerative disease that leads to premature death. Over the course of the illness, patients gradually lose motor function and become demented. Typical complications include aspiration pneumonia and sepsis due to dysphagia and inanition.

Differential diagnosis

Wilson's disease.
Sydenham's chorea.
Neuroacanthocytosis.
SLE.
Thyroid disease.

Etiology

• Neuropathologically, HD is characterized by selective neuronal loss in various brain regions, most prominently in the basal ganglia. The genetic abnormality in HD is an expansion of triplet nucleotide repeats (CAG) on chromosome 4. Persons affected with HD have greater than 39 repeats. The presence of 36–39 repeats is considered intermediate, and persons in this range may not exhibit signs of the disease. The relationship between CAG repeat length and clinical HD is loosely related by age of onset, with larger expanded alleles being associated with an earlier onset. However, the connection between CAG-repeat length and the neurodegenerative process remains obscure.

Epidemiology

• Estimated prevalence at 4–40:100,000 persons. Worldwide distribution, with isolated pockets of increased concentration.
• Age of onset is 35–45 y of age.
• The clinician should keep in mind that for each person with HD, there are typically four to five family members at risk for the disease.

Treatment

Diet and lifestyle management
• There is no proven therapy to treat this condition. Patients should be counseled as to the course of the illness and encouraged to refrain from stressful situations that could exacerbate chorea. Adequate diet and exercise are recommended.

Pharmacologic treatment
• The only proven therapies are by necessity palliative in nature and include symptomatic treatment of behavioral and emotional consequences of HD as well as treatment directed at chorea. With regard to psychiatric manifestations of HD, patients diagnosed with depression, mania, anxiety disorders, etc. should be approached no differently than those without HD.

• Concerning treatment of chorea in HD, it is clear that one of the signature features of HD is the progressive loss of motor skills, and also that adventitious movements can be somewhat ameliorated by the use of neuroleptics. However, because HD is a progressive disease, treatment directed at chorea will commonly require higher and higher doses of antichorea medications (eg, haloperidol). Benefits are temporary, and stopping neuroleptics once begun makes adaptation by the patients much more problematic, because these increasing doses of neuroleptics will often result in somnolence or other side effects. It is for this reason that treatment of the movement disorder is not recommended unless there is a severe impact on the patient's activities of daily living.

• In patients requiring treatment of their chorea, first-line drugs would include agents such as haloperidol or clonazepam. Dosage (see below) must be individually titrated, and patients should be closely monitored for side effects.

Standard dosage Haloperidol, 0.5–1.0 mg/d; increase as tolerated (generally no higher than 10 or 20 mg/d), divided two or three times daily.

Clonazepam, 0.5 mg two to three times daily, increase as tolerated.

Treatment aims
To provide education to patients and families, especially with regard to genetic counseling.
To appropriately identify and treat any associated psychiatric and behavioral components to the disease.

Prognosis
• HD is relentlessly progressive, resulting in loss of ability to provide self-care, ambulate, and ultimately, communicate. Patients eventually require skilled nursing care for management.

Follow-up and management
• Despite its progressive nature, the course may seem indolent at first. Patients should be seen at least one to two times per year routinely (more frequently should problems arise). Special care should be taken to ascertain the need for physical or occupational therapy, and speech or swallowing evaluations may be of benefit.

Support groups
• Patients and families should be referred to the following address, or to their local HD support group:
Huntington's Disease Society of America
140 22nd Street, 6th Floor
New York, NY 10011
Phone: 1-800-345-HDSA
E-mail: curehd@hdsa.ttisms.com

General references
Harper PS: Huntington's Disease: Major Problems in Neurology, vol 22. Philadelphia: WB Saunders; 1991.

Diagnosis

Definition
• Hypochondriasis is a preoccupation with the fear of having or the belief that one has a serious disease based on the person's interpretation of one or more physical signs or sensations. Although the belief is not of delusional intensity, the preoccupation or belief persists despite medical evaluation and reassurance.

Symptoms and signs
• The preoccupation with bodily symptoms causes clinically significant distress or impairment and lasts for at least 6 months. The preoccupation is typically with bodily functions, minor physical abnormalities, or vague and ambiguous physical sensations that the person attributes to the suspected disease.

Associated characteristics
• Hypochondriacal symptoms can be caused by another mental disorder (eg, major depression, dysthymia, or an anxiety disorder) and should respond to treatment for the primary condition.

• Hypochondriasis is more common in those who have suffered serious illness in the past, particularly in childhood, and those with ill family members.

• Individuals with this disorder typically resist referral to mental health settings.

Investigations
• Laboratory findings and physical examinations do not confirm the individual's preoccupation. There are no known routine laboratory tests to confirm the disorder.

Complications
Complications from repeated diagnostic procedures.

Medical problems missed due to cursory evaluations: of patients who have a history of multiple complaints in which previous studies have yielded no evidence of disease.

Strained social and family relationships.

Differential diagnosis
• The most important consideration in differential diagnosis is ruling out underlying medical conditions.
• Psychiatric conditions in the differential include major depressive disorder, dysthymic disorder, generalized anxiety disorder, panic disorder, obsessive-compulsive disorder, psychotic disorders, somatization disorder, factitious disorder, and malingering.
• Hypochondriacal concerns secondary to major psychiatric disorders are categorized with the primary disorder.
• Onset of increased health concerns in old age is likely due to a mood disorder.

Etiology
• The etiology of hypochondriasis is not known. Hypochondriasis does not seem to be more common in families of patients with hypochondriasis [1].

Epidemiology
• The prevalence of hypochondriasis in the general population is unknown. In general medical practices, 4%–9% of patients have hypochondriasis.
• The disorder is equally common in males and females.
• Although the disorder can begin at any age, onset is thought to be most common during the twenties.
• There appears to be no difference in prevalence based on socioeconomic status, education, or marital status.

Treatment

Pharmacological treatment [2]

• There is evidence that patients with uncomplicated hypochondriasis benefit from treatment with various psychotropic agents. It is unclear whether any particular drug has particular efficacy or whether nonspecific treatment effects are the primary cause of improvement.

• Patients who have comorbid psychiatric disorders often have improvement in their hypochondriacal symptoms when the comorbid condition is treated.

Selective serotonin-reuptake inhibitors (SSRIs) are commonly prescribed due to similarities between hypochondriasis and obsessive-compulsive disorder and numerous case reports that suggest preferential efficacy for SSRIs in hypochondriasis.

Nonpharmacologic treatment

Reassurance

• Physicians typically reassure patients in the face of negative clinical findings. In dealing with hypochondriacal patients, the physician's reassurance of the patient is more effective when it is directed at their relationship rather than at the clinical findings. For example, it is reassuring to some chronic patients to know that they will have a continuing relationship of trust and confidence with a physician that will be sustained regardless of the nature of their complaints [3]. Physician statements indicating that there is nothing wrong with a hypochondriacal patient typically increase the patient's fear and diminish their trust in the physician.

Cognitive-behavioral treatment

• Cognitive-behavioral treatment is a useful mode of therapy for patients willing to pursue formal psychological treatment.

Other information

• The majority of hypochondriacal patients are treated in the medical setting and they tend to resist mental health involvement.

• Psychiatric referral may be useful for help with evaluation of comorbid conditions, pharmacologic consultation, or formal on-going treatment. Success with such referrals may be increased by framing the referral as an adjunct to on-going medical treatment aimed to help the patient manage the stress of their illness.

Follow-up and management [4]

• The following recommended general management principles have been shown to be effective for managing somatizing patients and are appropriate for the care of hypochondriacal patients:

The patient should have one physician who is the major caregiver and who has primary responsibility for the patient.

The patient should be seen for regularly scheduled appointments for brief periods of time; avoid as-needed visits.

Perform physical examinations or partial examinations at each visit.

Look for signs of disease rather than relying on symptoms.

Diagnostic tests and surgical procedures should be avoided unless clearly indicated.

Avoid telling the patient "it's all in your head."

Treatment aims

To develop a trusting relationship between the patient and the primary physician, in which 1) the physician accepts the patient, and 2) the patient senses that the physician is dependable and will sustain the relationship.

Prognosis

• The course of hypochondriasis is usually chronic, with waxing and waning symptoms. Although some dispute this pessimistic prognosis, there are no long-term controlled clinical trials on which to make another judgement.

• Commonly cited favorable prognostic indicators include acute onset, absence of personality disorder, and the absence of secondary gain.

Key references

1. Noyes R, Holt C, Happel R, et al.: A family study of hypochondriasis. J Nerv Ment Dis 1997, 185:223–232.

2. Fallon B, Schneier F, Marshall R, et al.: The pharmacology of hypochondriasis. Psychopharmacol Bull 1996, 32:607–611.

3. Lipsitt D: Hypochondriasis and body dysmorphic disorder. In Treatments of Psychiatric Disorders ed 2. Edited by Gabbard G. Washington, DC: American Psychiatric Press; 1995:1783–1801.

4. Smith GR, Monson R, Ray D: Psychiatric consultation in somatization disorder. N Engl J Med 1986, 314:1407–1413.

General reference

American Psychiatric Association: Diagnostic and Statistical Manual of Mental Disorders ed 4. Washington, DC: American Psychiatric Press; 1994.

Diagnosis

General information

• Common inhalants abused today include solvents, aerosols, alkylnitrites, and nitrous oxide. Among these are varnish, paint thinners, lighter fluid, nail polish, room deodorizer, liquid incense, whipped cream dispensers, and additives for automobile engines.

• It is difficult to identify one particular effect or health consequence of inhalants because there are so many different types and each acts differently on the body.

Definition

• Patterns of abuse of inhalants may be classified into three types of increasing severity:

1. Experimenters who sample an inhalant a few times and then discontinue the practice.

2. Occasional or social users who use once a month or whenever the situation is conducive.

3. Daily or frequent users who are at the greatest risk of sustaining physical and psychologic damage according to their use.

Symptoms

Slurred speech and trouble walking a straight line as if intoxicated.

Temporary organic brain syndrome characterized by confusion, dizziness, inability to concentrate, lack of coordination, loss of memory, reduced inhibitions.

Illusions, hallucinations, and delusions may develop as the central nervous system becomes more affected.

Signs

Burns or frostbite at the nose and vocal cords.

Severe headaches.

Irritation of the respiratory tract.

Damage may occur in the central nervous system, peripheral nerves, kidneys, liver, and bone marrow.

• Physicians may see withdrawal in the form of sleep disturbance, nausea, shakes, diaphoresis, irritability, and abdominal and chest discomfort; these may last 2–5 days.

Investigations

• A detailed drug history is essential for all new patients in whom inhalant abuse is suspected and should include the following areas:

Family history of chemical dependency.

Age and onset of drug or alcohol use.

Amount and frequency of use.

Significant changes in life (familial, occupational, social).

Physical examination: should be included to look for physical manifestations of abuse.

Toxicology screen: may be administered according to the type of inhalant used.

• Physicians may want to call National Medical Services for further inquiry (1-800-522-6671).

Differential diagnosis

• Complications of inhalant abuse are often mistaken for primary instead of secondary diagnoses, eg, depression and mania.

• Antisocial personality disorder may exist comorbidly with inhalant abuse.

• Inhalant abuse usually exists along with other chemical abuse.

Etiology

• Risk factors for inhalant abuse include the following:

Those living in communities of low economic potential.

Children of alcoholics.

Those with limited education and unemployed individuals.

Children from dysfunctional families.

Adolescents.

Poor Hispanic youth.

Native Americans living on reservations.

Polysubstance drug abusers.

Epidemiology

• Approximately 5%–15% of all ages currently abuse inhalants.

• The most common age of abuse is 10–17 y of age

• A survey of high school students who reported solvent abuse found that 75% had inhaled a substance from a plastic bag, 50% had used paint, 40% glue, 37% gasoline, 27% nail polish, and 25% lacquer; 63% who abuse solvents also have antisocial personality disorder.

Complications

Cortical, cerebellar, and brain stem atrophy: have been reported among chronic users.

Sudden sniffing death: can occur with solvent and aerosol abuse; secondary to cardiac arrhythmias and cardiac arrest.

Nausea, dizziness, and weakness: may be caused by alkylnitrates.

Bowel and bladder dysfunction: may be caused by nitrous oxide.

Delirium, delusions, hallucinations, seizures, coma, respiratory depression, and death: are results of overdose.

Treatment

Diet and lifestyle
• Patients should avoid environments conducive to substance abuse (*eg*, bars, friends who use mood-altering substances).
• Regular exercise and balanced nutrition are recommended.

Nonpharmacologic treatment
• Management of inhalant abuse should include reassurance, elimination of unnecessary stimuli (*eg*, drug paraphernalia), protection from injury, and a supportive environment.
• Chemical dependency education may motivate the patient to remain abstinent.
• Referral to chemical dependency support groups, such as Narcotics Anonymous or Alcoholics Anonymous, is a foundation for effective treatment. Practitioners should have a list of referrals to locate the most effective program for the individual based on their personal needs.
• Associating physical problems (*eg*, confusion, inability to concentrate, hallucinations, headaches, delusions, and depression) with inhalant abuse may help in deterring further inhalant abuse.

Pharmacologic treatment
• The pharmacology of acute, high-dose exposure to inhalants is not well understood.
• Effective pharmacologic treatment for inhalant detoxification or abuse is not available.
• Treatment is basically supportive.

Treatment aims
To achieve complete abstinence from use of inhalants.
To identify other chemicals that may be used addictively.

Prognosis
• The high relapse rate is due to comorbid conditions that are commonly found with inhalant abuse.
• The individual has an increased chance of recovery from other problems such as depression, antisocial personality disorder, or alcoholism if treated at the same time.

Follow-up and management
Continued support from family and peers.
Periodic reviews of the need for maintenance counseling.
Continued monitoring for abuse of other substances.
Participation in 12-step support groups.

Other information
• Pharmacology and toxicology can be challenging because of the diversity of chemicals that may be used.
• Inhalant use seems to be an indication for an elevated risk of addiction to other substances on a lifetime basis.

General references
Dinwiddie S: *The Merck Manual.*
Ksir C, Oakley R: *Drugs, Society, and Human Behavior,* ed 6. St. Louis: Mosby-Year Book; 1993.
Milhorn T: *Chemical Dependence: Diagnosis, Treatment, and Prevention.* New York: Springer-Verlag; 1990.
Munoz A: *The Disease of Chemical Dependency.* Edited by Fowler N, Leighton L. Tuscon; 1991.

Diagnosis

Definition
• A syndrome of episodic dyscontrol of anger and aggression, resulting in assault against persons or property. By definition, it is a diagnosis of exclusion, and as such, there are few specific data on the disorder.

Symptoms and signs
• Aggressive outbursts may be preceded by a sense of tension or arousal that may be relieved after the episode.

• Physical examination may reveal "soft" neurologic signs: reflex asymmetries, mild hand-eye coordination defects, mirror movements.

• There may be signs of generalized anxiety or impulsiveness between episodes; patients are usually genuinely distressed and remorseful about their behavior.

DSM-IV diagnostic criteria
Several discrete episodes of failure to resist aggressive impulses that result in serious assaultive acts or destruction of property.

• The degree of aggressiveness expressed during the episodes is grossly out of proportion to any precipitating psychosocial stressors.

• The aggressive episodes are not better accounted for by another mental disorder (*eg*, antisocial personality disorder, borderline personality disorder, a psychotic disorder, a manic episode, conduct disorder, Tourette's syndrome, or attention-deficit–hyperactivity disorder) and are not due to the direct physiologic effects of a substance (*eg*, a drug of abuse, a medication) or a general medical condition (*eg*, head trauma, Alzheimer's disease).

Investigations
Detailed history: with attention to medical illnesses, developmental delays, head trauma, loss of consciousness.

Detailed neurologic examination.

Psychologic testing
Mini-mental State Examination.

Neuropsychological testing: may reveal subtle neurological abnormalities.

Part A and B of Trail Making Test.

Halstean-Reitan and Luria-Nebraska.

Aggression Rating Scales.

Overt aggression scale gives numeric score.

Laboratory studies
• No specific laboratory studies are recommended. Use them (*eg*, drug and toxicology screens) to rule out other disorders.

Screening tests
• Based on history, consider the following:

Magnetic resonance imaging to rule out mass lesions, bleeds, mesotemporal scarring.

Electroencephalography to rule out seizure.

Blood chemistry.

Complications
Comorbidity
Substance abuse and mood and anxiety disorders.

Behavioral outcomes
High rates of unstable interpersonal relationships; frequent legal entanglements.

• Males with intermittent explosive disorder are more likely to be encountered in forensic settings; females in psychiatric settings.

Differential diagnosis
Personality disorders include antisocial, borderline, narcissistic, obsessive, schizoid. Psychotic disorders include mania, conduct disorders, oppositional defiant disorders, attention deficit–hyperactivity disorder, substance intoxication or withdrawal (especially cocaine, PCP, and other stimulants), dementia, delirium, purposeful behaviors (eg, for monetary gain, revenge, or self-defense, to gain social dominance, express political views, or as part of gang activities), malingering, personality change due to a general medical condition (aggressive type), tumor, encephalitis, brain access, normal pressure hydrocephalus, subarachnoid hemorrhage, stroke, hypoglycemia, Tourette's disorder.

Etiology
• Cause is unclear. Theories include the following:
Psychosocial: a failure to develop frustration tolerance, self-control, and delay of gratification in childhood due to over- or undergratification; a failure to develop the potential for imitation and identification with the caregiver in early childhood.
Biologic: a defect in the serotonergic system, which acts as an inhibitor of motor activity; decreased 5-hydroxyindoleacetic acid level in cerebrospinal fluid of impulsive or aggressive patients; increase in postsynaptic 5-hydroxytryptamine$_2$ receptors; dysfunction in prefrontal cortex (noradrenergic, serotonergic); dysfunction in limbic or mesolimbic system (dopaminergic).

Epidemiology
Rare disorder; occurs more often in males than females.
Onset occurs in late adolescence to mid-third decade, with persistence into mid-life.
May remit in old age.
Acute onset without prodromal period.
Increased incidence in families with history of mood disorder, substance abuse.

Treatment

Diet and lifestyle
• Promote regular schedule of sleep and work; stress management.

Pharmacologic treatment
• There are no specific guidelines for the biologic treatment of intermittent explosive disorder; treatment recommendations are extrapolated from those of other disorders with aggressive or impulsive symptoms. Lacking controlled clinical studies, the most logical approach seems to be that of tailoring the use of pharmacologic agents to comorbid psychiatric conditions. In the absence of comorbid disorders, carbamazepine may be tried empirically. Before treatment, perform chemistry, liver function tests, complete blood count, electrocardiography; during treatment, serum Na$^+$ (can cause decreased Na$^+$ level) and complete blood count.

Beta-blockers
Standard dosage   Propanolol: begin at 20 mg daily to 3 times daily; increase by 60 mg every third day as tolerated to a maximum of 800 mg daily or to clinical efficacy; maintain dose for 6–8 weeks before concluding a treatment failure.

Contraindications   Certain cardiac disorders, diabetes, chronic obstructive pulmonary disease, asthma.

Special points   Monitor blood pressure while titrating dose.

Anticonvulsants
Standard dosage   Carbamazepine: begin at 200 mg daily in divided doses; increase by 100 mg twice weekly until side effects appear, then decrease by 200 mg; usual dosage range, 300–1600 mg daily (less in Asians and the elderly). Trough serum levels 4–12 mg/mL; follow every week for 2 months, every month for 6 months, for any change in dose.

Contraindications   History of hepatic, cardiovascular, or blood dyscrasia or hypersensitivity to any tricyclic compound.

Main side effects   Central nervous system and anticholinergic (dizziness, drowsiness, ataxia, headache, vision changes, others similar to cyclic antidepressants); monitor for hematologic effects (aplastic anemia, leukopenia, thrombocytopenia, agranulocytosis), and follow complete blood count every 2 weeks for 3 months, then every 3 months (controversial as to need).

Drug interactions   Induces metabolism of drugs via CTP 450 system.

Valproic acid
Standard dosage   Begin at 250 mg/kg/d, titrate to 750–3000 mg/d or serum level 50–100 mg/mL (trough); maintenance dose may be given in single daily dose.

Main side effects   Gastrointestinal (change in appetite), increased liver function tests, increased serum ammonia, menstrual disturbances, occasional central nervous system effects (*see* carbamazepine under Anticonvulsants); rare: hepatotoxicity, rash, platelet and clotting abnormalities.

Contraindications   Liver dysfunction, pregnancy.

Main drug interactions   Drugs that increase valproic acid levels: erythromycin, fluoxetine, phenothiazines, salicylates; valproic acid increases drug levels of alcohol, benzodiazepines, phenobarbital, phenytoin; others.

Laboratory tests   Before treatment: liver function tests, complete blood count; during treatment, perform same tests every month for 6 months, then every 6 months.

Treatment aims
To decrease frequency and severity of episodes and avoid harm to the patient and others.

Prognosis
• The course is generally episodic and chronic. The disorder usually continues into midlife, may spontaneously recede, but may again become prominent in old age, especially in the presence of a dementing illness.

Follow-up and management
For the acute phase: institute therapy; avoid harm to patients and others.
For chronic phase: medication monitoring, psychotherapy.

Nonpharmacologic treatment
Psychotherapy
• Aimed at teaching the patient how to recognize affect, especially anger, and to verbalize and express it appropriately; to identify and express fantasies surrounding rage.

General references
Bezchlibnyk-Butler JJ, ed.: *Clinical Handbook of Psychotropic Drugs*, ed 6. Hogrefe & Huber; 1996.

Denicoff KD, Meglathery SB, Post RM, Tandeciarz SI: Efficacy of carbamazepine compared with other agents: a clinical practice survey. *J Clin Psychiatry* 1994, 55:70–76.

Kavoussi R, Armstead P, Coccaro E: The neurobiology of impulsive aggression. *Psychiatr Clin North Am* 1997, 20:395–403.

Winchel RM, Yovell Y, Simeon D: Impulse control disorder, intermittent explosive disorder. In *Psychiatry*. Edited by Tasman, Kay, Lieberman. Philadelphia: WB Saunders; 1997.

Diagnosis

Definition
• Kleptomania is a compulsive and impulsive pattern of stealing items of little personal or monetary value.

Symptoms and signs
• Individuals with kleptomania report feelings of increasing tension prior to the theft and feelings of relief, pleasure, or gratification following the theft.

• Individuals with kleptomania often report monotony avoidance and discomfort and avoidance related to social activities and relationships.

• Family and friends may report suspicious behavior, secrecy, and observed anxiety in the individual with the disorder.

• The items that are stolen often have little personal or monetary value, and the individual with the disorder most often can afford the items.

DSM-IV diagnostic criteria
1. Recurrent failure to resist impulses to steal objects that are not needed for personal value or use or for their monetary value.

2. Increasing sense of tension immediately before committing the theft.

3. Pleasure, gratification, or relief at the time of committing the theft.

4. The stealing is not committed to express anger or vengeance and is not in response to a delusion or hallucination.

Investigations
Psychologic testing: Zuckerman Sensation Seeking Scale, Barrat Impulsivity Rating Scale.

Laboratory studies: none for clinical use.

Screening test: Minnesota Impulsive Disorder Interview.

Complications
Comorbidity
Major depression.

Bipolar affective disorder.

Compulsive buying.

Bulimia nervosa.

Generalized anxiety disorder.

Behavioral outcomes
Impairment in social network: due to frequent stealing from family and friends.

Difficulty with legal system: secondary to arrests due to shoplifting.

Impairment in occupational functioning: due to stealing from coworkers and reduced productivity due to distraction.

Differential diagnosis
Conduct disorder/antisocial personality disorder: stealing behavior is part of a larger tendency toward antisocial behavior.
Bipolar disorder: stealing behavior is a symptom of a manic episode in which the person engages in impulsive behavior.
Malingering: stealing is intentionally misrepresented as an uncontrollable impulse in order to avoid legal prosecution for shoplifting.

Etiology
• Etiology is uncertain; further research is required to determine specific biological and psychological risk factors for the disorder. Preliminary evidence suggests that dysregulation of the serotonergic system may be involved. Family studies indicate that individuals with kleptomania have family histories of mood disorders.

Epidemiology
• Kleptomania is rare in the general population, with a higher incidence in females than in males. Only 5% of shoplifters meet criteria for kleptomania. Prevalence rates may appear spuriously low due to the secret nature of the disorder.

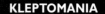

Treatment

Diet and lifestyle

• No specific dietary precautions are necessary. It may be helpful for the individual with kleptomania to initially refrain from environmental situations that promote stealing behavior (*eg*, trips to the mall at times of stress).

Pharmacologic treatment

• Comorbid disorders with specific target symptoms should be treated (*eg*, major depression). Pharmacologic treatment has varying results. Most research on drug effectiveness is based on case studies. Combination of drug treatment and psychotherapy may prove effective. The use of specific serotonin reuptake inhibitors may be the treatment of choice because of effectiveness in reducing impulsivity with few side effects.

Standard dosage	Fluoxetine, 20–60 mg.
	Fluvoxamine, 200–250 mg.
	Paroxetine, 10–60 mg.
	Sertraline, 25–200 mg.
Contraindications	Potential for drug interactions (*see* below).
Main drug interactions	Selective serotonin reuptake inhibitors (SSRIs) have potentially fatal interactions with monoamine oxidase inhibitors, and their co-consumption is contraindicated. In addition, many SSRIs have potentially serious interactions with mediations metabolized by the CYP450 enzyme system. Potential drug interactions should be reviewed before any of these medications are prescribed.
Main side effects	*SSRIs:* agitation, anxiety, sleep disturbance, tremor, sexual dysfunction (primarily anorgasmia), headache.

Nonpharmacologic treatment

Behavior therapy: little research has been done on the effectiveness of psychotherapeutic interventions for kleptomania; some uncontrolled anecdotal studies indicate effectiveness for cognitive behavioral interventions.

Stimulus control: individuals learn to monitor feelings of anxiety prior to stealing and develop alternative behaviors to substitute for stealing.

Covert sensitization: aversive images are paired with stealing so that stealing becomes aversive through classical conditioning.

Relaxation training: individuals are taught to reduce their levels of anxiety through alternative means than stealing.

Treatment aims
To achieve abstinence from stealing behavior.

Prognosis
• Remission of stealing behavior has been indicated with psychotherapeutic or pharmacologic interventions in fewer than 25% of cases.
• Response to pharmacologic agents requires at least 4 wk.

Other treatment options
• Hypnosis has been used, but little research has been conducted on its effectiveness.
• Electroconvulsive therapy has been used successively in a small number of cases.

Follow-up and management
• Little research has been conducted on long-term outcome of treatment for individuals with kleptomania. It has been shown that discontinuation of pharmacologic agents is associated with relapse.

General references
McElroy SL, Pope HG, Keck PE, *et al.*: Are impulse control disorders related to bipolar disorder? *Compr Psychiatry* 1996, 37:229–240.
McElroy SL, Keck PE, Phillips KS: Kleptomania, compulsive buying, and binge-eating disorder. *J Clin Psychiatry* 1995, 56:14–26.
McElroy SL, Keck PL, Pope HG, Hudson JL: Kleptomania: clinical characteristics and associated psychopathology. *Psychol Med* 1991, 21:93–108.

Diagnosis

General information
• There are three types of learning disorders—reading disorder, mathematics disorder, and disorder of written expression.

Symptoms and signs
Reading disorder
Inaccurate word recognition.

Inaccurate and slow oral reading.

Poor comprehension of written text.

Mathematics disorder
Mathematical ability substantially below that expected given the persons chronological age, IQ, and education.

Significant interference with academic achievement or activities of daily living that require mathematical ability.

Disorder of written expression
Writing skill substantially below those expected given the person chronological age, IQ, and education.

Significant interference with academic achievement or activities of daily living that require mathematical ability.

Complications (comorbidity)
Attention deficit–hyperactivity disorder.

Conduct disorder.

Internalizing disorders.

Difficulties with social competence.

Difficulties understand others' affective states.

Differential diagnosis
Normal variations in academic attainment.
Lack of opportunity for instruction, poor teaching.
Impaired vision or hearing.
NM
POD
Communication disorders.

Etiology
• Neuroanatomical studies have found evidence in support of a left hemisphere deficit.
• Genetic factors play a role; between 35%–40% of first-degree relatives of reading disabled children also have reading disabilities.
• In most cases, reading disabled children have a deficit in phonological processing skills.

Epidemiology
• ~5% of students in US public schools have a learning disorder.
• Between 60%–80% of individuals with reading disorder are boys

Treatment

Pharmacologic treatment
• Ritalin and Piracetan have been used with mixed results. In the absence of concurrent psychiatric disorder, the use of medication for remediation of reading disorders should be considered experimental.

Nonpharmacologic treatment

Educational remediation
• Most remedial efforts focus on direct instruction of component reading skills. An alternative approach is to avoid the area of weakness for reading-disabled individuals, namely auditoryphonological processes, by teaching reading through the usual route.

Psychosocial interventions
• Teachers, parents, and child should have an understanding of the presumed biologic and/or genetic basis of the learning disorder.

• Early intervention may minimize or avoid untoward sequelae such as low self-esteem or behavioral problems.

General references

Bryan T: Social problems and learning disabilities. In *Learning Disabilities*. Edited by Wong BY. San Diego: Academic Press; 1991:195–229.

Shepherd MI, Uhry JK: Reading disorder. *Child Adolesc Psychiatr Clin North Am* 1993, 2:193–208.

Torgesen JM, Wagner RK, Rashotte LA: Longitudinal studies of phonological processing and reading. *J Learn Disabil* 1994, 27:276–286.

Diagnosis

Symptoms and signs

• An episode of major depressive disorder (MDD) is characterized by the presence of depressed mood (or irritable mood in children and adolescents) or a loss of interest or pleasure in usual activities (persisting at least 2 wk) or both accompanied by four or more of the following: 1) significant change in appetite or weight (typically decreased, may be increased); 2) insomnia or hypersomnia; 3) psychomotor agitation or retardation (observable by others, rather than subjective); 4) fatigue or loss of energy; 5) feelings of worthlessness or excessive and inappropriate guilt; 6) diminished ability to think or concentrate, or indecisiveness; 7) recurrent thoughts of death, wishes to be dead (passive suicidal ideation), active plans for suicide, or a suicide attempt.

• Symptoms represent a change from previous functioning, cause clinically significant distress or impairment, are not due to the direct effects of a substance or a general medical condition, and cannot be better accounted for by bereavement (*see* Differential diagnosis).

• With single-episode MDD, there is no history of prior depressive, manic, mixed, or hypomanic episodes. It is not superimposed on a psychotic disorder.

• With recurrent MDD, there are two or more distinct episodes, with no history of prior manic, mixed, or hypomanic episodes. It is not superimposed on a psychotic disorder.

• The specify severity of MDD can be mild (just meets criteria), moderate, or severe (well exceeds criteria and causes marked impairment).

Subtypes of depression

Psychotic: in severe depression, delusions or hallucinations that may be mood-congruent (related to depressive themes) or mood-incongruent (not related to typical depressive themes, *eg*, delusions of external control); **atypical:** mood reactivity (mood improves with positive events), reversal of usual neurovegetative signs (*eg*, hypersomnia, increased appetite), leaden paralysis, long-standing pattern of interpersonal rejection sensitivity; **seasonal affective disorder (SAD):** regular occurrence of depressive episodes during a particular season (usually Autumn or Winter) for at least 2 years, with complete remission between episodes; **chronic:** episode meets full criteria continuously for at least 2 years; **catatonic:** immobility, excessive motor activity; negativism; mutism; bizarre posturing, stereotypes; echolalia, echopraxia (parroting examiner's words or actions); **melancholic:** total loss of pleasure or reactivity to pleasurable stimuli, early-morning awakening, diurnal variation (depression worse in the morning), anorexia, guilt, and psychomotor changes.

Investigations

Thorough history and complete mental status examination: necessary to establish the diagnosis and to rule out comorbid disorders (very common).

Recent physical and neurologic examination: in all patients but particularly in the elderly or when symptoms are consistent with physical illness.

Rating instruments: *eg*, Beck Depression Inventory, Zung Depression Scale, and Hamilton Rating Scale for Depression; helpful in quantifying severity of depression and serially following response to treatment.

Screening instruments: *eg*, the Prime MD; can help identify patients in a primary care setting who are in need of further evaluation.

Laboratory investigations: to rule out depression due to a medical condition (*eg*, endocrinopathy); prior to initiation of specific treatments (*eg*, tricyclic antidepressants, anticonvulsants, electroconvulsive therapy).

Suicide risk assessment: mandatory in all depressed patients; risk highest in those with prior attempts, concurrent substance abuse, social isolation, psychotic symptoms, and high degrees of expressed hopelessness or loss of future orientation; as a group, older divorced white males with alcohol dependence and history of violence have the highest risk of completed suicide; young females attempt suicide most frequently.

Differential diagnosis

Substance-induced mood disorder; mood disorder due to general medical condition, dementia; bipolar disorder, type I or II (depressed phase); schizoaffective disorder; schizophrenia; anxiety disorder with secondary depression; adjustment disorder with depressed mood; premenstrual dysphoric disorder; minor depression; recurrent brief depressive disorder; attention deficit–hyperactivity disorder; personality disorder; bereavement.

Etiology

Genetic: familial predisposition for mood disorders; first-degree relatives have 2–3 times the risk.
Biologic: perturbations in biogenic amine neurotransmitter systems; hypothalamic–pituitary–adrenal axis, circadian rhythms, and, sleep architecture may play a role.
Psychosocial: onset of depression often associated with stressful life events (especially losses); learned cognitive distortions may lead to misperceptions of environment and self-defeating behavior patterns that initiate and maintain depression; intrapsychic dynamics interact with all above factors to increase vulnerability.

Epidemiology

Female-to-male ratio, 2:1 (prevalence: 10%–25% women and 5%–12% men).
Community prevalence (1 mo), 2-5%.
Primary care outpatients, 5%–10%.
Medical inpatients, 10%–15%.
Cancer patients, 6%–39% (average, 31%).
Parkinson's patients, 21%–37% (avg 29%).
Stroke patients, 30%–50% (avg 38%).

Special cases

• Depression may overlap with symptoms and signs of physical illness (especially neurologic disorders); avoid undertreatment.
• Depression in elderly can present as multiple somatic complaints and social withdrawal with cognitive and functional declines with denial of depressed mood.

Complications

Suicide: ~15% of depressed individuals.
Death due to malnutrition and dehydration: usually seen in elderly patients.
Functional impairment: physical, social, and vocational morbidity equal to advanced coronary artery disease and more than in common chronic medical conditions.
Disruption of relationships: spouse, children, parents, friends, coworkers.

Treatment

Diet and lifestyle
• Reduce external stressors to the greatest extent possible. Get adequate exercise. Avoid substances of abuse, especially excessive alcohol use.

Pharmacologic treatment
• First-line treatment for major depression consists of combined pharmacologic and psychosocial therapeutic management for optimal response. Major depression is frequently recurrent; thus, treatment is divided into acute phase, continuation phase (to prevent relapse after full remission), and maintenance phase. Continuation-phase treatment at full therapeutic dosage is necessary for a minimum of 6 months after complete remission in order to decrease the likelihood of relapse. For patients with recurrent episodes or chronic depression, indefinite-maintenance pharmacologic and psychosocial therapeutic management may be indicated.

Standard dosage	Selective serotonin-reuptake inhibitors (SSRIs), *eg*, fluoxetine (20–80 mg), fluvoxamine (50–300 mg), paroxetine (20–50 mg), or sertraline (50–200 mg).
	Tricyclic antidepressants (TCAs), *eg*, desipramine (50–300 mg), nortriptyline (50–200 mg), amitriptyline (50–300 mg), or imipramine (50–300 mg).
	Other agents, *eg*, bupropion (200–450 mg), mirtazapine (15–45 mg), nefazodone (200–600 mg), venlafaxine (75–375 mg).
Contraindications	All agents are contraindicated with monoamine oxidase inhibitors (MAOIs); relatively contraindicated in pregnancy; greatest safety evidence is for nortriptyline and desipramine.
	SSRIs: avoid use with other serotonergic agents; high potential for drug interactions (*see* below).
	TCAs: contraindicated in acute recovery period after myocardial infarction; relatively contraindicated in ischemic heart disease and heart block, and narrow-angle glaucoma.
	Other agents: bupropion contraindicated in patients with seizure disorders, bulimia, or anorexia; nefazodone contraindicated with terfenadine, astemizole, cisapride.
Main side effects	All agents have a lower seizure threshold (TCAs more than SSRIs); most inhibit all phases of sexual response (bupropion and nefazodone the least).
	SSRIs: early (usually transient) anxiety, nausea, tremor, insomnia, sweating, diarrhea or constipation, anorexia, dizziness, drowsiness, anorgasmia.
	TCAs: anticholinergic effects, orthostasis, sedation, cardiac conduction changes.
	Other agents: bupropion causes agitation, insomnia, increased seizure incidence at doses >450 mg/d; mirtazapine causes sedation, weight gain; nefazodone causes dizziness; venlafaxine causes nausea, hypertension.
Main drug interactions	All agents have a potentially fatal interaction with MAOIs.
	SSRIs: potentially fatal serotonin syndrome can occur when combined with other serotonergic agents.
	TCAs: potentially fatal interaction with quinidine and procainamide.
	Also, hepatic enzyme inhibition may occur with SSRIs and nefazodone.

Treatment aims
To assure safety of patient during acute phase of depression, induce clinical remission, and prevent both relapse and recurrence of major depression.

Nonpharmacologic treatment
Inpatient treatment: necessary if safety cannot be assured in a less restrictive setting.
Electroconvulsive therapy.
Augmentation of pharmacotherapy.
Psychotherapy.
Bright light phototherapy.

Prognosis
• The initial response rate for a single depressive episode with an adequate therapeutic trial of a single antidepressant is 70%; ultimate response rate with all modalities is 90%. Treatment resistance should prompt reevaluation of diagnosis and treatment compliance.
• Lifetime risk of recurrence is 50% after first depressive episode, with up to 90% risk after three episodes.

Follow-up and management
Acute phase: with suicidal patients, dispense only a week's supply of medication when using agents with high toxicity in overdose (especially TCAs); weekly follow-up visits; safety plan of whom to call if suicidality increases.
Continuation phase: follow up at least monthly during first 8 wk of full remission and every 1–3 mo thereafter for medication checks.
Maintenance phase: with stable patients, follow up every 3–6 mo. Recurrences of depression are treated as new episodes.

General references
Diagnostic and Statistical Manual of Mental Disorders, ed 4. Washington, DC: American Psychiatric Association; 1994.

Practice Guideline for Major Depressive Disorder in Adults. Washington, DC: American Psychiatric Association; 1993.

Principles and Practice of Psychopharmacology, ed 2. Edited by Janicak PG, JM Davis, Preskorn SH, Ayd FJ. Baltimore, MD: Williams & Wilkins; 1997.

Wells KB, et al.: The functioning and well-being of depressed patients: results from the Medical Outcomes Study. *JAMA* 1989, 262:914–919.

Diagnosis

Definition
• Malingering is the intentional production of false or grossly exaggerated physical or psychologic symptoms. Unlike factitious disorders, malingering is motivated by external incentives (eg, avoiding military duty, garnering financial compensation, evading criminal prosecution, or obtaining drugs). Although malingering is not classified as a mental disorder, it may be a focus of clinical attention.

Symptoms and signs
• Like those with factitious disorder, individuals who malinger may engage in the following:

Total fabrications: eg, claiming falsely to have back pain.

Simulations: eg, grimacing in response to nontender palpation.

Exaggerations: eg, reporting occasional mild headaches as continual migraines.

Aggravations: eg, deliberately failing to take insulin for authentic diabetes.

Self-inductions: eg, surreptitiously taking thyroxine to mimic hyperthyroidism.

Investigations [1]
• Rarely is malingering proved conclusively in medical settings. Physicians must be circumspect in their approach to the patient and in documentation because malingering often becomes an issue in litigation. Diagnosis is rendered more challenging by the fact that the symptoms reported (eg, dizziness, pain, weakness) are usually difficult to quantify objectively.

• Common findings include the following:

1. Symptom reports and objective data (eg, from physical examination or laboratory tests) are incongruent.

2. Complaints intensify when the patient is asked directly about symptoms or when he/she is aware of being observed.

3. Response to treatment is nonphysiologic.

4. The patient is engaged in litigation or charged with a crime, is seeking disability funding, or is evidently pursuing other external goals.

5. The patient is uncooperative with diagnostic and treatment maneuvers.

Physical evidence (eg, pills or syringes) is discovered or the patient confesses.

• The Structured Interview of Reported Symptoms is useful in diagnosing malingered psychologic symptoms. The MMPI-2, cognitive batteries, and other measures are available to assess malingering in particular cases. For instance, discrepancies may be noted between MMPI-2 validity scales or among obvious/subtle clinical subscales. Physical tests (eg, electroencephalography) sometimes produce results that disconfirm the signs and symptoms being claimed.

Complications
Morbidity or mortality associated with self-induced illnesses.

Drug abuse or dependence: eg, opioids or benzodiazepines originally prescribed for malingered ailments.

Other iatrogenic complications.

Differential diagnosis
Authentic illness.

Factitious disorder: involves pursuit of psychologic gain rather than external incentives.

Somatoform disorder: patients do not intentionally mislead others.

Etiology [2]
Motivation for and potential availability of external gain.

Antisocial personality traits.

Epidemiology
• Malingering occurs in settings where external benefits can be accrued by illness. Among these are prisons, the military, courtrooms hearing personal or industrial injury disputes or criminal cases, and the offices of physicians performing disability evaluations.

• Malingering is more commonly seen in outpatient than inpatient settings.

• There is no known demographic pattern for malingerers. The behavior is determined more by setting than by personal characteristics.

Treatment [3]

Diet and lifestyle management
• The patient should be encouraged to consolidate his or her care at a single medical center to avoid doctor shopping, duplication of tests, and excessive prescriptions.

Pharmacological treatment
• There is no pharmacologic treatment for malingering.

Nonpharmacologic treatment
• The patient suspected of malingering usually should not be directly confronted. Instead, subtle communication can be used to indicate that others are aware of the deceptions.
• Alternatively, objective findings can be presented forthrightly to the patient without accusing the patient of deception.
• Face-saving maneuvers (eg, suggesting that patients with similar problems usually recover after a particular length of time) may be followed by perceptible improvement.

Treatment aims
To reduce the patient's dissimulation and medical or surgical overutilization.

Prognosis
• Patients intent upon acquiring external gains from illness will reemphasize or intensify their dissimulations until the goals have been achieved or the ruses uncovered. Some will progress from fabrication, simulation, or exaggeration to aggravation or self-induction.
• The tenacity of the malingering will increase if negative consequences are likely to follow disclosure (eg, a lawsuit will be filed by a previously-maligned employer).

Follow-up and management
• A disproportionate amount of time is involved typically when malingering is suspected due to the complexity of the diagnostic issues and legal or ethical considerations.
• Because there is no definitive intervention for malingering, clinicians should have modest expectations regarding their capacity to alter the course.
• Clinicians must also monitor their countertransference.
• In the forensic setting, a clear report of findings should be presented to the court and attorneys.

Key references
1. Ford CV, Feldman MD: Factitious disorders and malingering. In The American Psychiatric Press Textbook of Consultation-Liaison Psychiatry. Edited by Rundell JR, Wise MG. Washington, DC: American Psychiatric Press; 1996:533–544.
2. Ford CV: Lies! Lies!! Lies!!!: The Psychology of Deceit. Washington, DC: American Psychiatric Press; 1996.
3. Eisendrath SJ: Factitious disorders and malingering. In Treatments of Psychiatric Disorders. Edited by Gabbard GO. Washington, DC: American Psychiatric Press; 1995:1804–1818.

General reference
American Psychiatric Association: Diagnostic and Statistical Manual of Mental Disorders ed 4. Washington, DC: American Psychiatric Press; 1994.

Diagnosis

Definition

• Problems with marijuana can be categorized as either abuse or dependence.

• Dependence is characterized by several unsuccessful attempts to quit; reduction in social, occupational, recreational activities; tolerance; and the presence of withdrawal symptoms.

• Abuse is characterized by a maladaptive pattern of use lasting at least 1 month and occurring in either hazardous situations or despite having knowledge of a problem with the substance.

Symptoms and signs

Depression, anxiety, and personality disturbances: seen in some chronic users.

Loss of conventional motivation and inability to maintain long-term goals: "amotivational syndrome".

Shortness of breath: heavy users are at a particularly high risk for chronic asthma, bronchitis, emphysema, and possibly lung cancer.

Interference with complex mental functioning.

Mild paranoid feelings.

Conjunctival infection.

Increased appetite.

Dry mouth.

Tachycardia.

• Several questions were developed by Marijuana Anonymous to indicate problem use and to necessitate further evaluation on answering "yes." These questions include the following:

1. Has pot smoking stopped being fun?

2. Do you ever get high alone?

3. Do you smoke marijuana to avoid dealing with problems?

4. Do you become anxious or worry about getting more when your supply of pot is low?

Investigations

Detailed, specific alcohol and drug history: would be helpful in determining severity of the problem.

Family background history: would be helpful to determine any possible genetic predispositions.

Urine drug screen: can be used as an objective measure of marijuana in the system; because the half-life of THC (delta-9-tetrahydrocannabinol, the active ingredient in marijuana) is 20 days, and because up to 20% of metabolites stay in the body for 7 days, it may take up to 30 days for a single dose to be eliminated from the body.

• Speaking with a patient's family may also yield important information about changes in behavior, cognitive functioning, and mood.

Complications

Reduction in productivity at work.

Disruption in family functioning.

Use of other drugs.

Social attitude that marijuana is not dangerous or addictive.

Development of temporary sterility in chronic users.

Mild delirium or prolonged cannabis psychosis if used in very high doses.

Inflammation and other lung abnormalities indicating respiratory problems.

Higher risk of spontaneous abortions and still births.

Temporary increase in heart rate.

Differential diagnosis

• Symptoms of marijuana use can be mistaken for other drug problems, behavior problems, or simply lack of motivation. The physician at times may downplay the significance of negative consequences attached to marijuana abuse. Marijuana may also be mistaken for other psychiatric illnesses, eg, anxiety, depression, psychosis, or paranoia.

Etiology

• Some common predictors for possible problem marijuana use include the following:

Use of other drugs: marijuana is known as a "gateway" drug.

Male gender.

Low age of first use of cigarettes and alcohol.

Family history of addictions.

Young adults aged 18–25 y.

Epidemiology

• Marijuana is the illicit drug of choice among adolescents and adults.

• Marijuana is the fourth most commonly used psychoactive substance following alcohol, nicotine, and caffeine.

• One third of all Americans have tried marijuana at least once.

• Adolescent marijuana use is the best of all available predictors for cocaine use.

• The THC content in marijuana was ≤4% in 1967 and is now 10%.

• One "joint" is equivalent to four cigarettes in terms of tar consumption.

• Marijuana is only one form of cannabis (the plant that marijuana is derived from); other forms are hashish and hashish oil.

• The most common mode of marijuana self-administration is by smoking and inhaling.

• Marijuana can also be ingested.

Treatment

Diet and lifestyle

• No specific diet is indicated for treatment of chronic marijuana use. Lifestyle changes, however, are crucial for maintaining abstinence. These include changes in friends, establishing a support network, and abstinence from all other mood-altering substances.

Pharmacologic treatment

• No pharmacologic treatment is recommended for cannabis dependence or withdrawal.

Nonpharmacologic treatment

• For those who abuse marijuana or are dependent, a referral to a drug and alcohol treatment facility may be appropriate. Most programs subscribe to a 12-step model of treatment (based on Alcoholics Anonymous) and require total abstinence from all mood-altering substances. Building a support network through 12-step programs in the community is crucial. Generally, fear-based programs have not been effective in treating drug problems.

Treatment aims

To maintain abstinence from marijuana and all other mood altering substances because use of these may lead to relapse. To identify potentially dangerous relapse behavior.

Prognosis

• Factors that may positively influence maintenance of abstinence include involvement in a treatment program, support from family and friends, and being in a chemical- or drug-free environment.

Follow-up and management

• Aftercare meetings (support groups that meet regularly to discuss issues in recovery) are recommended following treatment to provide continued support.
• Primary care physicians should maintain contact with the patient on a regular basis in order to support and encourage the recovery process.

General references

Heit ML, Page R: Drugs, Alcohol, and Tobacco. Meeks Heit Publishing Company; 1995.

Johnson C, Simon C, Stacy A, Sussman S: Marijauna Use: Current Issues & New Research Directions. J Drug Iss, 26:695–733.

Miller N: Principles of Addiction Medicine, vol 1. 1995.

Gold MS: Marijuana. 1–5.

Wilkins JN, Gurelick DN: Management of phencyclidine, hallucinogen and marijuana intoxication and withdrawal. 1–10.

Diagnosis

Definition
• Narcissistic personality disorder is a spectrum of psychopathology of the self manifested by symptoms such as grandiosity in fantasy or behavior, a need to be admired, a lack of empathy, and feelings of specialness.

Symptoms and signs
• The narcissistic patient is characterized by beliefs and behaviors indicating a sense of specialness accompanied by a lack of empathy for others who are used as objects rather than as fellow human beings with feelings and needs. There is often envy of those who are more successful. Attitudes of entitlement lead to exploitation of others, resulting in little guilt or remorse. Unlike the sociopath, the narcissistic patient is fueled by thoughts of grandiosity and a need for admiration; such patients may be able to single-mindedly successfully pursue goals (eg, a career). The narcissist, feeling uniquely special and exaggerating achievements and abilities, may attempt to identify himself with only important people or prestigious institutions.

• Despite fantasies and attitudes of grandiosity, the narcissist is exquisitely vulnerable to criticism and may react with rage or marked feelings of humiliation and depression. Conversely, successes may be followed by an inflated sense of grandiosity and contempt or even sadistic behaviors toward others.

• A subtype of narcissistic pathology is the person who, while outwardly humble, secretly feels superior and contemptuous towards others (a "martyr"). Acts of apparent altruism are determined by personal needs rather than genuine empathy for others.

DSM-IV criteria
• A pervasive pattern of grandiosity (in fantasy or behavior), need for admiration, and lack of empathy, beginning by early adulthood and present in a variety of contexts, as indicated by five (or more) of the following:

1. Has a grandiose sense of self-importance (eg, exaggerates achievements and talents, expects to be recognized as superior without commensurate achievements).

2. Is preoccupied with fantasies of unlimited success, power, brilliance, beauty, or ideal love.

3. Believes that he or she is "special" and unique and can only be understood by or should associate with other special or high-status people (or situations).

4. Requires excessive admiration.

5. Has a sense of entitlement, ie, unreasonable expectations of especially favorable treatment or automatic compliance with his or her expectations.

6. Is interpersonally exploitative, ie, takes advantage of others to achieve his or her own ends.

7. Lacks empathy; unwilling to recognize or identify with the feelings and needs of others.

8. Is often envious of others or believes that others are envious of him or her.

9. Shows arrogant, haughty behaviors or attitudes.

Investigations
Psychologic testing: the Minnesota Multiphasic Personality Invenotory-2 and Millon Clinical Multiaxial Inventory-II are valid and reliable self-report instruments for personality disorders; the Structured Clinical Interview for DSM-IIIR Personality Disorders-II consists of a structured interview that also provides personality diagnoses.

Laboratory studies: none.

Differential diagnosis
Bipolar affective disorder, type II.
Cyclothymia.
Other cluster B personality disorders (antisocial, histrionic, and borderline).

Etiology
• No genetic studies demonstrating hereditability have been reported. Constitutional temperaments of high energy, tension, and conscientiousness have been suggested to predispose to narcissism. An increased familial incidence can be equally explained by environmental factors as to heredity.
• Psychodynamic explanations of narcissism revolve around issues of unmet basic childhood needs. The narcissist received inadequate empathy from parents who were preoccupied with their own situation (eg, careers or depression). The child experienced feelings of vulnerability from fear of failure or dependency, or environmental factors such as poverty.
• Sociologic explanations emphasize "the age of narcissism" characterized by a youth-oriented culture ("you only go around once"), consumerism, and a breakdown of the nuclear family.

Epidemiology
• Well-controlled epidemiologic studies of narcissistic personality disorder have not been completed. Estimates are that the prevalence is below 1% for the general population and that it is higher in men than women. The prevalence in the clinical population, particularly outpatient settings, is considerably higher; estimates range from 2%–16%.

Complications
Comorbidity: persons with narcissistic personality disorder may be more prone to major depression, particularly with occupational or interpersonal reverses (midlife crisis).
Behavioral outcomes: variable; some persons with narcissism are very successful occupationally; most are marginal or do poorly; most narcissists have troubled interpersonal and marital relationships.

Treatment

Diet and lifestyle

• Occupational goals should be commensurate with actual capabilities rather than fantasies and grandiose aspirations.

Pharmacologic treatment

• There is no specific pharmacologic treatment for narcissistic personality disorder. Psychotropic medications should be reserved for target symptoms of comorbid axis I disorders (eg, major depression).

Nonpharmacologic treatment

• Individual psychotherapy with a psychodynamic orientation is the primary treatment for narcissism. In an empathetic accepting environment, the patient is allowed to develop an idealizing transference toward the therapist. Subsequent interpretations focus on the patient's frustrations due to the therapist's inevitable empathetic failures and the patient's wishes for a more gratifying relationship. There is controversy as to the degree to which to confront the patient's narcissistic defenses (anger, envy), the need to be self-sufficient, and exploitation of others. A too active, or premature, confrontation may lead to narcissistic injury with a resultant compensatory increase in maladaptive defenses or an early flight from therapy.

• Group therapy may serve as a valuable adjunct to individual therapy but is rarely a primary treatment approach. The narcissist explores the effect of his behavior on others and practices empathy in response to the experiences of other group members. However, without individual therapy, the narcissist is likely to perceive intense competition with other group members for the therapist's attention and feel that his own needs for empathy are unmet.

• Behavioral therapy has not been shown to be useful.

Pitfalls

• Complications for psychotherapy include countertransference responses from therapists that result in behaviors and interpretations that are viewed by the patients as narcissistic injuries. The therapist may respond to the patient's arrogance, contempt, envy, or grandiosity with feelings of competitiveness or irritability. Periods of fatigue with decreased attention by the therapist or the need to cancel appointments may elicit angry responses from the narcissistic patient. Frequently these can be used in the service of the therapy, but at times, the anger may be so intense as to induce the patient to discontinue treatment.

Treatment aims

To achieve more realistic view of one's abilities.
To increase empathy for others.

Prognosis

Variable; milder forms of the disorder may improve with time, maturity, and fortuitous events such as favorable jobs or marriages; severe forms of narcissism are associated with occupation and interpersonal failure, which may intensify symptoms and, in the extreme, lead to occupational disability or suicide.

Follow-up and management

For the acute phase

• Psychotherapy for narcissistic pathology must be fairly intensive and lengthy. Psychotherapy sessions of ~1 h should be scheduled 1–3 times per week, and treatment may need to be extended for a several-year period.

For the continuation phase

• Even after the successful completion of psychotherapy, these patients remain at risk for reactivation of symptoms at times of loss or failures. The therapist should make him or herself available for as-needed therapy sessions because these relapses can often be addressed through relatively brief interventions.

General references

Cooper AM, Ronningstam E: Narcissistic personality disorder. In American Psychiatric Press Review of Psychiatry, vol 11. Edited by Tasman A, Riba MB. Washington, DC: American Press; 1992:80–97.

Groopman LC, Cooper AC: Narcissistic personality disorder. In Treatments of Psychiatric Disorders. Edited by Gabbard GO. Washington, DC: American Psychiatric Press; 1995:2327–2344.

Kernberg OF: Narcissistic personality disorder. In Psychiatry, vol 1. Edited by Cavenar J. Philadelphia: JB Lippincott; 1985:1–12.

Diagnosis

Definition

• Narcolepsy is a disorder of unknown etiology characterized by excessive sleepiness that typically is associated with cataplexy and other rapid eye movement (REM)–sleep phenomena, such as sleep paralysis and hypnagogic hallucinations [1].

Symptoms and signs [1,2,3]

Excessive daytime sleepiness: recurrent daytime naps or lapses into sleep that occur almost daily for at least 3 months.

Cataplexy: sudden loss of bilateral muscle tone with preservation of consciousness provoked by strong emotion.

Sleep paralysis: a transient inability to move or speak during the transition between sleep and wakefulness.

Hypnagogic hallucinations: vivid perceptual experiences occurring at sleep onset, often with realistic awareness of the presence of someone or something.

Disrupted nocturnal sleep.

Impaired memory/concentration.

Investigations

History: diagnosis is based on a thorough history to identify the typical signs and symptoms of narcolepsy and to rule out other causes of excessive sleepiness; all four symptoms of the narcoleptic tetrad are not required for diagnosis; sleepiness is usually the initial symptom and cataplexy may develop simultaneously or years later.

Overnight polysomnography followed by the Multiple Sleep Latency Test (MSLT): generally required for accurate diagnosis [1,3,4]; the MSLT is a laboratory-based procedure that provides an objective measure of sleep tendency and identifies abnormal sleep-onset REM episodes; most individuals with narcolepsy have mean sleep latency values of <5 minutes; two or more naps with entry into stage REM sleep is suggestive of narcolepsy, although other sleep disorders may be associated with this finding; overnight polysomnography often shows shortened sleep latency of <10 minutes, and sleep-onset REM periods are frequently seen (REM sleep appearing within 20 min of sleep onset); other sleep disorders (eg, obstructive sleep apnea syndrome and periodic limb movement disorder) may occur in patients with narcolepsy, and in some cases, these coexisting disorders must be treated first and followed by repeat evaluation for a definitive diagnosis of narcolepsy.

Laboratory blood work: generally not required for the diagnosis of narcolepsy.

Neuroimaging: indicated if there is clinical suspicion for increased intracranial pressure or intracranial mass.

HLA typing: shows the presence of HLA-DR2 and DQ1 (DR15 and DQ6 using newer nomenclature) in most cases; however, the presence of DR2 or DQ1 is neither necessary nor sufficient for the diagnosis of narcolepsy [1].

Complications

Accidents: due to excessive sleepiness or cataplexy may occur, and caution is urged regarding driving an automobile, operating heavy equipment, or during employment in certain jobs.

Depression: common among individuals with narcolepsy.

Impaired social function: may occur and include marital and interpersonal problems and loss of employment; deterioration in academic and social function may be particularly serious in children and adolescents with narcolepsy [3,4].

Differential diagnosis

For excessive sleepiness
Obstructive sleep apnea syndrome, periodic limb movement disorder, idiopathic hypersomnia, posttraumatic hypersomnia, insufficient sleep, sedating medications, drug withdrawal (particularly from stimulants), alcoholism, irregular sleep–wake schedule, circadian rhythm disorders, depression (especially atypical forms with hypersomnia), diencephalic lesions, obstructive hydrocephalus, encephalopathies, Prader–Willi syndrome, hypothyroidism.

Cataplexy
Atonic seizures, myasthenia gravis, hypotension, vertebrobasilar insufficiency, transient ischemic attacks, vestibular disorders, psychologic or psychiatric disorders, malingering.

Etiology

• The fundamental defect in narcolepsy is unknown. The physiologic signature of narcolepsy is an abnormal tendency for early entry into REM sleep. This early onset of REM appears to be part of a broader problem of impaired sleep–wake regulation [3]. Studies involving HLA indicate the presence of a narcolepsy susceptibility gene on chromosome 6, but environmental factors are also involved, as illustrated by monozygotic twins who are discordant for narcolepsy. Pharmacologic and pathologic studies in human and canine narcolepsy have demonstrated abnormalities in brain monoaminergic and cholinergic activity [3,4].

Epidemiology

• In North America, narcolepsy affects ~1:3000 individuals. Men and women are equally affected. Symptoms typically begin during the second decade of life, with peak incidence at 14 y of age. Symptoms may begin during childhood or well into adulthood [1].

Treatment

Diet and lifestyle

• Education of patient, family members, school personnel, and employer is important.

• Emphasize need for adequate nocturnal sleep. Occasionally, daytime naps are beneficial.

• Communicate with school personnel regarding diagnosis and treatment plans. Some students may require special adaptations such as untimed tests, longer times for completion of assignments, and scheduling more difficult classes during periods of maximal alertness.

• Avoid driving during periods of high risk for drowsiness or when not taking stimulants.

• Consider referral for counseling or psychologic therapy as needed for depression and adjustment problems.

• Avoid alcohol and sedating medications.

Pharmacological treatment

• Narcolepsy is a chronic, lifelong disorder that requires careful follow-up to monitor response to stimulant therapy and side effects and to monitor for emergence of other sleep disorders. The American Sleep Disorders Association appointed a task force to review the scientific literature regarding treatment [5], and practice parameters for the use of stimulants in the treatment of narcolepsy have been developed [6].

For treatment of sleepiness

• Begin with low dosages and titrate based on clinical response. Certain patients may require combinations of long- and short-acting stimulants.

Standard dosage	Pemoline, 18.75–150.00 mg/d, divided in 1–2 doses.
	Methylphenidate, 5–100 mg/d, divided in 1–4 doses.
	Dextroamphetamine, 5–100 mg/d, divided in 1–3 doses.
Main side effects	Appetite suppression, anxiety, tremor, racing thoughts, insomnia, headache.
Special points	In pediatric patients, stimulants can be used safely for treatment of narcolepsy in prepubertal children [6].
	In pregnant patients, stimulants should only be used during pregnancy when the potential benefits to the patient are judged to clearly outweigh the risks to the fetus. Most patients should be advised to reduce or discontinue stimulants during attempts at conception and for the duration of pregnancy [6].
	In nursing mothers, low doses of stimulants may be given to maintain wakefulness, but caution is urged [6].

For treatment of cataplexy

Standard dosage	Protriptyline, 5–30 mg/d in 1–3 doses.
	Imipramine, 25–200 mg/d in 1–3 doses.
	Clomipramine, 25–250 mg/d.
	Fluoxetine, 20–80 mg/d.
Special points	Abrupt withdrawal may induce rebound cataplexy.

Treatment aims
To educate patient and family about the disease.
To help family provide emotional, academic, and vocational support.
To administer pharmacotherapy for sleepiness and cataplexy.
The goal of treatment is to provide optimal alertness during key situations that require vigilance, and to minimize cataplexy.

Prognosis
• Narcolepsy is a chronic, lifelong condition that is treatable but not curable. There is significant variation in an individual's response to treatment with stimulants and anticataplexy medications.

Follow-up and management
• Long-term follow-up is important in monitoring response to stimulants and anticataplexy medications and in observing for emergence of other sleep disorders (eg, obstructive sleep apnea and periodic limb movement disorder). Decisions regarding driving and vocational choices should be individualized.

Key references

1. *International Classification of Sleep Disorders, Revised: Diagnostic and Coding Manual.* Rochester, Minnesota: American Sleep Disorders Association; 1997.

2. Yoss R, Daly D: Criteria for the diagnosis of the narcoleptic syndrome. *Proc Staff Meet Mayo Clin* 1957, 32:320–328.

3. Aldrich M: Narcolepsy. *Neurology* 1992, 42(suppl 6):34–43.

4. Guilleminault C: Narcolepsy syndrome. In *Principles and Practice of Sleep Medicine,* ed 2. Edited by Kryger M, Roth T, Dement W. London: WB Saunders; 1997:549–561.

5. Mitler M, Aldrich M, Koob G, Zarcone V: Narcolepsy and its treatment with stimulants. *Sleep* 1994, 17:352–371.

6. Standards of Practice Committee of the American Sleep Disorders Association: Practice parameters for the use of stimulants in the treatment of narcolepsy. *Sleep* 1994, 17:348–351.

Diagnosis

Symptoms and signs [1,2]

- All of the following are symptoms when associated with the use of neuroleptics:

Severe muscle rigidity.

Changes in consciousness.

Hyperthermia.

Confusion.

Diaphoresis.

Mutism.

Dysphagia.

Hypertension or hypotension.

Incontinence.

Elevated creatine phosphokinase (CPK).

Tachycardia.

Tachypnea or hypoxia.

Tremor.

Dysarthria.

Treatment with neuroleptics: within 7 days of onset (within 2–4 wk for depot neuroleptics).

- Symptoms usually evolve over 24–72 hours. The untreated syndrome lasts 10–14 days.

Investigations

Frequent monitoring of vital signs: to look for hyperpyrexia (100.4°–101°F), increased pulse and labile blood pressure, diaphoresis.

Complete blood count, serial CPKs, blood urea nitrogen and creatinine, electrolytes, liver function tests (LFTs): to rule out leukocytosis (with or without left shift), increased plasma myoglobin, increased CPK, myoglobinuria, increased LFTs, renal failure (occasionally), metabolic acidosis.

Complications

- The mortality rate for neuroleptic malignant syndrome (NMS) can reach 20%–30% or even higher when depot antipsychotic medications are involved.

- Complications may include aspiration pneumonia, renal failure, thrombophlebitis, thromboembolism, hepatorenal failure, cardiac arrest or failure, pulmonary edema, seizures, or sepsis.

Differential diagnosis [1]

Primary central nervous system disorders.

Infections (viral encephalitis, HIV, post- infectious encephalomyelitis).

Tumors.

Stroke.

Trauma.

Seizures.

Major psychoses (lethal catatonia).

Systemic disorders

Infections.

Metabolic conditions.

Endocrinopathies (thyroid storm, pheochromocytoma).

Autoimmune disease (systemic lupus erythematosus, porphyria).

Heat stroke.

Toxins (carbon monoxide, phenols, tetanus, strychnine).

Drugs (salicylates, stimulants, psychedelics, monoamine oxidase inhibitors, anesthetics, anticholinergics, alcohol or sedative hypnotic withdrawal, dopamine inhibitors and antagonists).

Etiology

- Disease is caused by the use of neuroleptics or sudden withdrawal of dopamine agonists (eg, L-dopa, carbidopa).
- Risk factors for NMS include the following [1]:

Found primarily in young and middle aged adults given neuroleptics but rarely in young children.

Slightly increased incidence reported in men.

Occurs independently of environmental heat or humidity.

Occurs across the neuropsychiatric diagnostic spectrum.

Potential increased risk in patients with psychomotor agitation, electrolyte imbalance, dehydration, previous episodes of NMS, increased rate of neuroleptic dosing, parenteral medication, high-potency neuroleptics.

Individual susceptibility.

Epidemiology [1]

- The incidence ranges from 0.02%–3.23%. This range reflects differences in diagnostic criteria, survey techniques, patient population, clinical settings, and treatment practices. Later studies with decreased incidence may reflect earlier recognition and reduction in risk factors.

Treatment

General information

• Neuroleptic malignant syndrome is a medical emergency [1]. The first step in treatment is cessation of neuroleptics and rapid initiation of intensive medical support. The status of fluid replacement, cardiac, respiratory, and renal functions should be monitored. Some patients may require transfer to an intensive care unit. The patient must be cooled (cooling blankets and sponge baths), and the symptomatic treatment of fever should be monitored along with vital signs, electrolytes, fluid balance, and renal output.

Pharmacologic treatment [3]

• The following drugs may be helpful:

Standard dosage   Dantrolene (a skeletal muscle relaxant), start at 1 mg/kg i.v. or orally, then 1–10 mg/kg/d in 4 divided doses (infuse i.v. over 1 h).

                     Bromocriptine, 7.5–60 mg/d orally in 3 divided doses.

• Treatment usually lasts between 5–10 days with the goal of symptom resolution.

• Antiparkinsonian drugs (*eg*, amantadine) may reduce muscle rigidity.

Treatment aims

To obtain remission of symptoms and reestablish the patient's physical health.

Other treatment options

• Benzodiazepines may be useful in controlling agitation or reversing catatonia.
• Anticholinergic drugs may worsen delirium or contribute to hyperthermia.
• Some have reported that lisuride, nitroprusside, muscle relaxants, and calcium channel blockers may be useful.
• Electroconvulsive therapy has also been reported with favorable outcomes [1].

Prognosis

• The risk of recurrence is ~30% in some studies. Some patients may be inherently predisposed.

Follow-up and management

• Low-potency drugs may be less likely to cause recurrence. At least 2 wk should elapse after complete recovery from NMS prior to reintroduction of neuroleptics [1]. Gradual titration of low doses of low-potency neuroleptics may be the safest way to proceed with treatment. Although atypical agents (*eg*, clozapine, risperidone, and olanzepine) may lessen the risk, further study is indicated.

Key references

1. Caroff SN, Mann SC: Neuroleptic malignant syndrome. *Contemp Clin Neurol* 1993, 77:185–203.

2. Kaplan HI, Sadock BJ, Greb JA: *Synopsis of Psychiatry*, ed 7. Baltimore: Williams & Wilkins; 1994.

3. Schneiderhan ME, Marken PA: An atypical course of neuroleptic malignant syndrome. *J Clin Pharmacol* 1994, 34:325–334.

Diagnosis

Definition
• Nicotine is the psychoactive agent in tobacco. Continued use usually leads to addiction, creating tolerance, physical dependence, and withdrawal symptoms.

• All elements of drug addiction exist in tobacco use.

• The smoker's behavior is controlled by seeking and taking the psychoactive drug nicotine, despite the fact that most would like to quit and believe in related health hazards.

• A unique feature of nicotine addiction is that most tobacco smokers are willing to openly describe their behavior, which produces ideal intervention opportunity.

Signs and symptoms
• Although initial exposure may have unpleasant effects (eg, nausea, vomiting, and pallor), tolerance develops rapidly.

• Most smokers report pleasurable effects, including arousal, relaxation, improved attention span and performance of tasks, and relief of negative emotions.

• Withdrawal symptoms include craving a cigarette, irritability, anxiety, impatience, anger, difficulty concentrating, increased appetite, and sleep disturbances.

• Withdrawal symptoms begin within a few hours of last cigarette, peak in first 2–3 days of cessation, and gradually subside over several weeks.

• The prominent signs of withdrawal are decreased heart rate and electroencephalographic changes.

Investigations
• Must have a system in place to identify all tobacco users at every visit.

• Consider tobacco status as part of vital signs (eg, "tobacco use" status stickers on patient charts or inclusion of "tobacco use disorder" on active problem list).

The Fagerstrom Test for Nicotine Dependence [1]: assists in establishing level of physical dependence (see table); a correlation exists between high levels of dependence (score >6) and severity of withdrawal symptoms, difficulty with abstinence, and relapse.

The Fagerstrom Test for Nicotine Dependence*

1. How soon after you wake up do you smoke your first cigarette?
   <5 min (3)   6–30 min (2)   31–60 min (1)   >61 min (0)
2. Do you find it difficult to refrain from smoking in places where it is forbidden (eg, church, library, movie theater)?
   Yes (1)   No (0)
3. Which cigarette would you hate most to give up?
   First morning cigarette (1)   Any other cigarette (0)
4. How many cigarettes per day do you smoke?
   >31 (3)   21–30 (2)   11–20 (1)   <10 (0)
5. Do you smoke more frequently during the first hours after waking than during the rest of the day?
   Yes (1)   No (0)
6. If you are so ill that you are in bed most of the day, do you still smoke?
   Yes (1)   No (0)

* Scores in parentheses.

Etiology
• Nicotine is the agent in cigarettes responsible for addictive properties.

• Dependence occurs via increased expression of brain nicotine receptors, changes in brain glucose metabolism, and release of catecholamines.

• Positive reinforcement occurs with delivery of nicotine via cigarettes. Negative reinforcement occurs via withdrawal symptoms during attempts to quit.

Epidemiology
• Prevalence of cigarette smoking among adult Americans peaked at 40% in 1965 and dropped to 26% by 1992 due to public awareness of health hazards.

• Prevalence declined from 1965 to 1992 in men (from 50% to 28%) and in women (from 32% to 24%).

• More young women than men have started smoking.

• Prevalence of smoking is lower in college graduates (14%) compared with adults with less than 12 y of education (32%).

• Because black Americans consistently smoke at higher rates than white Americans, smoking prevalences by the year 2000 are projected to be 34% in blacks compared with 29% in whites.

Complications

Dangers to user
Fatal fires, peptic ulcer disease, Burger's disease, asthma, heart disease, stroke, lung cancer, chronic obstructive pulmonary disease, other pulmonary complications (including pneumonia and influenza), impotence (in men), reduced fertility (in women), impaired ability to sustain lactation (in women), impaired cognitive performance, early menopause (in women), oropharyngeal cancers, gum recession, cataracts, impaired wound healing, immune suppression, impaired mucociliary clearance, earlier development of pneumonia in HIV-infected individuals, synergy with radon and asbestos in causing lung cancer, reduced athletic performance, wrinkles.

Dangers to persons near user
Fatal fires, bronchitis and pneumonia (in small children), asthma, middle ear infections (in small children), reduced athletic performance, reduced performance on standardized achievement tests, low-birth-weight babies, sudden infant death syndrome.

Treatment

Diet and lifestyle

• Patients should 1) gather support of family, friends, and coworkers; 2) remove cigarettes from daily environment; 3) anticipate difficult situations and plan a nonsmoking coping mechanism.

• Eighty percent of smokers gain weight after quitting; however, most gain less than 10 pounds.

• Those who are at higher risk of major weight gain are women, black Americans, people older than 55 years of age, and heavier smokers.

• Encourage a balanced, low-fat diet and regular exercise to help minimize weight gain.

• Stress positive effects of cessation of smoking.

Pharmacologic treatment

• Nicotine replacement therapy should be offered to all patients who smoke more than 10 cigarettes per day because it is proven to increase cessation success rates.

Transdermal nicotine patches

• **Habitrol, Nicoderm, and ProStep are for 24-hour use; Nicotrol is for 16-hour use.**

Standard dosage	if 5–10 cigarettes per day, use midrange dose (10–14 mg/d)
	If >10 cigarettes per day, use heaviest dose of given brand (precise patch dosages vary among manufacturers).
Contraindications	Unstable angina, myocardial infarction or revascularization procedure within prior 4 weeks, serious arrhythmias.
Main drug interactions	There are no adverse interactions to nicotine replacement; however, absence of smoking decreases metabolism of many drugs, including caffeine and theophylline, requiring dose reduction.
Special points	Choose hairless site and change site each day; will require 2–3 days to achieve maximum systemic levels; may consider supplementation with chewing gum during this time.

Chewing gum (polacrilex)

Standard dosage	If <20 cigarettes per day or if Fagerstrom score <6, use 2-mg stick.
	If >20 cigarettes per day or if Fagerstrom score >6, use 4-mg stick.
Contraindications	Pregnancy category C, cardiovascular problems (as with transdermal nicotine patches).
Main drug interactions	As with transdermal nicotine patches.
Main side effects	Jaw fatigue, hiccoughs, belching, nausea.
Special points	Use ~1 stick of gum per hour; must chew and "park" between cheek and gums every 15–30 minutes.
	Acidic beverages decrease absorption.

Buspropion

Standard dosage	Begin at 150 mg/d given as a single dose in the morning; if adequately tolerated, increase to 300 mg/d given in 2 divided doses.
Contraindications	Patients with seizure disorders and patients taking Wellbutrin and Wellbutrin SR should not take buspropion (Zyban); because buspropion is associated with dose-dependent seizures, do not prescribe >450 mg/d.

Treatment aims

To ensure that every patient who smokes is provided with effective cessation intervention at every visit. To maintain patient abstinence.

Prognosis

• Only 2%–3% of all smokers quit successfully each year.

• 90% of those who quit did so without formal treatment but required several cycles of quitting and relapse before succeeding.

• Most attempts at quitting fail within 2 wk; 70% of smokers who quit relapse within 3 mo.

Other treatment options

Nicotine nasal spray: available in 1997. Nicotine inhaler: approved for marketing by Food and Drug Administration. Long-term nicotine maintenance: use devices that deliver nicotine without other toxic substances in tobacco products (Premier and Eclipse).

Follow-up and management

• Follow up within first week after quitting.

• Second follow-up should be within first month after quitting and should focus on relapse prevention and emphasize the successful quitter. Discuss benefits and problems associated with continued cessation.

Key reference

1. Heatherton TF, Kozlowski LT, Frecker RC, Fagerstrom KO: The Fagerstrom Test for Nicotine Dependence: a revision of the Fagerstrom Tolerance Questionnaire. *Br J Addict* 1991, **86:**1119–1127.

General references

The Agency for Health Care Policy and Research's Smoking Cessation Clinical Practice Guideline. *JAMA* 1996, **275:**1270–1280.

Arnsten JH: Treatment of nicotine dependence in the primary care setting. *Primary Psychiatry* 1996, **3:**27–30.

OBSESSIVE–COMPULSIVE DISORDER

Diagnosis

Definitions

- Obsessive–compulsive disorder (OCD) is a common affliction consisting of pathologic obsessions and compulsions.
- Obsessions (from the Latin *obsidere*, meaning "to besiege") are recurrent troubling thoughts or concerns that the patient perceives as distressing, excessive, or absurd at least some time during the illness; they are "ego alien" (*ie*, not perceived as something the person wants to do).
- Compulsions (from the Latin *compulare*, meaning "to force") are ritualistic actions or thoughts that the patient usually repeats in response to obsessive worries. Similar to obsessions, compulsions are thought to be senseless, or excessive, but unless the patient performs them, there is a distressing build up of discomfort (either anxiety or tension). Compulsive rituals are something that an individual is *compelled* to perform, not truly voluntary.
- Obsessions are distinguished from preoccupation, and compulsions are distinguished from purposeful rituals and routines, which are not only experienced as voluntary but often accompanied by a sense of "right" or even pleasure.

Signs and symptoms

- Up to one third of patients may have only covert "mental" compulsive rituals, and some claim only to have obsessions. Compulsions without obsessions are uncommon but not rare.
- Most patients have multiple obsessions and compulsions, and there is a tendency for them to shift with time. A person who was once a washer may only check years later. In the majority of patients, the severity of OCD symptoms tend to wax and wane over time; adolescence and the postpartum period are often accompanied by exacerbation.
- Obsessions and compulsions are very common in the general population; to qualify as the disorder, these symptoms must be so severe that they interfere with function, or cause notable distress.

Common obsessions
Contamination, pathological doubt, somatic, needs for symmetry, aggressive or violent thoughts, abhorrent sexual thoughts, senseless words or tunes.

Common compulsions
Washing or decontaminating, checking, counting, need to ask or confess, repeating reassuring words or actions, rearranging for symmetry or precision, hoarding.

Investigations

- There are no tests or procedures at present that establish the diagnosis of OCD, which is made largely on the clinical presentation.

Complications

Commonly comorbid conditions
Episodic major depression: seen in a majority of patients; primary OCD symptoms frequently exacerbate during depression; **Tourette syndrome:** OCD and Tourette's syndrome may be manifestations of a more general condition; **simple phobias; panic disorder; agoraphobia; separation anxiety disorder; social phobia; "body dysmorphic disorder":** difficult to distinguish from somatic concerns in OCD; **Tricotillomania:** hair pulling; **Anorexia nervosa.**

- Substance abuse is common, especially during OCD exacerbation. Substance abuse secondary to OCD (*ie*, self-medication) needs to be distinguished from primary substance abuse accompanying OCD. Research suggests that the former is more common than the latter and may remit with effective OCD treatment.

Differential diagnosis
- Aside from the common comorbid disorders (see Complications) that can exist without OCD, the conditions most commonly confused with OCD are the impulse control disorders.
- Obsessive–compulsive personality disorder has neither obsessions nor compulsions but is characterized by preoccupation with orderliness, perfectionism, and control. Any personality type can be seen in OCD.

Epidemiology and course
- OCD has been described in clear, unmistakable terms from ancient times and has been seen in all cultures and ethnic groups studied to date. The prevalence in the general US population (1%–3%) seems very similar to that in most countries studied.
- Most OCD patients have at least minor manifestations in early childhood. Before puberty, boys may have a higher incidence of pathology reaching diagnostic criteria; by adulthood, the sexes have similar rates.
- Family history is often positive for OCD, Tourette's syndrome, Sydenham's chorea, or one of the other comorbid conditions listed in the Complications section. Sporadic cases in adulthood often have a neurologic lesion (eg, lacunar stroke) in cerebral regions associated with abnormal activity in typical OCD patients.
- Once OCD is established, it tends to be a lifelong condition.

Etiology
- There is general agreement that OCD is a condition with a neurologic underpinning, although its exact nature is unknown. Functional neuroimaging studies of OCD have consistently implicated dysfunction in a brain system that involves the paralimbic prefrontal cortex, basal ganglia, and thalamus. Likewise, neurologic conditions that mimic OCD have pathology in this same system. This brain system seems important in the mediation of many complex behavioral sequences that are carried out in a semiautomatic fashion in everyday life.
- In the last several years, genetic, brain imaging, and phenomenologic studies have suggested that OCD may be related to both Tourette's syndromes and Sydenham's chorea. The neurotransmitters serotonin and dopamine play important roles in such corticobasal ganglionic systems.

Treatment

Pharmacologic treatment

Selective serotonin-reuptake inhibitors

• Selective serotonin-reuptake inhibitors (SSRIs) are the only group of medications with clearly demonstrated efficacy in OCD. No one SSRI is consistently better than another in OCD; however, given individuals may respond much better to one agent than another. If the first one fails, try another. Once started, SSRIs should be continued long term unless behavior therapy is successful. Relapse is common on discontinuation of SSRIs, even after years of decreased symptoms.

Standard dosage	Nontricyclic SSRIs: fluoxetine (40–80 mg), paroxetine (40–60), fluvoxamine (150–300), sertraline (150–200), citalapram (40–60).
	Tricyclic SSRIs: clomipramine (150–250).
Contraindications	Fluoxetine (the SSRI with the largest data base) is generally considered safe during pregnancy. There is significant risk of major OCD relapse in the postpartum period; if SSRIs have been stopped during pregnancy, they should be restarted right after delivery.
Main side effects	Jitters, over- or under-stimulation, anxiety, appetite changes, sweating (all tend to diminish with time). Start patient on low dose (*eg*, 10 mg fluoxetine) and raising slowly as tolerated because it increases tolerance. Trazodone (25–100 mg every bedtime) helps with SSRI-induced sleeplessness. Delayed orgasm is common in both men and women but may respond to bupropion (75–200 mg/d) added to SSRI.
Special points	All require at least 2-3 months at an adequate dose to judge efficacy. Most patients show little response in first month. Major task in therapy is keeping patient taking medication long enough to see response; supportive psychotherapy is always indicated.
	Important to stop substance abuse for maximal effects. These agents also don't work as well if the patient is slightly hypothyroid (check thyroid-stimulating hormone).
	In children: The same drugs are indicated, but dosage is different (*eg*, fluoxetine & paroxetine, 1 mg/kg/d; fluoxetine, 3 mg/kg/d; clomipramine, 3 mg/kg/d [*warning*: this is a tricyclic; electrocardiography monitoring required]. Fluoxetine, fluvoxamine and paroxetine seem well-tolerated in children and are probably the agents of choice.

Adjunctive medications

• Pimozide, thiothixene, or haloperidol (1–6 mg/d) are especially useful for tics and OCD if there is history of Tourette's syndrome or multiple motor tics.

• Olonzapine (2.5–5.0 mg/d) or risperidone (1–3 mg/d) are especially useful for patients with intense horrible thoughts as obsessions; also useful in the rare patient with comorbid schizophrenia.

• Benzodiazepines (*eg*, clonazepam [0.5–1.0 mg three times daily] or lorazepam [1–2 mg three times daily]) are often used for temporary relief of general anxiety, but patients may use it to avoid unpleasant tasks, and there is some evidence that these drugs may interfere with learning of the type needed in behavior therapy; may potentate substance abuse in some patients.

• Aside from its use for sexual side effects (*see* SSRIs), bupropion (75–450 mg/d in divided doses) often seems to potentate subjective "energy" in OCD patients.

• Trazodone (25–100 mg every bedtime) helps with sleep and overagitation early in the course of SSRI therapy.

Treatment aims
To diminish symptoms and enhance patient strategies to cope with residual pathology, so life function and personal satisfaction are achieved; it is rare for presently available treatments to abolish the symptoms of OCD.

Prognosis
• Typically, patients with OCD who receive proper intensive treatment have good responses, although 6 mo is not an unusually long time to achieve adequate results.

Other treatments options
Behavior therapy: deconditioning, cognitive techniques are helpful.
Experimental neurosurgical procedures: several show promise for severe, refractory OCD.
Family therapy: family education is always indicated; other family work aimed at reintegration may be indicated after symptoms are lessened.
Vocational rehabilitation: is often needed.

Support organizations
Obsessive–Compulsive Foundation, Inc.
9 Depot Street
P.O. Box 70
Milford, CT 06460-0070
Phone: (203) 878-5669
Fax: (203) 874-2826
E-mail: jphs28a@prodigy.com
Internet:
http://pages.prodigy.com/alwillen/ocf.html

General references
Baxter LR, Saxena S, Brody AL, *et al.*: Brain mediation of obsessive-compulsive disorder symptoms: evidence from functional brain imaging studies in the human and non-human primate. *Semin Clin Neuropsychiatry* 1996, 1:32–47.

Jenike MA, Baer L, Minichiello WE: *Obsessive-Compulsive Disorders: Practical Management*, ed 3. Mosby: St Louis; 1998.

Diagnosis

Definition

• The individual with obsessive-compulsive personality disorder (OCPD) demonstrates a long-standing pattern of perfectionism, rigidity, and controlling behaviors toward others that adversely affects efficiency and productivity and renders these individuals unable to enjoy novelty, pleasures, or open debates.

Symptoms and signs

General traits

Perfectionistic, obstinate, parsimonious, perseverating, "anal," overly disciplined; main focus on maintaining control of self and others: pays precise attention to bowel habits, time, routines, lists; maintains excessive orderliness; overly resistant or deferential to authority, morally rigid, harshly critical of mistakes in self and others, inflexible about bending rules or laws; leads dull life, leisure seen as "waste of time," focus of hobbies on accomplishment or gains, lives below means; enjoys rituals, predictability: spontaneity and change cause anxiety; angry when lacks control; handles by suppressing and ruminating over some detail or becoming righteously indignant over minor matter of principle.

Occupational dysfunction

• OCPD is adaptive: employees are dutiful, work long hours, rarely take vacations.

• Potential dysfunctions include falling behind due to perfectionistic need to redo tasks, failing to make decisions when no procedure available, being unable to compromise, wasting time on procedures or detail, being unable to delegate, insisting on being "right," being unable to see viewpoint of others, damaging own interests out of "principle."

Social dysfunction

Usually in stable marriage, has few friends; formal, stiff, even at passionate moments.

Mental status examination

• Neat appearance, meticulous dress, constricted affect, serious mood, expressionless speech lacks expression, carefully chosen wording; thought processes are impaired; gives excessive details that may be circumstantial, machine-like responses (continues a response to the end, ignoring cues to stop or change subject).

DSM-IV diagnostic criteria

• OCPD is indicated by the presence of four or more of the following:

1) Rigid preoccupation with rules, details, schedules to such an extreme that end point of activity is neglected; 2) perfectionism to a degree that interferes with completing tasks; 3) excessive devotion to work or productivity to the exclusion of leisure and social activities; 4) inflexibility or excessive conscientiousness about moral and ethical issues; 5) "pack rat" syndrome (inability to discard useless objects); 6) reluctance to delegate tasks unless they are done exactly patient's way; 7) hoarding of money for future catastrophes or miserly spending style; 8) stubbornness and rigidity.

Investigations

History: obtain developmental history and history of adult social and occupational functioning; observe manner in interview; obtain history from family members when possible; rule out comorbid psychiatric conditions, predisposing medical conditions (ie, head trauma), and substance abuse.

Testing and questionnaires: Minnesota Multiphasic Personality Inventory and Millon Clinical Multiaxial Inventory administered by a psychologist can suggest clustering of personality traits; physician-rated questionnaires such as Structured Clinical Interview for DSMIII-R Personality Disorders (SCID-II) and the Personality Disorder Examination are valid and useful; the patient-rated Personality Diagnostic Questionnaire-Revised and the SCID-II self-report questionnaire are also available.

Differential diagnosis

• Obsessive-compulsive traits are common, generally adaptive, and flexible when necessary as opposed to OCPD, which is characterized by inflexible behaviors and social or occupational impairment.

• In some cultures, it is normal to follow certain rituals in a rigid fashion or to focus excessively on work or productivity.

• Obsessive-compulsive disorder is marked by intrusive obsessions and repetitive compulsions.

• Rule out narcissistic or schizoid personality disorders and personality change due to medical condition or substance abuse.

Etiology

• Genetic studies show role for inheritance.

• Cultures that emphasize strong work ethic or personal restraint may have higher prevalence of OCPD.

• Psychodynamic theories include:
Freud: child's failure to resolve issues arising when aggressive impulses conflict with socialization by parents leads to fixation or regression to the anal phase. Erikson: autonomy versus shame—child's strong emotions are consistently criticized (rather than validated) by parent; child protects self by distancing himself from emotions or true dependency needs and gets validation by becoming "hyperproductive"; fails to develop through subsequent phases of maturity.

Epidemiology

• The prevalence in the general population is 1.0%–1.7%; 3%–10% in mental health settings; male-to-female ratio, 2:1.

• The prototypical patient is the oldest child, white, married, employed, male.

Complications

• Poor adaptation to change can lead to depression at times of crisis, particularly during late middle age. OCPD patients are prone to psychosomatic conditions, anxiety disorders, phobias, and obsessions and compulsions. Paranoid and schizoid personality disorders and delusional disorder can coexist with OCPD.

• "Type A" personality features put the patient at risk for cardiovascular disease.

• Emotional unavailability or controlling behaviors lead to strained relationships with spouse or children.

• Occupational failures and personal despair over lost opportunities later in life are common.

Treatment

Diet and lifestyle management

• Persons with OCPD often lead healthy, well-regulated personal lifestyles and may be "health nuts." Patients may need education on risks of burnout from overwork and failure to take vacations.

Pharmacologic treatment

• OCPD is not generally responsive to medications; biologic treatments at best are adjunctive to therapy and do not address the underlying character problem.

• Selective serotonin reuptake inhibitors (eg, fluoxetine, sertraline, or paroxetine) can act nonspecifically to increase sense of well-being, improve stress tolerance, and diminish anger.

• If true obsessions or compulsions develop, medications used for OCPD (eg, fluoxetine, paroxetine, fluvoxamine, or clomipramine) can reduce symptoms.

• If depressive symptoms are present or develop secondarily, standard antidepressants are helpful.

• For excessive anxiety, buspirone can be used; benzodiazepines such as alprazolam or clonazepam can be used on an as-needed or short-term basis; long-term use carries a risk for dependence.

Nonpharmacologic treatment

Psychodynamic psychotherapy: Long-term insight-oriented psychotherapy or psychoanalysis are the treatments of choice for this condition; nondirective discussion and free association allow the expression of spontaneity and feelings, minimizing intellectualization; short-term insight-oriented therapy can help patient with a more circumscribed problem (ie, conflict with superior at work, inability to complete a specific project).

Gestalt therapy.

Cognitive-behavioral therapy: can address patient's perfectionistic self statements and directly modify subsequent pathologic behaviors.

Group therapy: patient sees how behaviors affect others in therapeutic setting; validation by group facilitates change.

Pitfalls

• Like OCPD patients, most clinicians have obsessive-compulsive traits that have allowed them to succeed and isolate affect (suppress emotions) in professional settings to maintain appropriate clinical distance. Because of this similarity or identification with the patient, the clinician is cautioned to:

• Avoid struggle for control of treatment or sessions. Instead focus away from battles or challenges onto feelings, or discuss the process of battling as part of the treatment. For example, the clinician might say, "What kind of reaction do you expect when you insist on taking the medicine I prescribe according to your own rules; do you do this in other situations?"

• Avoid colluding with patient in over-intellectualizing problems while avoiding dealing with feelings. This merely reinforces the patient's pathologic defensive functioning.

• Understand one's self well enough to control natural tendency to devalue, criticize, or feel belittled by the patient.

Treatment aims

To help patient directly identify dependency needs or anger so he can relax controlling defenses and become more emotionally available in relationships and freer to focus on productive tasks at work.

Prognosis

• Course is variable: some individuals may evolve naturally or with therapy into more open-minded feeling people; others may continue to function adequately occupationally but their emotional life may be barren; these individuals are at risk for developing axis I disorders such as depression, particularly at times of unexpected changes or loss.

• A minority of these patients are in the prodromal stage of schizophrenia, or are paralyzed by their condition to the extent that they become occupationally disabled.

Follow-up and management

For the acute phase

• Develop an alliance with patient that is accepting, noncritical, respectful. Help patient identify and explore affects that underlie rigidity.

For the continuation phase

• Constructively point out how behaviors may be hurting patient's own interests. Support patient in efforts to change undesirable behaviors. Medications prescribed for stress symptoms can sometimes be tapered after 4–6 mo with maintenance of treatment gains. Psychotherapy may take many years.

General references

American Psychiatric Association: Diagnostic and Statistical Manual of Mental Disorders, ed 4. Washington, DC: American Psychiatric Association; 1994.

Nigg JT, Goldsmith HH: Genetics of personality disorders: perspectives from personality and psychopathology research. Psychiatry Bull 1994, 115:346–380.

Perry CJ, Vaillant GE: Personality disorders. In Comprehensive Textbook of Psychiatry, ed 5. Edited by Kaplan H, Sadock B. Baltimore: Williams & Wilkins; 1989: 1352–1387.

Widiger TA, Sanderson CJ: Personality disorders. In Psychiatry, vol 2. Edited by Tasman A, Kay J, Lieberman J. Philadelphia: W.B. Saunders; 1997:1291–1317.

Diagnosis

Symptoms and signs
- Withdrawal syndrome occurs on the discontinuation or significant reduction in opioid use. In addition, the administration of an opiate antagonist precipitates a characteristic abstinence syndrome. Some reliable early signs of the withdrawal syndrome are increased resting respiratory rate, rhinorrhea, lacrimation, and perspiration. Continued withdrawal symptoms include anxiety, dysphoria, sleep difficulties, and flulike symptoms.
- Tolerance is characterized by the development of significant tolerance to opioids; the patient may show very few signs of drug use and may appear to function normally even after the administration (or reported consumption) of very large doses. Tolerance to the side effects of opioids may develop unevenly, eg, a person may become largely tolerant to the euphoric and depressant effects and yet still have constricted pupils and constipation.
- Persistent acute intoxication may include atropine-like side effects, including constricted pupils, decreased respiratory rate and depth, hypotension, bradycardia, and decreased body temperature.
- Opioid overdose includes moderate to severe respiratory depression, and may include significant central nervous system (CNS) depression or coma. In addition, a person in overdose will have pinpoint pupils and may have direct evidence of drug use, eg, needle marks or soft tissue infection.
- Drug-seeking behavior is characterized by significant time spent on drug acquisition activities (eg, visiting multiple medical facilities, doctor shopping, and emergency room hopping), development of new and increasingly severe physical symptoms that are not supported by other data, and self-reports of allergy or negative effects from other nonopioid treatment options.
- Continued use of opioids is defined as continuous use despite negative side effects or consequences that are directly associated or exacerbated by the continued use. Opioids are often used in larger amounts or for a longer period than was prescribed, planned, or medically necessary.
- Significant life changes are associated with opioid use or acquisition.
- Important social, occupational, or recreational activities may be reduced in quality or quantity because of opioid use.
- Failure to control use despite attempts to reduce the amounts of opioids used. There may be a desire to control use accompanied by hopeless resignation to long-term use.

Differential diagnosis
Dependence on other drugs, especially CNS depressants.
Hypoglycemia.
Head trauma.
Severe infection.
Fluid and electrolyte abnormalities.

Etiology
- Those at higher risk include the following:
Any person with significant use of opioids over time.
Young white adults.
Health care professionals and others with easy access.
Persons with chronic pain.
Persons with a family history of substance dependence.

Epidemiology
Most prevalent in the 25–45-y age range. Largely unrecognized in the higher socioeconomic population.

Other information
- The occurrence of tolerance and withdrawal symptoms are variable and do not themselves imply addiction.
- Take note of any of the following to diagnose opioid addiction: adverse associated consequences, loss of control of use, and preoccupation with obtaining opioids.

Investigations
- A detailed opioid use history is essential. The history should include the following factors:

Amount, route (i.v., smoked, ingested), and frequency of current use.

Age and reason for initial use.

Concomitant substance abuse: eg, alcohol, other CNS depressants.

Family history of substance dependence.

Changes in role functioning (occupational, social).

- No routine laboratory studies are available to diagnose dependence; toxicology reports may be used to verify self reports of current use.

Complications
- Many complications of opioid dependence are caused by unsanitary intravenous administration; however, smoking or ingesting opiates also have significant complications. The most common severe complications are bacterial or viral endocarditis, hepatitis, and HIV infection. Other complications include chronic constipation, pulmonary problems, arthritic conditions, and neuralgic disorders.
- The most serious overdose complication from opioids is death from respiratory depression. General supportive therapy must be instituted to ameliorate morbidity and prevent mortality, including assessment and clearance of airway, support of ventilation as needed, assessment and support of cardiac function, and intravenous access and fluids.

Treatment

Diet and lifestyle
• Patients desiring treatment for opioid dependence should be committed to abstinence from opioids. Most positive outcomes result from a commitment to abstinence from all mood-altering substances because of the risk of cross-tolerance and secondary dependence.

• Early recovery requires an environment safe from protected abstinence.

Pharmacologic treatment
• Clinical management of opioid withdrawal can be extremely difficult. Close supervision with frequent physician contact is a requirement. To legally use an opioid drug to treat dependence and manage withdrawal symptoms, the existence of a physiologic opioid dependence must be established. (Physicians treating dependence should be fully aware of federal, state, and local regulations regarding pharmacologic intervention and maintenance programs for opioid dependence.)

For substitution and detoxification

Standard dosage	Methadone, propoxyphene napsylate, or the opioid of dependence: after an effective withdrawal-suppressing dose is established, reduce progressively by no more than 20% each day.
	Clonidine, 0.2 mg orally every 4 hours up to 1.2 mg daily; maintain for 4 days, then reduce by 25% daily for 3 days.
Contraindications	*Methadone, or propoxyphene napsylate, or the opioid of dependence*: suicidal ideation; extreme caution in patients taking any CNS depressant, including alcohol.
	Clonidine: should be used with caution in patients with severe coronary insufficiency, recent myocardial infarction, cerebrovascular disease, or chronic renal failure.
Main drug interactions	*Methadone, propoxyphene napsylate, or the opioid of dependence*: opiate antagonists, all CNS depressants.
	Clonidine: tricyclic antidepressants may decrease the effects; may enhance effects of CNS depressants.
Main side effects	*Methadone, propoxyphene napsylate, or the opioid of dependence*: respiratory depression, sedation, nausea, vomiting.
	Clonidine: dry mouth, sedation, dizziness due to orthostatic hypotension.
Special points	*Methadone, propoxyphene napsylate, or the opioid of dependence*: supportive therapy; treatment program or self-help group attendance is mandatory.
	Clonidine: does not reduce psychologic drug craving; monitor for hypotension.

For opioid overdose

Standard dosage	Naloxone, 0.4 mg–2.0 mg i.v.; repeat at 2–3-minute intervals if desired improvement in respiratory status is not obtained.
Contraindications	Preexisting cardiac disease; not effective for decreased respiratory function due to nonopioids.
Main side effects	Abrupt reversal of depressed symptoms that may cause immediate withdrawal symptoms.
Main drug interactions	Competes with all opioids for receptor sites.
Special points	Recovery can be dramatic; severe withdrawal symptoms may begin immediately; patient may become agitated or combative.

Treatment aims
To manage major withdrawal symptoms.
To encourage abstinence from opioid use.
To prevent relapse.

Prognosis
• Outcomes vary widely and are dependent on severity of illness, social support, and type of treatment received.

Follow-up and management
• The primary goal of follow-up is the prevention of relapse into dependence.
• Management of pain and other symptoms must be accomplished with nonopioid alternatives.
• Watch for symptoms of cross-addiction to nonopioid mood-altering substances.

Other treatment options
Behavioral therapy.
Therapeutic communities.
Rapid detoxification under anesthesia.
Maintenance therapy (methadone).
Levomethadyl acetate and buprenorphine (maintenance).

Nonpharmacologic treatment
• Referral to a chemical dependency treatment program or an appropriate referral to self-help support groups (eg, Narcotics Anonymous) is the primary method of treatment.
• The physician or a colleague, social worker, or addictions counselor should be aware of locally available resources and appropriate programs for individual patients based on patient preferences, availability, and costs.

General references
The Merck Manual. Merck & Co; 1992.

Diagnostic and Statistical Manual of Mental Disorders, ed 4. Washington, DC: American Psychiatric Association; 1994.

The Principles of Addiction Medicine. The American Society of Addiction Medicine; 1994.

Gold MS: ASAM. 1994.

Diagnosis

Symptoms and signs

Negativistic behavior.

Anger, resentment.

Spitefulness, vindictiveness.

Active defiance.

Deliberately annoying behavior.

Temper tantrums.

Investigations

Interview with the child or adolescent.

Family history.

School information.

Standard parent and teacher rating scales.

Psychologic testing.

Physical evaluation.

Complications

Chronic course.

Conduct disorder: may result.

Adult passive–aggressive personality disorder.

School problems.

Differential diagnosis

Normal oppositional behavior (common 18–36 mo).

Attention deficit–hyperactivity disorder (ADHD).

Conduct disorder.

Mental retardation.

Depression.

Schizophrenia.

Organic mental disorders.

Etiology

Lax parental discipline patterns.

Unduly harsh or restrictive parental discipline patterns.

Inconsistent.

Parent unavailability.

Parents who are poor role models with regard to their own attitude toward authority.

Difficult child temperament.

Epidemiology

Prevalence, 65% general child and adolescent population.

Male predominance, 2:1.

Treatment

Pharmacologic treatment

• There is no medication for pure oppositional defiant disorder.

Psychostimulants: for comorbid ADHD.

Lithium: for mood disorder.

Antidepressants: for underlying depression.

Antipsychotic medication: for comorbid psychiatric disorder.

Nonpharmacologic treatment

Behavior therapy.

Family interventions: parental guidance, training, and therapy.

Individual or group psychotherapy.

School interventions.

Residential and day treatment programs.

General references

Hales R, Yudofsky S (eds): *Synopsis of Psychiatry.*
DC: American Psychiatric Press; 1996.

Kaplan H, Saddock B (eds): *Comprehensive
Textbook of Psychiatry*, ed 5. Baltimore: Williams
& Wilkins, 1989.

Diagnosis

Symptoms and signs

Persistent or recurrent delay in (or absence of) orgasm following normal sexual excitement.

• The symptom must cause significant distress or relationship problems to be classified as a female orgasmic disorder (FOD). Symptom may be lifelong or acquired, generalized or specific to a situation or partner. Orgasmic ability is often present during masturbation.

• It is generally considered rare to be anorgasmic during masturbation but fairly common to be anorgasmic during intercourse.

• Many women do not experience orgasm without clitoral stimulation; the need for clitoral stimulation does not suggest FOD.

• Lifelong, generalized subtypes of FOD are considered the most severe types but possibly the most treatable.

Investigations

History: the diagnosis is made from history.

Physical evaluation: to rule out possible contributory or causative medical factors (*eg*, abnormal genital anatomy, endocrinopathy, neuropathy, and medication use).

Psychologic assessment and testing: may reveal characteristics, behaviors, or disorders that may be contributing to the intensity, duration, or frequency of orgasmic difficulties; screening for depression, anxiety, and relational problems is particularly important.

Assessment of the patient's (and partner's) understanding of normal sexual anatomy and function.

Complications

Sexual inadequacy: in anorgasmic females; the patient's partner, similarly, may feel that he or she is at fault for failing to provide adequate sexual stimulation or satisfaction.

Relationship problems: may cause, contribute, or result from FOD.

Psychologic difficulties (especially depression and anxiety): may cause, contribute, or result from FOD.

Differential diagnosis

• FOD differs from female sexual arousal disorder in that the female reports being aroused but unable to achieve orgasm with a partner.

• FOD may lead to hypoactive sexual desire disorder or sexual aversion disorder.

Etiology

• The cause is often unclear in a particular individual. Sufficient mental and physical erotic input may result from one or more following:

Psychologic factors (eg, anxiety, relationship problems).

Unhealthy attitudes toward or inadequate knowledge about sexual function.

History of sexual trauma.

Insensitivity, impatience, or lack of understanding by the partner with regards to the patient's needs and preferences.

Poor communication between the couple.

Medications (especially most antidepressants and some antihypertensives) that cause anorgasmia.

Hormonal variations.

Alcohol or drug use.

Epidemiology

• Prevalence figures vary considerably, most indicating that 15%–50% of women in their 30s fail to regularly reach an orgasm during intercourse. Because orgasmic capacity in women increases with age, the disorder is more common in younger women. Many females increase their orgasmic capacity as they become more knowledgeable (and comfortable) about their sexuality and sexual stimulation [1,2,3].

Treatment

Diet and lifestyle
• Alcohol and drug use may play a role and should, therefore, be minimized.

Pharmacologic treatment
• Bupropion is being studied as a drug to increase orgasmic response but is currently unproven for this indication.

Nonpharmacologic treatments
• Treatment will most likely include the following components:

1. Education for female and her partner regarding sexual anatomy and normal sexual function.

2. Enlistment of the partner's cooperation, understanding, and patience.

3. Increasing patient's ability to feel comfortable with her body in the presence of a partner.

4. Sex therapy: may include sensate focus exercises, relaxation therapy, increased awareness that orgasmic capacity should not be used as a measure of "success" for a sexual encounter or that a very satisfactory sexual relationship can exist in the absence of orgasms for one or both of the partners, guided/directed masturbation, sharing of pleasure points with her partner, and discovering variations of stimulation to enhance sexual experiences.

5. Addressing relationship problems and conflicts over intimacy and sexuality.

6. Addressing sexual abuse or sexual trauma. Treatment of individuals who have been sexually traumatized or abused is difficult and best undertaken by a clinician who has the experience and time necessary to help the patient safely and successfully resolve these traumatic experiences.

7. Bibliotherapy: many helpful books (see General references) are available to help the woman become more comfortable with and knowledgeable about her sexuality.

8. Psychotherapy: generally assumes that all females are biologically capable of attaining orgasm; treatment goals include becoming comfortable with nudity and genitalia, feeling safe in her relationship, and focusing on the receipt of pleasure that is free of guilt or expectations.

Treatment aims
To address medical problems that may contribute to FOD.
To increase sexual satisfaction by means of enhancing and accepting one's sexuality.

Prognosis
• Good prognosis is associated with lifelong, generalized FOD
• Fair to good prognosis is associated with acquired and situational FOD.

Key references
1. Heiman J, LoPiccolo J, LoPiccolo L: Becoming Orgasmic Englewood Cliffs, NJ: Prentice Hall; 1988.

2. Kelly MP, Strassberg DS, Kircher JR: Attitudinal and experimental correlates of anorgasmia. Arch Sex Behav. 1990, 19:165–177.

3. Kinsey AC, Pomeroy W, Martin C, Gebhard P: Sexual Behavior in the Human Female. Philadelphia: WB Saunders; 1953.

General references
Barbach L: For Yourself. New York: Signet Books; 1973.

Barbach L: For Each Other New York: Signet Books; 1984.

Heiman J, Grafton-Becker V: Orgasmic disorders in women. In Principles and Practices of Sex Therapy Edited by Leiblum S, Rosen R. New York: The Guilford Press; 1989.

Hendrix H, Harville: Getting the Love You Want New York: Harper & Rowe; 1988.

Hendrix H, Harville: Keeping the Love You Find New York: Harper & Rowe; 1990.

Levine SB: Sexual Life New York: Plenum Press; 1992.

Masters WH, Johnson VE: Human sexual inadequacy. Boston: Little, Brown; 1976.

McCarthy B, McCarthy E: Sexual Awareness (1984). New York: Carrol & Graf Publishers; 1984.

McCarthy B, McCarthy E: Intimate Marriage (1992). New York: Carrol & Graf Publishers; 1992.

O'Conner D: How to Make Love to the Same Person for the Rest of Your Life and Still Love It. Doubleday & Company, Inc.: New York; 1995.

Rosen RC, Beck JG: Patterns of Sexual Arousal New York: The Guilford Press; 1988.

Diagnosis

Symptoms and signs

Persistent or recurrent delay in (or absence of) orgasm following normal sexual excitement despite sustained erectile function.

• The symptom must cause significant distress or relationship problems to be classified as male orgasmic disorder (MOD). Symptom may be lifelong or acquired and generalized or specific to a situation or partner [1].

• Frequently individuals will experience no orgasm with their partners but may experience orgasms during masturbation or sleep.

• There is no consensus regarding the objective criteria to determine "delayed" orgasm. Proposed criteria include time to ejaculation, man's perception, couple's perception, man's feeling of not being in control of timing.

Investigations

History: the diagnosis is made from history.

Physical evaluation: to rule out possible contributory or causative medical factors (*eg*, abnormal genital anatomy, endocrinopathy, neuropathy, and medication use).

Psychologic assessment and testing: may reveal characteristics, behaviors, or disorders that may be contributing to the intensity, duration, or frequency of orgasmic difficulties; screening for depression, anxiety, and relational problems is particularly important.

Assessment of the patient's (and partner's) understanding of normal sexual anatomy and function.

Complications

Sexual inadequacy: in anorgasmic males; the patient's partner, similarly, may feel that he or she is at fault for failing to provide adequate sexual stimulation or satisfaction.

Relationship problems: may cause, contribute, or result from MOD.

Psychologic difficulties (especially depression and anxiety): may cause, contribute, or result from MOD.

Differential diagnosis

• MOD differs from male sexual arousal disorder in that the male reports being aroused but unable to achieve orgasm with a partner. Varying degrees of delayed (but not completely inhibited) ejaculation are common.

Etiology

• The cause is often unclear in a particular individual. Sufficient mental and physical erotic input may result from one or more following:

Psychologic factors (eg, anxiety, relationship problems).

Unhealthy attitudes toward or inadequate knowledge about sexual function.

History of sexual trauma.

Insensitivity, impatience, or lack of understanding by the partner with regards to the patient's needs and preferences.

Poor communication between the couple.

Medications (especially most antidepressants and some antihypertensives) that cause anorgasmia.

Hormonal variations.

Alcohol or drug use.

Epidemiology

• Anorgasmia is much less common in males than females, affecting ~1%–2% of men who are otherwise capable of normal sexual activity. Prevalence estimates may be low because many males are reluctant to report this problem and may present for treatment only at the demand of their partners who want to become pregnant [1].

Treatment

Diet and lifestyle

• Alcohol and drug use may occasionally play a role and should therefore be minimized.

Pharmacologic treatment

• Bupropion is being studied as a drug to increase orgasmic response but is currently unproven for this indication.

Nonpharmacologic treatment

• Educating both the patient and partner about his own pleasure points, sexuality, and sexual needs and desires is helpful.

• Underlying psychologic and relationship conflicts should be sought and explored. If fear of impregnation is present, the patient may need education about contraception.

• Patient and partner should be educated regarding adequate foreplay and the need for patience and understanding between the couple during sexual relationships.

• The couple should be aware that orgasmic capacity should not be used as a measure of "success" for a sexual encounter and that a very satisfactory sexual relationship can exist in the absence or orgasms for one or both of the partners.

• There are many helpful books available to help men become more comfortable with and knowledgeable about their sexuality [4].

Prognosis

• Prognosis is largely dependent upon identification and correction of underlying causative or contributory psychologic and relationship factors.

Key references

1. Appelbaum B: Retarded ejaculation: a much misunderstood syndrome. In *Principles and Practices of Sex Therapy* Edited by Leiblum S, Rosen R. New York: The Guilford Press; 1989

2. Zelbergeld B: *The New Male Sexuality*. New York: Bantam Books; 1992.

3. Levine SB: *Sexual Life*. New York: Plenum Press; 1992.

General references

• *See* General references for Orgasmic disorder, female.

PANIC DISORDER

Diagnosis

Symptoms and signs

Prodrome: 10 minutes of rapidly increasing symptoms of fear and "a sense of impending doom and death").

Confusion and inability to concentrate.

Tachycardia, palpitations, dyspnea, and sweating.

Stammering, impaired memory.

Concern about cardiac or respiratory death: syncope occurs in 20% of patients.

Inability to pinpoint a cause.

• Symptoms can appear unexpectedly, disappear rapidly or slowly (usually last 20–30 min).

• Panic disorder can manifest itself with or without agoraphobia (the fear of being outside the home alone, in a crowd, in a line, on a bridge, or in a bus, train, or car).

Investigations

History: other family members with panic disorder suggest a four-to-eight times greater probability.

Complications

Normal activities restricted.

Avoidance: *eg,* driving a car, going to the store.

Depression.

Alcohol and other substance abuse.

Suicide: increased risk.

Family, school, work affected.

Differential diagnosis

Cardiovascular diseases (eg, anemia, congestive heart failure, angina, hypertension, myocardial infarction, paroxysmal atrial tachycardia).
Pulmonary diseases (eg, asthma, hyperventilation, pulmonary thromboembolism).
Neurologic diseases (eg, epilepsy, transient ischemic attack, Meniere's).
Endocrine diseases (eg, Addison's, Cushing's, diabetes mellitus, hyperthyroid, hypoparathyroid, menopause, premenstrual syndrome).
Drug intoxication (eg, amphetamine, amyl nitrite, anticholinergics, cocaine, marijuana, nicotine).
Drug withdrawal (eg, alcohol, antihypertensives, opiates, sedative-hypnotics).

Etiology

• Neurotransmitters (eg, norepinephrine, serotonin, γ-aminobutyric acid) have been implicated.
• Locus ceruleus, median raphe nucleus, limbic system, prefrontal cortex, and temporal lobes implicated.
• Precipitants (pancogens) include carbon dioxide, sodium lactate, yohimbine, fenfluramine, cholecystokinin, caffeine, and isoproterenol.
• Cognitive-behavioral–therapy anxiety is a learned response.
• The "psychoanalytic theory" proposes that there is an unsuccessful defense against anxiety-producing stimuli.

Epidemiology

• Lifetime prevalence is 1.5%–3.0%.
• Females are 2–3 times more likely to suffer from this disorder.
• Often there is a recent history of divorce or separation.
• Disorder usually begins in young adulthood (mean age, 25 y).

Treatment

Diet and lifestyle
• Decrease caffeine intake and nicotine, alcohol, and marijuana use.

Pharmacologic treatment

Standard dosage	Selective serotonin-reuptake inhibitors (SSRIs), start with ~25% the usual antidepressant dose and titrate higher (if necessary) by approximately this same dose every 2 weeks.
	Tricyclic antidepressants, dosing similar to SSRIs.
	Monoamine oxidase inhibitors, *eg*, phenelzine (45–90 mg/d).
	Benzodiazepines, *eg*, alprazolam or clonazepam (1–4 mg/d).
Special points	*SSRIs*: Doses exceeding standard antidepressant doses are not usually required.
	Benzodiazepines: Dependence is a concern; thus, drug must be slowly tapered when discontinuing treatment.

Nonpharmacologic treatment
Cognitive-behavioral therapy.

Family and group therapy.

Relaxation therapy.

Respiratory training: to control hyperventilation.

Treatment aims
To provide education about death, the nature of symptoms, and the effects of caffeine, stress, etc.
To eliminate or decrease symptoms sufficiently to permit normal functioning and activities.

Prognosis
• Treatment yields dramatic improvement.
• Some patients are symptom free (30%–40%); many have mild symptoms (50%).
• Significant symptoms remain in 10%–20% of patients.

Follow-up and management
• Most patients require at least 8–12 mo of treatment.

General references
Barlow DH: Cognitive-behavioral approaches to panic disorder and social phobia [abstract]. *Bull Menninger Clin* 1992, 56(suppl):A14.

Comprehensive Textbook of Psychiatry, 6th edition, Harold Kaplan and Benjamin Sadock, Williams & Wilkins; 1995.

Consultation Psychiatry, ed 2. Edited by Wise M, Rundell J: Washington, DC: American Psychiatric Association; 1994.

Keller MB, Hanks DL: Course and outcome in panic disorder. *Prog Neuro Psychopharmacol Biol Psychiatry* 1993, 17:551–570.

Psychiatry: Current Clinical Strategies. Edited by Hahn R. Laguna Hills, CA: CCS Publishing; 1997.

Psychiatry: House Officer Series, ed 5. Edited by Tomb D. Baltimore: Williams & Wilkins; 1995.

Klerman GL: Panic disorder: strategies for long-term treatment. *J Clin Psychiatry* 1991, 52(suppl):2.

Diagnosis

Definition

• Paranoid personality disorder (PPD) is a pattern of pervasive distrust and suspiciousness of others such that their motives are interpreted as malevolent. It begins in early adulthood and is present in a variety of contexts.

Symptoms and signs

Projection and externalization of blame; social isolation; cold, unfeeling aloofness; mandatory autonomy and personal control; control over others; centrality: perceiving self as center of others' concern; ideas of reference; guarded secretiveness; argumentativeness; complaining; stubbornness; poor sense of humor; an inability to relax; hostility; sarcasm; litigiousness; grandiosity; attraction to manifestations of power and rank; attraction to political and religious groups who share perceptions and perspectives; rare brief psychotic episodes in response to stress; sometimes predates Axis I psychotic disorders; often occurs together with schizoid, schizotypal, narcissistic, borderline, or avoidant personality disorders.

DSM-IV diagnostic criteria

• Paranoid personality disorder does not occur exclusively during the course of schizophrenia, a mood disorder with psychotic features, or another psychotic disorder, and it is not caused by the direct physiologic effects of a general medical condition.

• The disorder is indicated by the presence of four or more of the following symptoms:

1. Suspects, without sufficient basis, that others are exploiting, harming, or deceiving him or her.

2. Is preoccupied with unjustified doubts about the loyalty or trustworthiness of friends or associates.

3. Is reluctant to confide in others because of unwarranted fear that the information will be used maliciously against him or her.

4. Reads hidden demeaning or threatening meanings into benign remarks or events.

5. Persistently bears grudges, ie, is unforgiving of insults, injuries, or slights.

6. Perceives attacks on his or her character or reputation that are not apparent to others and is quick to react angrily or to counterattack.

7. Has recurrent suspicions, without justification, regarding fidelity of spouse or partner.

Investigations

Minnesota Multiphasic Personality Inventory-2: cluster A personality disorders typically are reflected in elevations of scales 6 (paranoia), 8 (schizophrenia), and 0 (social introversion); a low score on scale 6 may reflect a highly paranoid individual who is attempting to escape detection.

Millon Clinical Multiaxial Inventory-III: scale P specifically measures for PPD.

Rorschach: useful in detecting mild thought disorders and emotional trait characteristics.

Complications

Comorbidity

Alcohol and other substance abuse or dependence; major depression; panic disorder; agoraphobia; obsessive-compulsive personality disorder.

Behavioral outcomes

Divorce and marital discord; interpersonal conflict, "feuds," lawsuits; possible violence at home or in the workplace.

Differential diagnosis

Disorders of persistent psychotic symptoms (eg, delusional disorder, persecutory type; schizophrenia, paranoid type; mood disorder with psychotic features).
Personality change due to a general medical condition (eg, early frontal lobe dementia, hyperthyroidism-induced PPD).
Paranoid traits associated with chronic substance use.
Paranoid traits associated with the development of a physical handicap (eg, hearing loss).
Other personality disorders (eg, schizotypal, schizoid, borderline and histrionic, avoidant, antisocial, narcissistic, adaptive paranoid).

Etiology

• Etiology is not established.
• Some evidence exists indicating a relationship to the "schizophrenia spectrum" of disorders:
Schizophrenia and other psychotic disorders (more prevalent among relatives of those with PPD).
PPD (more prevalent among relatives of those with schizophrenia; even higher prevalence among relatives of those with delusional disorder).
• PPD and schizophrenia possibly are associated with major affective disorders; one large study found a higher family relationship of PPD to probands with unipolar major depression (2.9%) than those with schizophrenia (1.7%); another study demonstrated increased family risk for schizophrenia and related disorders (including PPD) among those with major affective disorders, and the reverse (increased family risk for major affective disorders) among those with schizophrenia and related disorders.
• The disorder's pervasive defense mechanism of projection suggests a developmental psychodynamic pathogenesis.

Epidemiology

• The estimated prevalence in the general population is 0.5%–2.5%; within the psychiatric inpatient settings, 10%–30%; within outpatient mental health clinics, 2%–10%.
• PPD is more common in men than in women.

Treatment

Pharmacologic treatment

• Low-dose neuroleptic medication is of dubious benefit.

• One study combining phenothiazenes and lithium demonstrated no benefit.

• Comorbid conditions, such as depression or anxiety, should be conventionally treated.

• Prescriptions may provoke autonomy and control issues, which could threaten the therapeutic alliance.

Nonpharmacologic treatment

Psychotherapy

• Considerations influencing psychotherapy:

externalization of blame and egosyntonic nature of traits counter any perception of need for therapy; distrust of others opposes capacity for alliance; threats of harm to the therapist may arise; and because paranoid patients may sue the therapist, diligence is a must regarding confidentiality and other therapeutic duties, standards, and records.

• Beneficial techniques in establishing trust include 1) listening empathetically; 2) avoiding familiarity, humor, and the questioning of beliefs (do not dispute false beliefs, but do not agree with them either); 3) allowing the patient to make the decisions whenever possible; 4) avoiding reference to patient information that patient has not personally disclosed; 5) giving letters or forms about the patient to the patient for him or her to forward; 6) and guarding against your own impatience with defensive projections and argumentativeness during therapy.

Behavioral therapy

• Behavioral therapy is contraindicated by paranoid dynamics.

Cognitive therapy

• Nondirective cognitive techniques are useful. Basic issues of beliefs, assumptions, and automatic thoughts are exceedingly delicate.

Family therapy

• There is a risk of undermining the individual therapy alliance.

Group therapy

• There is a potential opportunity for social insight and skills and a risk of provocation of paranoid defenses or regression.

Treatment aims

To provide crisis stabilization and situational support.
To stabilize interpersonal reality perceptions.
To stabilize mood and self-worth.
To insure maximal psychosocial functioning.

Prognosis

Generally poor.
• Paranoid dynamics usually preclude long-term treatment.
• Psychologic insight is rarely acquired.
• Treatment benefit is stabilization and support for most cases.

Other treatments

Self-help groups: usually too threatening.
Day treatment programs: beneficial for some.
Partial hospital programs: useful for crisis support.
Acute inpatient treatment: only for overt endangerment.
Long-term inpatient treatment: virtually never needed.

Follow-up and management

• There is no "acute phase" to the disorder of personality, and its "trait" nature confers long-term perspective.
• More favorable prognosis is gained by long-term therapy process.

General references

Diagnostic and Statistical Manual of Mental Disorders, ed 4. Washington, DC: American Psychiatric Association; 1994.

Klein DF, Gettelman R, Quitkin F, et al. (eds): *Diagnosis and Drug Therapy of Psychiatric Disorders: Adults and Children*, ed 20. Baltimore: Williams & Wilkins; 1980.

Treatments of Psychiatric Disorders, ed 2. Edited by Gabbard GO. Washington, DC: American Psychiatric Press; 1995.

Treatment outlines for paranoid, schizotypal, and schizoid personality disorders. *Aust N Z J Psychiatry* 1990, 24:339–350.

Diagnosis

Symptoms and signs
• Idiopathic Parkinson's disease (IPD; paralysis agitans) is a clinical diagnosis.

The "classic triad"
Paucity of movement (bradykinesia): necessary to the diagnosis.

Muscle stiffness ("lead-pipe rigidity"): velocity independent.

Resting 4–5-Hz hand tremor ("pill rolling"): common (in 70% of patients) but not necessary to make the diagnosis.

Other associated signs and symptoms
Asymmetric presentation; festinating gait; stooped posture; "masked face" or "reptilian stare"; decreased volume of voice (hypophonia); small handwriting (micrographia); axial/postural instability; orthostatic hypotension; lip, jaw, or foot tremor; chronic constipation; muscle cramps; painful limb posturing (dystonia); loss of olfaction; depression (in 40% of patients); dementia (in 40% of patients).

Investigations
Trial of levodopa/carbidopa
• If the signs and symptoms are consistent with IPD, a trial of levodopa/carbidopa is warranted. Most patients with IPD respond to carbidopa/levodopa, and those that do not may have a variant of parkinsonism.

Other investigations
• Other investigations (*ie*, blood tests or imaging) are usually reserved for patients that have an atypical presentation.

Fluoro-dihydroxyphenylalanine ([18F]-DOPA) positron-emission tomography (PET) scan: used in some institutions to help verify the diagnosis, but its cost effectiveness has been debated; a definitive diagnosis of IPD can be made at autopsy; microscopically, neuronal degeneration and cytoplasmic inclusions (Lewy bodies) are seen in catecholamine-producing, pigmented areas of the brain such as the substantia nigra and locus ceruleus.

Ceruloplasmin and serum and urine copper levels: to rule out Wilson's disease if the patient is <60 years of age before onset of symptoms.

Ophthalmologic examination (slit lamp): may also be warranted to determine the presence of Kayser–Fleischer rings

Cranial magnetic resonance and other imaging studies: may suggest atypical parkinsonian variants; progressive supranuclear palsy (PSP) usually is associated with a severely atrophied midbrain, whereas the pons and cerebellum are usually affected in olivopontocerebellar atrophy.

Complications
All patients
Increased injury or death: from falls secondary to postural instability.

Increased risk of suicide: in patients with depression.

Death: due to dehydration, malnutrition, and infections in later stages of disease.

Patients on carbidopa/levodopa
• Parkinson patients on carbidopa/levodopa for extended periods of time may eventually develop the following motor complications:

"Wearing-off" phenomenon: therapeutic efficacy of levodopa/carbidopa doses decreases with prolonged use.

"On-off" phenomenon: abrupt clinical changes relating to fluctuations in concentration of levodopa in brain; when "on," patients obtain therapeutic benefit; "off" refers to being below the therapeutic window for carbidopa/levodopa, resulting in the sudden onset of bradykinesia and rigidity.

Dyskinesia: presence of involuntary writhing movements when above the therapeutic window for carbidopa/levodopa.

Differential diagnosis
Neurodegenerative disorders
Parkinson's plus syndromes, PSP, corticobasal ganglionic degeneration, multisystem atrophy, olivopontocerebellar atrophy, striatonigral degeneration, Shy–Drager syndrome, Huntington's disease (rigid variant), Wilson's disease, pallidal degenerations, Alzheimer's disease, diffuse Lewy body disease

Secondary parkinsonism
Vascular disease, postencephalitic, post-traumatic, hydrocephalus, space-occupying lesions, drug- or toxin-induced parkinsonism, antidopaminergic drugs, dopamine receptor antagonists, dopamine depletors, MPTP, carbon monoxide, manganese.

Epidemiology
• IPD is rare <50 y of age.
• Incidence ranges from 4.5–21.0:100,000 population; greater in whites than in Asians (2-3.3:1) or in blacks (4:1).
• Prevalence is greater in men than women.

Etiology
• IPD is a neurodegenerative disease associated with decreased amounts of brain monoamine neurotransmitters, especially dopamine. There is no known cause of IPD, but 5%–40 % of IPD patients have a positive family history for Parkinsonism, suggesting a genetic component.
• Factors statistically associated with increased risk of developing IPD include history of head trauma, exposure to heavy metals (manganese, iron), living on a farm or in a rural residence, history of long-term well-water exposure, herbicide or pesticide exposure (dieldrin), working in the steel or wood pulp industries, excessive emotional stress, having a shy or depressed personality.
• Factors statistically associated with decreased risk of developing IPD include consumption of vitamin E, supplemental multivitamins, cod liver oil, tocophereol, alcohol, tobacco.

Treatment

Diet and lifestyle

• There are no special recommendations. Dietary issues primarily revolve around the use of pharmacotherapeutic agents (*see* Pharmacologic treatment).

Pharmacologic treatment

• Carbidopa/levodopa is the most commonly used and most effective drug; however, it may only have 10–20 years of useful efficacy.

• Younger patients (<65 y of age) should be treated initially with a dopamine-receptor agonist (*eg*, bromocriptine, pergolide, pramipexole, ropinirole), amantadine, or a monoamine oxidase inhibitor (*eg*, selegiline).

• Tremors may be treated with an anticholinergic agent (*eg*, trihexyphenidyl or benztropine mesylate). Carbidopa/levodopa doses may have to be added and increased with disease progression. If motor fluctuations develop on carbidopa/levodopa, dopamine-receptor agonists or catechol-O-methyl transferase inhibitors (*eg*, tolcapone, entacapone) may be added and carbidopa/levodopa doses decreased, if possible.

Standard dosage	Carbidopa/levodopa, 25 mg/100 mg (or 10 mg/100 mg, 25 mg/250 mg, 25 mg/100 mg CR, 50 mg/200mg CR) three times daily or more.
	Bromocriptine, 1.25 mg twice daily or more.
	Pergolide, 0.5-1.0 mg/d to three times daily.
	Pramipexole 0.125-1.500 mg three times daily.
	Ropinirole 0.25-8.00 mg three times daily.
	Amantadine, 100 mg/d to twice daily.
	Selegiline, 5 mg to twice daily.
	Trihexyphenidyl, 1-10 mg/d.
	Benztropine mesylate, 0.5-2.0 mg/d to twice daily.
	Tolcapone, 100-200 mg three times daily.
	Entacapone 200 mg three times daily.
Contraindications	Dopamine-replacement therapies should not be given to overtly psychotic individuals or those with malignant hypertension. Anticholinergics should be avoided in the elderly. Avoid antidopaminergic drugs (*ie*, most neuroleptics and antinausea medicines) in patients with IPD.
Main side effects	*All dopamine-replacement therapies*: nausea, visual hallucinations, orthostatic hypotension.
	Bromocriptine, pergolide: retropulmonary fibrosis.
	Pramipexole, ropinirole: transient somnolence.
	Anticholinergics: drooling, confusion.
	Tolcapone: chronic diarrhea.
Main drug interactions	Potentially fatal interaction occur between monoamine oxidase inhibitors and antidepressants.
Special points	*All dopamine-replacement therapies*: (*ie*, carbidopa/levodopa, bromocriptine, pergolide, pramipexole, ropinirole) should be given with food, started at a low dose, and increased slowly. For example, start carbidopa/levodopa 25/100 at a half-tablet at breakfast and increase every 5–7 days by half-tablet intervals to each meal up to a total dose of 2 tablets three times daily before reassessment. Increase as needed until clinical efficacy or side effects are seen. Dopamine-replacement–induced nausea is treated by taking medications with food, adding extra carbidopa (available only from the manufacturer) or domperidone (available only in Canada and Europe).

Treatment aims

To obtain relief of symptoms without development of side effects.
To maintain the highest level of function.

Prognosis

• IPD is a progressive but treatable disease. Pharmacologic therapies are tried first, and surgical options used as a last resort. Parkinson variants have a worse prognosis and either respond poorly or not at all to standard pharmacologic therapies. There is no cure.

Follow-up and management

• After starting patients on carbidopa/levodopa 25/100, it will take ~2 mo to taper up to a dose of two tablets three times daily, and the patient should be seen at that time. When a patient is on a stable treatment regimen, routine clinic visits should be done every 6–12 mo.

Other treatment options

• Dyskinesia can be treated surgically by stereotaxic pallidotomy. Tremor can similarly be treated stereotaxically with thalamotomy or deep brain thalamic stimulation. Experimental treatments include deep brain stimulation to the pallidum or subthalamic nucleus and striatal implants of fetal mesencephalic tissue (although reported to produce benefits, many of these therapies are being actively investigated for safety and efficacy).

General references

Harris EC, Barraclough BM: Suicide as an outcome for medical disorders. *Medicine* 1994, 73:281–296.

Janko, Shannon: Parkinsonism and Parkinson's disease. *Nurse Practitioner Forum* 1996, 7:174–178.

Jankovic J, Tolosa E (eds): *Parkinson's Disease and Movement Disorders.* Williams & Wilkins: Baltimore; 1993.

Tanner, *et al.*: Epidemiology and genetics of Parkinson's disease. In *Movement Disorders.* Edited by Watts RL and Koller WC. New York: McGraw-Hill; 1997:137–152.

Weiner WJ, Lang AE (eds): *Movement Disorders: A Comprehensive Survey.* New York: Futura Publishing Co.; 1989.

Diagnosis

Definition

• Pathological gambling is the persistent, recurrent, and maladaptive gambling behavior that disrupts personal, family, and vocational pursuits.

• The addictive paradigm is defined as pursuit of an aroused or euphoric state through gambling, tolerance (increased amounts and odds), and withdrawal (restlessness, dysphoria) on cessation.

• Four phases describe the condition:

1. Winning: fantasies of omnipotence, escape-seeking.
2. Losing: "chasing" efforts to win back losses.
3. Desperation: to restore losses and regain euphoria.
4. Hopelessness: accepts impossibility of regaining losses, but continues to seek the arousal.

DSM-IV diagnostic criteria

• This disorder of persistent and recurrent maladaptive gambling behavior is indicated by five (or more) of the following:

1. Is preoccupied with gambling (eg, preoccupied with reliving past gambling experiences, handicapping or planning the next venture, or thinking of ways to get money with which to gamble).
2. Gambles increasing amounts of money to achieve desired excitement.
3. Has repeated unsuccessful efforts to control, cut back, or stop gambling.
4. Is restless or irritable when attempting to cut down or stop gambling.
5. Gambles as a way of escaping from problems or of relieving a dysphoric mood (eg, feelings of hopelessness, guilt, anxiety, depression).
6. After losing money, often returns to get even ("chasing" one's losses).
7. Lies to family members, therapist, or others to conceal the extent of gambling.
8. Has committed illegal acts such as forgery, fraud, theft, or embezzlement to finance gambling.
9. Has jeopardized or lost a significant relationship, job, or educational or career opportunity because of gambling.
10. Relies on others to relieve desperate financial situations caused by gambling.

• In addition, gambling behavior is not better accounted for by manic episode.

Investigations

Psychologic testing

MMPI-2: scales 4 (psychopathic deviate) and 9 (hypomania) are often elevated in those with history of impulsivity; problems with impulse control are likely when scale 4 is 10 or more T points higher than scale 3 (hysteria).

Millon Clinical Multiaxial Inventory-III expected scale elevations: 5, narcissistic; 6A, antisocial; 6B, sadistic; 7, compulsive; C, borderline.

Screening tests

South Oaks Gambling Screen: Illinois Institute for Addiction Recovery, Peoria, IL 61614; phone: 1-800-522-3784; website: www.addictionrecov.org/southoak.html.

Gamblers Anonymous' Twenty Questions: website: www.gamblersanonymous.org/20questions.html.

Complications

• **Comorbidity:** substance addiction, mood disorders, anxiety disorders, attention deficit disorder, compulsive sexual behavior, bulimia, compulsive buying.

Behavioral outcomes: suicide; divorce; bankruptcy; criminal behaviors.

Medical complications: hypertension; peptic ulcer disease; irritable bowel syndrome; migraine headache syndrome.

Differential diagnosis

Social gambling: limited time, limited losses. Professional gambling: limited risks, disciplined.
Gambling problems not meeting criteria: usually brief compulsion to win back losses.
Manic episode.

Etiology

None established.

• Some theories include sensation-seeking behavior due to norandrenergic or dopaminergic deficits, eg, increased cerebrospinal fluid MHPG; subnormal plasma MHPG; increased urinary excretion of norepinephrine and metabolites; decreased cerebrospinal fluid homovanilic acid and other dopamine metabolic products; increased D_1 and D_2 receptor genetic variants.

• The obsessive-compulsive spectrum includes the following serotonergic aberrations: lowered platelet MAO; neuroendocrine response deviations to intravenous clomipramine and intravenous CPP; and "the gambling personality" (risk-taking and excitement-seeking), described as highly competitive, energetic, restless, easily bored, overly concerned with approval of others, generous to the point of extravagance, and compulsive in other areas (eg, work).

Epidemiology

• In the United States, $17 billion is spent on legal gambling; 48 states have some form of legalized gambling.

• The onset of pathological gambling occurs usually in adolescence or early adulthood.

• Parents of pathological gamblers have increased pathological gambling and alcohol and drug abuse.

• In the general population, 80% of adults have gambled; 1%–3% are pathological gamblers.

• Male-to-female ratios: pathological gamblers, 67% and 33%; attendees of Gamblers Anonymous, 96% and 4%.

• The estimated pathological gambling-related indebtedness among men is $50,000–$90,000; among women, $15,000.

• 15%–20% of pathological gamblers have attempted suicide.

Treatment

Pharmacologic treatment

• There is no established treatment of choice.

• Administer serotonin reuptake inhibitor medications (clomipramine and fluvoxamine reported).

• Noradrenergic and dopaminergic data cited above raise possibilities, but no clinical trials exist.

• Treat comorbid conditions.

Standard dosage None established.

Fluvoxamine, 100–300 mg (mean dose, 220 mg) reported effective in one study.

Special points Disinhibiting medications (*eg*, benzodiazepines, barbiturates, and opiates), alcohol, and any other substances of abuse should be avoided.

Nonpharmacologic treatments

Gamblers Anonymous

• Gamblers Anonymous (GA) is a 12-step recovery program active since 1957.

• The characteristics of the compulsive gambler as defined by GA include an inability and unwillingness to accept reality ("the escape into the dream world of gambling"), emotional insecurity ("emotionally comfortable only when 'in action'"), immaturity ("a desire to have the good things in life without any great effort"), and a need to feel all-powerful.

• According to GA, a person stops gambling through a progressive character change and by following the GA recovery concepts.

• GA is sufficient treatment alone for many gamblers; however, some people are resistant to 12-step precepts (confrontation of denial is key), groups are still small and few in number, and availability of sponsors may be limited.

Gamblers Anonymous International Service Office: PO Box 17173, Los Angeles, CA 90017; phone: 213-386-8789; website: www.gamblersanonymous.org/about.html; e-mail: isomain@gamblersanonymous.org.

For family and spouses (Gam-Anon)

• Gam-Anon coordinates with GA but is independent both organizationally and financially to help family members change their own lives as means of dealing with the effect of gambling addiction within the home. They provide comfort to members, help family members extend encouragement and understanding to the GA member, and provide spiritual growth through the 12-step approach.

Gam-Anon International Service Office: PO Box 157, Whitestone, NY 11357; phone: 718-352-1671; website: www.gamblersanonymous.org/gamanon.html.

Psychotherapy

Crisis support is avaiable for mood problems (especially suicidal ideation), family system distress, legal and financial problems, structure for time and cash access, and relapse prevention and self-control strategies.

Treatment aims

Cessation of gambling and recovery from comorbid conditions.

Prognosis

• Posttreatment relapses: ~45% in 12 mo. Drop-out rates are high in both clinical settings and GA.

Follow-up and management

For the acute phase: medication interventions include weekly monitoring until response is seen; weekly GA; individual and family therapy.
For the continuation phase: no objective data exist.

Other therapeutic concerns

Comorbid conditions: eg, alcoholism.
Psychodynamic issues: personalized meaning of gambling and money beyond the issues of stimulation and arousal gratification; self-deceptions and issues of omnipotence versus inadequacy; any childhood trauma.
Behavioral approach: imaginal desensitization.
Inpatient treatment for suicidal states or inability to stop gambling despite outpatient efforts.

Other support groups

• The National Council on Problem Gambling, Inc. (PO Box 9419, Washington, DC 20016; phone: 800-330-8739; website: www.ncpgambling.org/) is a nonprofit agency that links state councils and affiliates and offers a resource catalog, training, and conferences.

General references

Comprehensive Textbook of Psychiatry, ed 6. Edited by Kaplan HI, Sadock BJ. Baltimore: Williams & Wilkins; 1995.

DeCaria CM, Hollander E, et al.: Diagnosis, neurobiology, and treatment of pathological gambling. *J Clin Psychiatry* 1996, 57 (suppl 8):80–83.

Diagnostic and Statistical Manual of Mental Disorders, ed 4. Washington, DC: American Psychiatric Association; 1994.

Hollander E, Wong C, Kelly A: *Monograph for New Developments in the Treatment of OCD*. New York: MBL Communications; 1997.

Diagnosis

Symptoms and signs of intoxication

Symptoms and signs of intoxication by stage

Category	Stage I	Stage II	Stage III
Central nervous system	Conscious	Stupor to mild coma; seizures	"Eyes open coma," seizures
Pain response	Blunted	Deep pain intact	Deep pain absent
Motor system	Ataxia, muscle rigidity, grimacing	Muscle rigidity, muscle twitching	Generalized myoclonus; opisthotonic or decerebrate posturing
Eye signs	Horizontal nystagmus	Nystagmus (any direction), corneal reflex loss, disconjugate gaze	Nystagmus, absent corneal reflex, disconjugate gaze, ptosis
Vital signs	Mildly increased	Moderately elevated	Hyperpyrexia, blood pressure spikes, periodic breathing, apnea
Deep tendon reflexes	Increased	Increased	Absent
Autonomic signs	Nausea, vomiting, diaphoresis, lacrimation	Protracted vomiting, diaphoresis	Diaphoresis, flushing, hypersalivation

Symptoms and signs of withdrawal
• Physiologic withdrawal is not common and does not require medical management when it does occur.
• Depression, irritability, and craving are the most common symptoms.

Investigations
Drug screen: can be helpful.

Complete blood count with differential: leukocyte count may be increased.

Urinalysis: may indicate myoglobinuria.

Liver enzymes: may be elevated.

Electroencephalograpm: may show diffuse theta activity with periodic slow-wave complexes.

Complications
Malignant hyperthermia.

Aspiration pneumonia.

Pulmonary edema.

Status epilepticus.

Self-inflicted injuries.

Acute venal tubular necrosis.

Acute hepatic necrosis.

High output cardiac failure.

Hypertensive encephalopathy.

Intracranial hemorrhage.

Treatment

Diet and lifestyle

- Recovery from PCP dependence requires a lifestyle change in order to achieve and maintain abstinence.
- Abstinence from all mood-altering drugs is recommended.

Pharmacologic treatment

- Treatment should take place under close observation in a quiet, safe environment, with reduced external stimuli.
- Stage I intoxication is best treated nonpharmacologically; stage II and III intoxication, when indicated.

Antihypertensives

Standard dosage	Hydralazine, 5–20 mg i.v.
	Propranolol, 1 mg i.v. every 30 minutes (8 mg total).
	Diazoxide, 300 mg i.v.
Contraindications	Known hypersensitivity.
Main drug interactions	None.

Benzodiazepines

Standard dosage	Diazepam, 10–30 mg orally or 2.5 mg i.v. (25 mg total).
	Lorazepam, 2–4 mg i.m. as needed.
Contraindications	Known hypersensitivity.
Main drug interactions	Synergistic central nervous system depression with sedative-hypnotics.

Adjunctive medications

Furosemide: 20–40 mg i.v. every 6 hours to increase urinary output.

Naloxone: 0.4 mg i.v. if respiratory rate is <12/min.

Aminophylline: 250 mg i.v. for bronchospasm.

Ascorbic acid: 0.5–105 mg every 4–6 hours as needed to reduce urine pH to <5.5 to aid PCP clearance.

Treatment aims

- Observe until all symptoms have resolved.
- Reduce PCP-induced psychotic behavior.
- Keep patient from self-harm.
- Prepare patient for possible prolonged psychiatric sequence.

Prognosis

Good, with aggressive medical management.

Follow-up and management

- PCP tends to be the longest acting of any abused drug. The entire picture may take up to 6 wk to clear. Long-lasting psychiatric sequelae can include anxiety, depression, and psychosis. Flashbacks are rare. Treatment for most sequelae is psychosocial. Antipsychotic medications may be necessary for psychosis.
- All PCP-dependent individuals should be referred to treatment and support groups to aid in maintaining abstinence.

Other information

- The risk for prolonged psychiatric reactions depends on the following: The patient's premorbid psychopathology. The number of prior exposures to the drug. The history of multiple drug use.

General references

Carroll ME, Comer SD: Phencyclidine and the hallucinogens: *Topics in Addiction Medicine* 1995, 1–10.

Milhorn TH: *Chemical Dependence* New York: Springer Verlag; 1990:242–252.

Wilkins JN, Gorelick DA: Management of phencyclidine, hallucinogen and marijuana intoxication and withdrawal. *Topics in Addiction Medicine* 1995, 1–9.

Diagnosis [1,2]

Symptoms and signs
• This disorder involves sexual arousal associated with recurrent fantasies, urges, or behaviors of sexual acts with children (generally considered ≤13 y of age). Individuals must meet the following criteria for diagnosis:

Significant distress or impairment in functioning due to fantasies, urges, or actual behaviors.

Symptoms present for ≤6 months.

Individual is at least 16 years of age and at least 5 years older than the child.

• Diagnostic criteria have been questioned for their applicability to the heterogeneous nature of pedophiles and child molesters. At present, the individual may be a child molester and not meet criteria for pedophilia.

• Many convicted child molesters deny recurrent urges or fantasies involving children. It has been suggested that individuals having fantasies, urges, or any sexual behavior involving children receive treatment.

• Pedophiles are frequently categorized as incest-only or nonfamilial subtypes. Pedophiles are also categorized according to their preferred victims (*eg*, girls, boys, or both).

Investigations
Laboratory investigations: none are indicated.

Psychologic testing: may identify additional psychiatric disorders and paraphilias contributing to the severity and likelihood of pedophilic behavior.

Penile plethysmography: may offer additional information to establish arousal associated with this behavior; this measure may result in false-negative information; the ethical use of this measure has been questioned, particularly for the use of identifying adolescents or juveniles who sexually abuse children.

Complications
Legal implications of behavior: sexual activities involving children and child pornography are illegal; in addition, the individual may commit other crimes in an effort to locate, obtain, and maintain a victim.

Substance abuse or dependence: the most common problem associated with child molestation has been identified as substance use; in particular, specific abuse incidents are often preceded by substance use.

Impaired social or sexual functioning: pedophiles may only be able to achieve sexual arousal through deviant activities; these fantasies, urges, and behaviors are likely to strain social and sexual relationships with adults and result in further emotional loneliness; because the individual may distort his or her perceptions to allow commission of the deviant behavior, they may also have other interpersonal styles that impair appropriate relationships.

Differential diagnosis
Obsessive-compulsive disorder (OCD): some individuals with OCD have fears that they might abuse children or that they have abused children; in general, however, these individuals are not fantasizing about children and have never acted on the obsessions, but rather have intense fears that they may or may have acted on the urges; the image or urge is often viewed as repugnant to the individual, and is not considered sexually arousing.

Etiology
• No single etiologic theory appears to account for the heterogeneity of pedophiles. Most clinicians and researchers accept that a combination of factors is likely to be involved, including low empathy with victims of sexual abuse, low self-esteem, high rates of cognitive distortions (eg, denial, minimization), poor parent-child relationship, neglect, hostility, physical abuse within family, history of childhood sexual victimization, poor social or interpersonal skills, lack of intimacy, loneliness, classic and operant conditioning (eg, deviant fantasies, urges, or behaviors are paired with sexual arousal [classic conditioning], which is inherently positive [operant conditioning]).

Epidemiology
• Onset is assumed to begin during adolescence, although some information suggests that urges are not present until adulthood for certain pedophiles.
• Abusers are typically male, with a subset of female abusers.

Other information
• Related paraphilias include the following:
Urophilia (sexual arousal associated with urinating on someone or being urinated upon).
Coprophilia (sexual arousal associated with defecating on someone or being defecated upon).
Hypoxyphilia (sexual arousal associated with oxygen deprivation; may result in injury or death, usually by accident; has been associated with other masochistic behaviors, transvestitism, and self-observation; reported deaths include individuals ranging from 10–60 y of age, usually males).
• Risk factors for engaging in deviant behavior include the following:
Being in a situation where abuse could occur.
Persistent drunkenness.
Emotional upset.
Stressful situations.

Treatment [1–3]

General information
• Most clinicians prefer a combination of various psychologic and medical treatment interventions. Hormonal treatment may not be considered an ethical option for prepubescent offenders. Mentally handicapped individuals are likely to receive minimal benefit from psychologic treatment.

Pharmacologic treatment
Psychotropic medication
• Most medications given for paraphilias are thought to work by treating the "obsessional nature" of the disorder, and by taking advantage of the sexual side effect profile of these medications. Other medications have been reported in case studies and are potentially beneficial for unspecified reasons.

• Appropriate dosage has not been determined. It is generally accepted that medications will be prescribed similarly to treatment of obsessive-compulsive disorder or depression, and adjusted until symptoms are controlled or side effects intolerable.

• Selective serotonin reuptake inhibitors generally have fewer side effects and may be considered first-line agents, especially for patients on few or no other medications.

Standard dosage   Fluoxetine, 20–80 mg/d.

Paroxetine, 20–60 mg/d.

Fluvoxamine, 50–300 mg/d.

Sertraline, 50–200 mg/d.

Clomipramine, 150–300 mg/d.

Hormonal agents
• Antiandrogens have been shown to be effective in suppressing sexual urges, but they also may truncate an individual's sexual life; sooner or later the individual may wish to stop them.

Medroxyprogesterone acetate: lowers testosterone levels and has demonstrated efficacy for decreasing sexual urges, fantasies, and behaviors for most paraphilias.

Cyproterone acetate (in Canada): blocks the action of testosterone and has demonstrated efficacy in treatment of paraphilias.

Long-acting gonadotropic hormone-releasing hormone agonists: have recently shown efficacy in paraphilic populations; these agents result in decreased secretion of luteinizing hormone and follicle-stimulating hormone that result in lowered testosterone secretion.

• Usually symptoms of the paraphilia rapidly recur on discontinuation of psychotropic medications or hormonal agents.

Nonpharmacologic treatment
• Cognitive-behavioral therapy may include the following:

Behavior therapy: to reduce inappropriate sexual arousal and increase appropriate sexual arousal.

Challenging distorted thinking and beliefs: especially those concerning justification for the paraphilic behavior.

Social skills training, assertiveness training, communication skills training.

Relapse prevention: to help identify vulnerable thoughts or situations and intervene to prevent or stop the behavior by using various cognitive skills and behavioral skills.

Treatment aims
To reduce or eliminate pedophilic behavior (child molestation).
To reduce or eliminate pedophilic fantasies or urges.
To increase, if possible, sexual arousal associated with appropriate stimuli.

Prognosis
• Male-victim offenders may have higher recidivism rates than female-victim nonfamilial offenders.
• Poor prognosis is associated with individuals having low empathy for their victims.
• Most prognostic indicators are associated with details of the individual's past (eg, number of victims) rather than treatment or future occurrences.
• Prediction of likelihood of abusing again is most significantly related to the individual having the opportunity to abuse (ie, if the individual is in a situation where he/she can abuse a child, it is likely that he or she will abuse the child.)

Follow-up and management
• Relapse prevention is necessary for any individual who has committed child molestation.
• It is recommended that individuals be supervised extensively.
• Vulnerable situations, behaviors, and moods should be identified and coping skills examined to prevent individuals from being in situations that might facilitate deviant behavior.

Key references
1. Laws DR, O'Donohue W: *Sexual Deviance.* New York: Guilford Press; 1997.
2. Elliot M, Browne K, Kilcoyne J: Child sexual abuse prevention: what offenders tell us. *Child Abuse Negl* 1995, 19:579–594.
3. Kafka MP: A monoamine hypothesis for the pathophysiology of paraphilic disorders. *Arch Sex Behav* 1997, 26:343–358.

General reference
Becker JV, Quinsey VL: Assessing suspected child molesters. *Child Abuse Negl* 1993, 17:169–174.

Diagnosis

Definition
• Pica is defined as eating nonnutritive material for at least 1 month, which must be inappropriate for the patient's stage of development.

Symptoms and signs
• The criteria for pica are not met if the person is eating nonnutritive substances as a part of a cultural rite or practice. Substances could include such things as paint, plaster, string, hair, cloth, dirt, animal feces, stones, and paper. Signs and symptoms of anemia, zinc, and iron deficiency often occur with clay and starch ingestion.

Investigations I
Serum iron and zinc levels.

Complete blood count.

Lead levels and hemoglobin.

Complications
Intestinal obstruction: can occur with ingestion of hair, stones, or gravel.

Iron, zinc, and lead poisoning. can occur.

Differential diagnosis
Failure to thrive.
Schizophrenia.
Autism.
Psychosocial dwarfism.
Anorexia nervosa
Klein–Levin syndrome.

Etiology
Nutritional deficiency.
Familial links.
Parental neglect (oral needs).

Epidemiology
Children between 1–6 y of age, 10%-32%.
Children >10 y of age, 10%.
Institutionalized children and adolescents, 5%
Males–to–female ratio, 1:1.
More children than adults.
Pregnant females favor clay.

Treatment

Diet and lifestyle
• Family support is thought to play a significant role in the treatment.

Pharmacologic treatment
Symptomatic treatment: for poisoning.

Nonpharmacologic treatment
Psychosocial therapy.

Environmental protection.

Behavioral therapy.

Family education and guidance.

Treatment aims
To eliminate psychosocial stressors and symptomatic treatment.

Prognosis
Usually will disappear by adolescence
Among the mentally retarded the process may go on for years
After a pregnancy is completed this phenomenon will usually disappear

General references
Kaplan H, Saddock B (eds): *Synopsis of Psychiatry*, ed 7. Baltimore: Williams & Wilkins; 1994.

Blinder Bl, Chaitin B, Goldstein R: *The Eating Disorders Pergamon*, New York: 1987.

Diagnosis

Symptoms and signs [1]

• Postpartum mood disorder (PPMD) can present as major depressive, manic or mixed episode of major depressive disorder or bipolar disorder. The onset is usually within 4 weeks postpartum.

Mood lability and fluctuating course.

Psychomotor agitation.

Suicidal ideation.

Obsessional fears of harming the child.

Persecutory delusions about the infant: can occur with psychosis.

Guilt.

Insomnia: even when time is available to sleep.

Decreased concentration.

Anxiety.

Difficulty bonding with child.

Crying spells.

Investigations

Screening for postpartum: Edinburgh Postnatal Depression Scale [2].

Laboratory investigations: no specific lab tests are routinely indicated; however, tests to rule out mood disorders secondary to other causes may be indicated based on patient's history and symptoms (*eg*, delirium, alcohol or drug abuse, or endocrine disturbance [especially thyroid]).

Complications

Impairment of bonding to child and care of child.

Impairment of social, familial, occupational functioning.

Suicide risk.

Infanticide risk: with delusional illness.

• Postpartum psychosis is an emergency, requiring hospitalization and aggressive treatment with psychotropics and/or electroconvulsive therapy.

Differential diagnosis

Postpartum delirium.

Maternity blues (lasts <2 wk after child-birth; >60% of new mothers have it).

Postpartum minor depression (2–5 symptoms of major depression or symptoms secondary to stressors).

Postpartum brief psychotic disorder.

Etiology

Biologic factors: familial; major fall in gonadal hormones PP and the potential effects on neurotransmitters.

Psychosocial factors: major life changes with childbirth including changing roles for patient.

Other risk factors: prior mood disorder (especially prior to PPMD or premenstrual dysphoric disorder), family history of mood disorder (especially bipolar disorder), maternity blues (15%–20% continue into PPMD), depression and anxiety during pregnancy, recent adverse life event, marital discord or lack of social support.

Epidemiology

• Incidence of postpartum nonpsychotic mood disorder is 10%–15% as index episode of a mood disorder. It is higher in adolescent mothers.

• Incidence increases to 25% with past history of a mood disorder and is greater if there is a history of bipolar disorder.

• Incidence increases to 35% with past history of PPMD and is greater if there is a history of psychotic mood disorder.

• Incidence of postpartum psychosis is 1–2:1000 births (>70% are mood disorders).

Treatment

Diet and lifestyle.
- Adequate self-care is encouraged, including diet and sleep.
- Recruitment of family and social support is important.

Pharmacologic treatment [3]

For unipolar depression

Standard dosage	Selective serotonin reuptake inhibitors [SSRIs], DOSAGE or
	Secondary amine tricyclics, DOSAGE.
Contraindications	Pregnancy category C.
Main side effects	*SSRIs:* gastrointestinal (*eg*, anorexia, diarrhea), sexual dysfunction, agitation, insomnia.
	Secondary amine tricyclics: anticholinergic effects, cardiac dysrhythmia (higher levels or underlying cardiac disease).
Main drug interactions	*SSRIs:* Monoamine oxidase inhibitors (MAOIs); hepatic cytochrome P_{450} isoenzyme inhibition caused by SSRIs may lead to various drug interactions.
	Secondary amine tricyclics: MAOIs.

For bipolar disorder

Standard dosage	Lithium, DOSAGE (titrate to therapeutic blood levels).
	Valproic acid, DOSAGE (titrate to therapeutic blood levels), or
	Carbamazepine, DOSAGE (titrate to therapeutic blood levels).
Contraindications	*Lithium:* major renal disease, in nursing mothers because infant levels are 33%–50% of mother's level (*see* Main drug interactions below); pregnancy category D.
	Valproic acid: hepatic disease; pregnancy category D
	Carbamazepine: past bone marrow depression; pregnancy category C.
Main side effects	*Lithium:* diarrhea, tremors; caution with concomitant diuretic use.
	Valproic acid: gastrointestinal distress, sedation.
	Carbamazepine: sedation, unsteadiness.
Main drug interactions	*Carbamazepine:* possibly MAOIs.

For psychotic symptoms

Standard dosage	Neuroleptics, *eg*, haloperidol (5–15 mg/d).
Contraindications	Pregnancy category C.
Special points	*Neuroleptics:* Neuroleptic malignant syndrome with hyperpyrexia, autonomic instability, muscle rigidity.

Although newer psychotropic agents may have lesser side effects or more specificity, there is relatively limited experience with these agents; thus, their efficacy and safety (*eg*, long-term effects of neonatal exposure) are not well established in postpartum disorders. See product literature for cautions concerning breast-feeding mothers because they may cause infant side effects.

Treatment aims
To effectively treat the mood disorder.
To restore normal functioning.

Nonpharmacologic treatment
Interpersonal psychotherapy: for 12 wk to address the various role changes and interpersonal conflicts that may arise in the postpartum time and to empower the patient to seek viable solutions to her problems.
Electroconvulsive therapy: for severe depression with suicidality or psychosis may be safer and give a faster treatment response; it may also be preferred in some cases in which breast feeding is desired.

Prognosis
- PPMD increases the likelihood of future postpartum and nonpostpartum mood episodes especially if past postpartum psychotic episodes occurred (*see also* Epidemiology).
- Consider prophylactic postpartum treatment with lithium or anticonvulsant if history of postpartum bipolar disorder or antidepressants if history of postpartum unipolar depression.

Follow-up and management
- Closely follow up every 1 2 wk, depending on severity until symptoms improve significantly.
- Continue treatment for at least 1 y after remission. Risk period is up to 2 y postpartum.

Key references
1. *Diagnostic and Statistical Manual of Mental Disorders,* ed 4. Washington, DC: American Psychiatric Association; 1994.
2. Cox JL, Holden JM, Sagovsky R: Detection of postnatal depression: development of the 10-item Edinburgh Postnatal Depression Scale. *Br J Psychiatry* 1987, 150:782–786.
3. Stowe ZN, Nemeroff CB: Women at risk for postpartum-onset major depression. *Am J Obstet Gynecol* 1995, 173:639–645.

Diagnosis

Signs and symptoms

Painful reexperiencing of event.

Pattern of avoidance.

Emotional numbing.

Relatively constant hyperarousal.

Panic attacks and/or dissociation states.

Illusions and hallucinations: possible.

Attention impairment.

Aggression, violence, poor impulse control, depression, and substance-related disorders.

Distress in social, occupational, and familial functions.

• Symptoms may occur months or years after event and last at least 4 weeks.

• Risk factors include assault, combat experience, concentration camps, natural catastrophes, rape, serious accidents.

Investigations

Minnesota Multiphasic Personality Inventory: elevated Sc, D, F, and Ps scores.

Rorschach: aggression and violent material.

Diagnostic Interview Scale.

Complications

Suicide: increased rate

Distress to others in social network.

Impairment in occupational function.

Differential diagnosis

Head injury.
Epilepsy.
Substance-related disorders, including alcohol.
Anxiety disorders.
Pain disorder.
Personality disorder (especially borderline).
Factitious disorder.
Malingering.

Etiology

Subjective response to stressor.
Vulnerability (childhood trauma, personality disorders [eg, borderline, paranoid, dependent, antisocial]).
Inadequate support system.
Genetic predisposition.
Stressful life changes.
Secondary gain: money, sympathy, dependence.
Excessive alcohol use.
Hyperactivity.

Epidemiology

Lifetime prevalence, 9%
Lifetime prevalence of exposure to a traumatic event, 39%
Percentage of patients receiving treatment, 5%
Lifetime prevalence for male Vietnam vets, 30%
Lifetime prevalence for female Vietnam vets, 26%

Treatment

General information
• The patient should be engaged in therapy as soon as possible after the event.

Diet and lifestyle
Healthy nutritious diet.

Rest and exercise.

Pharmacologic treatment
• Antidepressants, especially selective serotonin-reuptake inhibitors (*eg*, fluoxetine, paroxetine, sertraline, fluvoxamine) and monoamine oxidase inhibitors (phenelzine, tranylcypromine) are often helpful.

• Other potentially useful agents include carbamazepine, valproic acid, beta-blockers, clonidine, lithium, and benzodiazepines.

Nonpharmacologic treatment
Group and individual therapy.

Psychotherapy.

Hypnosis.

Support groups.

Destigmatization and desensitization.

Treatment aims
To establish support.

To promote acceptance of event.

To provide educational information.

To meet health needs.

Follow-up and management
• For pharmacologic treatment, treat patients for 8 wk with maintenance for 1 y.

• For nonpharmacologic treatment, treat patients for at least 1 y.

• Hospitalization may trigger reoccurrence of posttraumatic stress disorder (eg, nightmares, flashbacks, and episodes).

• Seventy percent to 80% of patients drop out of therapy or are noncompliant.

General references
Consultation Psychiatry, ed 2. Edited by Wise M, Rundell J. Washington, DC: American Psychiatric Association; 1994.

Gersons BPR, Carlier IVE: Post-traumatic stress disorder: the history of a recent concept. *Br J Psychiatry* 1992, 161:742–748.

Paige SR, Reid GM, Allen MG, Newton JEO: Psychophysiological correlates of posttraumatic stress disorder in Vietnam veterans. *Biol Psychiatry* 1990, 27:419–430.

Psychiatry, ed 5. Edited by Tomb D. Baltimore: Williams & Wilkins; 1995.

Synopsis of Psychiatry. Edited by Kaplan H, Sadock B. Baltimore: Williams & Wilkins; 1995.

Tomb D: The phenomenology of post traumatic stress disorder. *Psychiatr Clin North Am* 1994, 17:237–250.

Diagnosis

Symptoms

Mental retardation: mild in 60% of patients; moderate in 30%.

Hypotonia, developmental delay: early feeding difficulties secondary to hypotonia

Self-injurious behavior: *eg*, picking at skin.

Speech delay, articulation problems, hypernasal speech.

Food-related behavior problems: *eg*, excessive appetite, absence of satiation, obsession with eating; usually starting in early childhood.

Other behavior problems: *eg*, perseveration, poor control of temper; become more frequent in later childhood.

High pain threshold.

Signs

Infantile hypotonia: with initial failure to thrive

Morbid obesity: onset usually midchildhood.

Short stature: postnatal onset.

Small hands and feet.

Facies.

Almond-shaped eyes.

Upslanting palpebral fissures.

Strabismus.

Hypogonadism: micropenis and cryptorchidism; hypogonadotropism with delayed puberty, infertility

Hypopigmentation.

Esotropia, myopia.

Investigations

Genetic

• In 100% of Prader–Willi syndrome cases, the cause is an alteration of the PWS/AS gene locus at chromosome 15q11-13.

• In 70%, there is a loss of the paternally contributed critical region (diagnosed by cytogenetic or FISH studies of chromosome 15).

• In 25%, there is maternal uniparental disomy of chromosome 15 (diagnosed by DNA methylation studies).

• In 5% of patients, there is a chromosomal translocation or abnormality (diagnosed by chromosomal karyotyping).

• Blood should be sent for routine high-resolution banded-chromosome analysis and for DNA diagnostic studies by a laboratory specializing specifically in diagnosing this syndrome.

Other

• Secondary endocrinopathies should be screened for follicle-stimulating and leutinizing hormones (hypogonadotropism) and glucose (diabetes mellitus).

Complications

Early hypotonia and late morbid obesity: *eg*, sleep apnea, type II diabetes mellitus.

Osteoporosis: in most adults and teens.

Differential diagnosis
Albright hereditary osteodystrophy.
Bardet–Biedl syndrome.
Laurence–Moon–Biedel syndrome.
Cohen syndrome.

Etiology
• The cause is an alteration of the PRS/AS gene locus at chromosome 15q11-13. This is an "imprinted" region that requires properly functioning genes from both maternal and paternal lines.

Epidemiology
• Occurs in ~1:10,000 newborns in equal frequency in both sexes, with ascertainment bias toward male diagnosis.

Treatment

General information

- Management of Prader–Willi syndrome differs for infants, children, and adults.
- In adults, psychosis, obsessive–compulsive behavior, and mood disorders occur in increased frequency; management of these disorders in Prader–Willi syndrome is the same as for the general population.

Diet and lifestyle

Infants
Special feeding techniques: due to hypotonia.

Children
Nutritional counseling: caloric intake of 1000–1200 kcal/d.

Appropriate educational services.

Adults
Diet and exercise control: obesity is the major cause of morbidity and mortality.

Optimal living and employment situations: promote optimal behavior and weight control; affected individuals usually require a sheltered employment environment. Issues of guardianship should be investigated.

Pharmacologic treatment

Children
Deficient sex hormone replacement.

Calcium supplementation: for osteoporosis.

Growth hormones: trials currently ongoing.

Psychopharmacologic agents: trials are ongoing.

Nonpharmacologic treatment

Infants
Early-intervention physical therapy.

Screening for strabismus.

Children
Speech therapy.

Endocrinology evaluation.

Adults
Genetic counseling.

Treatment aims
To increase functioning and quality of life of affected individual and family.
To screen for and treat secondary medical problems.

Prognosis
- Morbidity and mortality are secondary to complications of early hypotonia (aspiration) or late morbid obesity (coronary artery disease, hypertension, diabetes, sleep apnea)

Follow-up and management
- Lifelong follow-up of medical and behavioral problems is necessary.

Support Groups
- Prader–Willi Syndrome Association (US) 2510 S. Brentwood Blvd., Suite 220 St. Louis, MO 63144-2326 Phone: 800-926-4797 Internet: http://athenet.net/-pwsa_usa/index.html
- PWS International Information Forum 40 Holly Lane Roslyn Heights, NY 11577 Phone: 800-358-0682
- The Prader–Willi Connection http://www.pwsyndrome.com
- Prader–Willi Foundation on the Internet http://ww.prader-willi.inter.net
- Genline: Prader–Willi Syndrome http://www.hslib.washington.edu/genline/pws.html

General references
Diagnostic testing for Prader-Willi and Angleman syndromes: report of the ASHG/ACMG Test and Technology Transfer Committee. *Am J Hum Genetics* 1996, 58:1085–1088.

Greenswag LR, Alexander RA (eds): *Management of Prader-Willi Syndrome*, ed 2. New York: Springer-Verlag; 1995.

Nicholls RD. New insights reveal complex mechanisms involved in genomic imprinting [editorial; comment]. *Am J Hum Genetics* 1994, 54:733–740.

Robinson WP, Bottani A, Xie YG, *et al.*: Molecular, cytogenetic, and clinical investigations of Prader-Willi syndrome patients. *Am J Hum Genetics* 1991, 49:1219–1234.

Diagnosis

Definition [1,2,3]

• The diagnosis of premature ejaculation (PE) has been complicated by various definitions. Partner satisfaction, number of thrusts, absolute time, and voluntary control have all been used as primary criteria. The DSM-IV definition of a "persistent or recurrent ejaculation with minimal sexual stimulation before, on, or shortly after penetration and before the person wishes it," is a clinically useful but ambiguous definition. Further research is needed to delineate specific subtypes, which undoubtedly comprise this heterogeneous population.

• The DSM-IV further suggests that the clinician take into account factors that affect duration of the excitement phase (eg, age, novelty of the sexual partner or situation, and recent frequency of sexual activity). The disturbance must cause marked distress or interpersonal difficulty and not be due exclusively to the direct effects of a substance (eg, withdrawal from opioids).

Lifelong versus acquired PE

• One should determine whether the condition is lifelong or developed after a period of normal functioning. Acquired forms are more often seen in older men and are frequently associated with erectile dysfunction. Lifelong PE is more common in younger men who are often less sexually experienced.

Global versus situational PE

• Some people may only have difficulty with a certain partner, type of partner, or specific sort of sexual activity, yet they may function normally with masturbation, other partners, or other activities. Situational PE may be more likely to have psychologic etiologies, but organic processes can still be contributing factors. Global dysfunction may result from either psychogenic or organic processes.

PE due to psychologic factors versus combined factors

• This is a difficult distinction to make, and undoubtedly, most cases are due to combined factors to some degree.

Investigations

Assessment for organic causes: although there are no specific tests for the condition, patients should have a general history and physical to help rule out organic causes (see Differential diagnosis); urology referral may be indicated if additional signs or symptoms of genitourinary system dysfunction are present.

Assessment for psychopathology: screen for other major psychiatric disorders; depressive and anxiety disorders are most commonly associated; psychiatric referral may be indicated depending on severity of symptoms.

Complications [4]

Relationship stress.

Impairment of procreation.

Exacerbation of any comorbid psychiatric conditions.

Differential diagnosis [4]

Organic injuries and illnesses: cardiovascular disease, diabetes, generalized neurologic disease, localized sensory impairment, trauma to sympathetic nervous from abdominal aortic aneurysm surgery, pelvic fractures, urologic pathology, prostatic hypertrophy, prostatitis, urethritis, arteriosclerosis, polyneuritis, local genitourinary disease, opioid withdrawal.

Less likely causes: spurious polycythemia, polyneuritis.

Relationship issues: discrepancy between partners in preferred latency to ejaculation.

Poor information: undereducated regarding "normal" latency to ejaculation that ranges from 5–15 min.

Etiology [1,4]

• Most researchers support the division of this heterogeneous population into at least two basic types: one predominantly biogenic and the other predominantly psychogenic. The current literature does not support a definitive causal factor. Limited data suggests that the following variables are associated with PE (although the direction of these relationships is controversial):

High levels of sexual anxiety.

Greater penile sensitivity.

A highly excitable bulbocavernosus reflex.

Typically younger, less experienced men and men who have sex infrequently.

Overarousal.

Lack of awareness of ejaculatory inevitability ("point of no return"); recent evidence contradicts this theory.

Inability or failure to monitor sexual arousal.

• Some theorists have suggested that males who make efforts to masturbate very quickly may increase their likelihood of PE. Evidence for this theory is mixed.

Epidemiology [1,4]

• With a 29% US prevalence, PE is the most common male sexual dysfunction.

• In Western cultures today, as many as 60% of men wish to prolong latency to orgasm. Interestingly, women who rapidly attain orgasm are not considered to have any dysfunction.

• Historically, rapid orgasm for males may have been considered a positive trait.

Treatment

Pharmacologic treatment [5]

Standard dosage	Selective serotonin-reuptake inhibitors (SSRIs), *eg*, sertraline (50–200 mg/d [mean dosage, 141 mg/d]), fluoxetine (20 mg every other day), or paroxetine (20–40 mg/d).
	Clomipramine, 50 mg/d.
Contraindications	*SSRIs*: relate mainly to potential drug interactions (*see* below).
	Clomipramine: recent myocardial infarction, ischemic heart disease, heart block.
Main side effects	*SSRIs*: gastrointestinal upset, anorexia, vomiting, diarrhea, agitation, insomnia, sexual dysfunction.
	Clomipramine: cardiac dysrhythmias (high levels or underlying cardiac disease), anticholinergic effects (*eg*, dry mouth, orthostasis, constipation, urinary retention), lower seizure threshold.
Main drug interactions	*All agents*: potentially fatal interaction with monoamine oxidase inhibitors; potentially fatal interaction with antiarrhythmic agents; serotonergic crisis (hypertension, hyperpyrexia, seizures) possible in patients on other serotonergic medications.
	SSRIs: hepatic cytochrome P_{450} isoenzyme inhibition, yielding a large number of potential drug interactions.
Special points	*SSRIs*: generally have fewer side effects and may be considered first-line agents, especially for patients on few or no other medications.
	Some patients report decreased intensity of orgasm and decreased desire as well as delay of orgasm.
	Following drug therapy alone, female partners are less likely than males to be satisfied with treatment outcome [2].

Treatment aims
To increase capacity for and enjoyment of sexual functioning.
To reduce level of distress or interpersonal difficulties primarily by helping them delay ejaculation.

Prognosis [4,5]
• With behavioral therapy alone, long-term outcome is questionable, although short-term outcome is positive. Initial-outcome studies of pharmacologic treatments appear promising; long-term–outcome studies are pending.

Follow-up and management
• Dosages of medicines should be titrated slowly in order to find the lowest effective dose. Different agents, even from the same class, may be tried because individual tolerance to side effects is highly variable.

Nonpharmacologic treatment [4]

Behavioral therapy: traditional modality that utilizes the stop/start and squeeze techniques; has been the gold standard for over twenty years.

Couples therapy: may be indicated in some cases, especially acquired PE; a significant number of men with PE have a sexually dysfunctional partner; however, sometimes there is no clear relationship between sexual and dyadic problems.

Education: most patients should receive some form of education about normal human sexuality; for mild cases, this may be all that is necessary; for more severe cases, further education within the context of one of the therapies above may be indicated.

Key references
1. Grenier G, Byers ES: Rapid ejaculation: a review of conceptual, etiological, and treatment issues. *Arch Sex Behavior* 1995, 24:447–473.
2. *Case Studies in Sex Therapy* Edited by Rosen RC, Leiblum SR. New York: The Guiliford Press; 1995.
3. *DSM-IV* Washington, DC: APA; 1995.
4. Metz ME, Pryor JL, Nesvacil LJ, *et al*.: Premature ejaculation: a psychophysiological review. *J Sex Marital Ther* 1997, 23:3–23.
5. Balon R: Antidepressants in the treatment of premature ejaculation. *J Sex Marital Ther* 1996, 22:85–96.

Diagnosis

Symptoms and signs [1]

• In most menstrual cycles, dysphoric symptoms (*eg*, depressed mood, anxiety, mood swings, irritability) have occurred during the 1–2 weeks before menses. Symptoms of premenstrual dysphoric disorder (PMDD) abate over menses, with no symptoms in the week after menses.

• In order for PMDD to be diagnosed, there must be 1) significant interference with school, work, or social activities or relationships; 2) confirmation by prospective, daily symptom logs over at least 2 symptomatic cycles; and 3) at least 4 of the following symptoms:

Decreased interest in activities.

Increased or decreased appetite with cravings for sweets or salt.

Decreased concentration.

Decreased energy.

Increased or decreased sleep.

Feeling overwhelmed/out of control.

Physical symptoms: *eg*, breast pain, bloating, headaches.

Investigations

Scales: some form of prospective, rating log of the endorsed premenstrual syndrome (PMS) symptoms must be kept to confirm time of occurrence of symptoms with respect to the menstrual cycle [2].

Laboratory and physical examinations: none routinely indicated; physical evaluation and investigations may be indicated to rule out other medical illnesses that may mimic PMS physical symptoms (*eg*, hypothyroidism, endometriosis, anemia).

Screen for comorbidity of depressive and anxiety disorders.

Complications

Increased risk of future mood disorders especially depression.

Increased risk of future reproductively-related mood disorders: *eg*, PPMD, perimenopausal depression.

Impairment in occupational or social functioning and family or social relationships.

Differential diagnosis

PMS (more common, transient syndrome associated with mild physical and psychologic symptoms that occur before and during menses).
Premenstrual exacerbation of current psychiatric disorders (especially mood, anxiety, or other disorders [*eg*, eating disorders, personality disorders]).
Premenstrual exacerbation of current medical disorders (*eg*, hypothyroidism, endometriosis, anemia, and migraine).

Etiology

Genetic vulnerability (familial).
Serotonergic dysregulation.
Gonadal hormone dysregulation.
Stress (current or earlier in life).
• Risk factors for PMDD include:
Prior episodes of mood or anxiety disorder (particularly depression).
Prior episodes of reproductively related mood disorder (*eg*, postpartum mood disorder [PPMD]).
Family history of mood disorder, including reproductively related disorders (*eg*, depression, PMDD, PPMD).

Epidemiology

• Percentage of women who meet criteria for PMDD is 3%–8%.
• Percentage of women with PMDD who have past history of depressive illness is 30%–70%.
• Symptoms can be present from menarche to menopause, but they usually occur in 30s and 40s and may worsen with age.

Treatment

Diet and lifestyle

Education: retiming of symptoms to menstrual cycle and their variable presence and severity over time; diet and exercise should be optimized (*see* below).

Diet: decrease refined sugars, salt, caffeine, and alcohol; consume small and frequent meals; increase complex carbohydrates.

Regular aerobic exercise: throughout menstrual cycle.

Stress management: to attempt to decrease potential stressors as feasible, especially premenstrually.

Pharmacologic treatment [3]

• Medication is targeted at the predominant problematic symptoms for the duration needed.

During premenstrual and luteal phases only

• Alprazolam may be adequate for treating symptoms of irritability, mild depression, anxiety, and insomnia during the premenstruum, with tapering off over menses.

Standard dosage	0.25–0.50 mg three times daily.
Contraindications	May have potential drug interactions secondary to inhibition of hepatic cytochrome P_{450} isoenzyme system; pregnancy category D.
Main side effects	Sedation, fatigue.
Special points	Use caution when escalating alprazolam in patients with a history of alcohol or drug abuse.

Throughout menstrual cycle

• Selective serotonin-reuptake inhibitors have been uniquely effective for treatment of moderate to severe depression and other mood symptoms that may last for 1–3 weeks of the cycle.

Standard dosage	Fluoxetine 20–60 mg,
	Sertraline 50–150 mg, or
	Paroxetine 10–30 mg.
Contraindications	May have potential drug interactions secondary to inhibition of hepatic cytochrome P_{450} isoenzyme system; pregnancy category C.
Main side effects	Nausea, cramping, diarrhea, agitation, insomnia, sexual dysfunction.
Main drug interactions	Monoamine oxidase inhibitors.

Treatment aims

To eliminate symptoms or diminish them to the degree that they do not cause significant impairment of occupational, social, and relationship functioning.

Prognosis

• The natural course of this disorder without treatment is the presence or absence of symptoms for months to years at a stretch, with onset or offset potentially linked to times of reproductive hormone flux, stress, or other factors.
• Symptom severity appears to be absent or diminished during anovulatory cycles.

Follow-up and management

• Efficacy of each treatment trial should be assessed over 2–3 cycles using daily rating logs of symptoms.
• Effective treatment should be continued for 6 mo or more, depending on continued presence of symptoms.

Key references

1. *Diagnostic and Statistical Manual of Mental Disorders*, ed 4. Washington, DC: American Psychiatric Association; 1994.
2. Chandraiah S: Premenstrual syndrome. In *Women's Medicine*. Edited by Blackwell RE. Cambridge, MA: Blackwell Science, Inc; 1996.
3. Yonkers KA, Brown WA: Pharmacologic treatment for premenstrual dysphoric disorder. *Psychiatr Ann* 1996, 26:586–589.

Diagnosis

Definition

• Psychotic depression is a form of major depression seen as a distinct subtype or even a separate illness because of its differences in severity, outcome, biologic abnormalities, and effective forms of treatment [1,2]. Psychosis can be seen in episodes of either unipolar or bipolar (manic–depressive) depression.

Signs and symptoms

• An episode meets DSM-IV criteria for major depression if the following are present:

1. Predominantly depressed mood or loss of interest and pleasure

2. Fatigue, thoughts of death or suicide, appetite disturbance, sleep disturbance, worthlessness or guilt, and poor concentration (at least three must be present).

3. Psychotic signs: delusions and/or hallucinations with occasional disorganization of thought processes (eg, loose associations); based on their compatibility with depressive thinking and mood, delusions and hallucinations can be mood congruent (eg, the belief that one has committed an unforgivable sin) or mood incongruent (eg, the belief that one's actions are controlled by space aliens).

• Risk factors include previous episodes of major depression with psychosis, depression in a bipolar patient, and family history of depression with psychosis or other psychotic disorders.

Investigations

General history, physical examination: to rule out medical illnesses (causative or comorbid); substance abuse and dependence should be ruled out and should be treated even if not the cause of illness per se.

Interview with the patient, family members, or other informants: to make sure psychosis is not underdiagnosed in patients with depression.

History of mania or hypomania: should be sought because psychosis is common in bipolar depression.

Complications

Suicide: may be more likely than in depression overall [2].

Potential harm to others: especially if patient has the delusion that others are also hopeless or doomed, and especially if the patient experiences auditory hallucinations encouraging harm to others.

Functional impairment: long-term disability; more likely than in depression without psychosis; patients with psychotic depression may have more impairment on neuropsychologic tests [3].

Differential diagnosis

Schizoaffective disorder (distinguished by persistence of psychosis when depression is in remission).

Schizophrenia with depressive symptoms (post-psychotic depression seen in some schizophrenic patients).

Depression caused by a medical or neurologic illness (eg, severe hypothyroidism, AIDS, stroke).

Depression caused by or complicated by substance intoxication or withdrawal.

Dissociative disorders (eg, posttraumatic stress disorders) producing hallucination-like phenomena and coexisting with depression.

Etiology

• A specific cause is not known.

• A genetic vulnerability to psychosis may be inherited separately from liability to depression.

• Biologic abnormalities seen in depression overall are more common in psychotic depression.

• Hypercortisolemia and dexamethasone nonsuppression are likely [4].

• Altered monoamine (serotonin, topapamine, and norepinephrine) neurotransmission has been hypothesized in all mood disorders. Evidence exists for specific dopaminergic abnormalities in psychosis.

Epidemiology

• Major depression is seen in 6%–18% of the population (lifetime prevalence).

• Psychotic features are seen in 14%–25% of patients with major depressive episodes.

• Male-to-female ratio is 1:2 for depression overall and roughly the same for depression with psychosis.

Treatment

Diet and lifestyle
• Avoid alcohol and drugs of abuse. Maintain physical activity and self-care activities.

Pharmacologic treatment
• This illness requires biologic treatments. Antidepressants alone have been relatively ineffective, as have antipsychotics alone [5]. Accepted treatments include combinations of both agents at therapeutic doses.

• Tricyclic antidepressants (eg, amitriptyline, imipramine, or desipramine [~150 mg/d and up], or nortriptyline [to obtain blood levels of 50–150 mg/mL]) in combination with conventional antipsychotics (eg, phenothiazines or haloperidol [5–15 mg/d]) have been used since the 1960s. These agents frequently cause serious adverse effects (eg, orthostatic hypotension, anticholinergic effects, sedation, and cardiac conduction delays with tricyclics; acute extrapyramidal effects and tardive dyskinesia with long-term use of neuroleptics).

• Most clinicians now prefer to combine newer antidepressants (eg, the selective serotonin-reuptake inhibitors [fluoxetine, sertraline, and paroxetine], bupropion, venlafaxine, nefazodone, or mirtazepine) with newer antipsychotics (eg, risperidone, quetiapine, or olanzepine) to take advantage of the more benign side-effect profiles of each class. These combinations have been found effective in a clinical experience, but rigorous controlled studies have yet to be performed.

• Patients whose depressive episode is part of a bipolar disorder need a mood stabilizer (eg, as lithium, carbamazepine, or valproate) titrated to therapeutic blood levels.

Nonpharmacologic treatment
• Electroconvulsive therapy (ECT) is a useful treatment option not only for medication-resistant episodes but as a first-line treatment [1]. A full course of ECT (usually 6–12 treatments) often brings about a faster remission than medication, and with appropriate modification (muscle relaxation, oxygenation, monitoring), is quite safe. ECT is especially useful when the psychotic depressive episode is complicated by intense suicidality, agitation, stupor, dehydration, or malnutrition from poor oral intake.

• Because of the overall severity of the illness and the risk of suicide, hospitalization is generally preferred for initiation of treatment and stabilization.

• Psychosocial therapies are most useful after the acute episode has been treated. Issues that can impede full recovery or predispose to relapse (eg, demoralization, poor interpersonal skills, poor insight into the illness, and family problems) should be considered.

Treatment aims
To obtain a full remission of symptoms.
To prevent relapse.

Prognosis
• Recovery is likely with aggressive treatment, but long-term outcome is not as favorable as in nonpsychotic depression.
• Prognosis is better for patients with mood-congruent psychotic symptoms than for those having mood-incongruent delusions or hallucinations.
• Recurrence of depression after recovery is likely. Not all these recurrences will also be psychotic, but psychosis during a recurrence is more common in patients who have had a previous psychotic episode than in those who have never been psychotic.

Follow-up and management
• Intensive follow-up treatment is important because the relapse rate is high.
• Maintenance with antidepressants at therapeutic doses is a cornerstone, and patients who have had several episodes may respond to prophylactic lithium even if they have never had a manic episode.
• Long-term treatment with antipsychotic medication is desirable only when symptoms cannot be adequately controlled with antidepressants alone.

Key references
1. Coryell W: Psychotic depression. *J Clin Psychiatry* 1996, 57(suppl 3):27–31.
2. Dubovsky S, Thomas M: Psychotic depression: advances in conceptualization and treatment. *Hosp Community Psychiatry* 1992, 93:1189–1198.
3. Jeste DV, Henton SC, Paulsen S, *et al.*: Clinical and neuropsychological comparison of psychotic depression and schizophrenia. *Am J Psychiatry* 1996, 153:490–496.
4. Nelson JC, Davis JM: DST studies in psychotic depression: a meta-analysis. *Am J Psychiatry* 1997, 154:1497–1503.
5. Spiker DG, Weiss JC, Dealy RS, *et al.*: The pharmacological treatment of delusional depression. *Am J Psychiatry* 1985, 142:430–436.

Diagnosis

Definition
• Pyromania is an impulse control disorder that leads to the recurrent deliberate and purposeful setting of fires in the absence of an ulterior motive, involving tension release or urge gratification and a fascination or attraction to fires and their aftermath.

Symptoms and signs
• Some patients report prolonged advance preparation before the act, thereby suggesting a "compulsive" component.

• Remorse may be present or absent.

DSM-IV diagnositc criteria
1. Deliberate and purposeful fire setting on more than one occasion.

2. Tension or affective arousal before the act.

3. Fascination with, interest in, curiosity about, or attraction to fire and its situational contexts (*eg*, paraphernalia, uses, consequences).

4. Pleasure, gratification, or relief when setting fires, or when witnessing or participating in their aftermath.

5. The fire setting is not done for monetary gain (*ie*, as an expression of sociopolitical ideology, to conceal criminal activity, to express anger or vengeance, to improve one's living circumstances, in response to delusion or hallucination, or as a result of impaired judgement [*eg*, in dementia, mental retardation, substance intoxication]).

6. The fire setting is not better accounted for by conduct disorder, manic episode, or antisocial personality disorder.

Investigations
Psychologic testing
Minnesota Multiphasic Personality Inventory-2: scales 4 (psychopathic deviate) and 9 (hypomania) are often elevated in those with history of impulsivity; problems with impulse control are likely when scale 4 is 10 or more T points higher than scale 3 (hysteria).

Millon Clinical Multiaxial Inventory-III: expected scale elevations include scale 5 (narcissistic), 6A (antisocial), 6B (sadistic), 7 (compulsive), C (borderline).

Complications
Comorbidity
Alcoholism and other drug abuse.

Personality disorders other than antisocial: usually pyromania laden with insecurity and narcissistic issues.

Affective and anxiety disorders: obsessive-compulsive spectrum?

Other tension-discharging behaviors: stealing, running away, truancy, sexual activity, psychosexual dysfunction, resentment of authority figures.

• Meeting the criteria for pyromania does not exclude a second diagnosis.

Behavioral outcomes
• This disorder is the most endangering to lives and property of all the impulse-control disorders.

• Some patients have set fires within their institutional placement.

• Justice system actions are common; court-mandated treatment arrangements are often important in case management.

Differential diagnosis
• Rule out other causes of fire-setting as follows:
A specific purposeful motive (criterion E), eg, profit, sabotage, revenge, concealment of crime, political statement.
A developmental experimentation of childhood (criterion E)
A consequence of impaired judgement (criterion E), eg, influence of delusions or hallucinations, dementia or mental retardation, substance intoxication (very common).
Another mental disorder in which fire-setting might be an associated feature (criterion F), eg, conduct disorder, manic episode, antisocial personality disorder.

Etiology
• There is no known etiology, but preliminary evidence of biologic factors exist:
Low cerebrospinal fluid 5-hydroxyindoleacetic acid level.
Low cerebrospinal fluid MHPG.
Reactive hypoglycemic traits.
Brain and electoencephalographic abnormalities (scant reports).
• Factors often associated include poor academic performance, learning disabilities, attention-deficit disorders, speech problems, visual and other physical defects, enuresis, cruelty to animals.
• Increased prevalence in family history exists for alcoholism, divorce, lower income, increased frequency of adoptions.

Epidemiology
• The average number of those arrested who are <10 y of age is 7%; 11–15 y of age, 43%; 16–25 y of age, 15%; >26 y of age, 35%.
• Most fire-setting does not qualify for pyromania.
• Approximately half of arson arrests in the United States are individuals under age 18, usually associated with conduct disorder, attention deficit hyperactivity disorder or adjustment disorder.
• Approximately 90% of pyromania occurs in males.
• The prevalence within the general opulation appears to be rather rare, but the majority of arson cases are never resolved.
• The prevalence within the clinical psychiatric population has been estimated to be from 2%–15%.

Treatment

General information

- Treatment success is difficult to validate because of the waxing and waning intermittent course of illness, incomplete criminal justice measurements, suspect reliability of self-reporting, and inconsistent and uncontrolled methods of outcome evaluation in the clinical literature.
- Promote awareness of the consequences of fire-setting at both cognitive and affective levels ("overt sensitization"—visiting scenes of fires and burn units with the therapist).
- Promote heightened awareness of affect signals and recognition of prodromal arousal states.
- Treat comorbid conditions (*eg*, alcoholism, sexual conflict issues).
- Pay attention to any history of childhood trauma or abuse.
- Pay attention to the symbolic meaning of fire and fire-setting in the patient's case.
- Provide insight, object relations, and a sense of self and self-esteem.

Diet and lifestyle

- Supervise and instill accountability in patient.
- Provide structured living arrangements and interpersonal conflict management. Favor impulse avoidance.
- Teach supportive techniques, including problem-solving, social skills enhancement, and time scheduling.

Pharmacologic treatment

- Controlled pharmacologic treatment studies are lacking.
- No treatment approach has been shown to be superior to any other.
- The biological observations cited above offer a basis for treatment trials with selective serotonin reuptake inhibitors, antidepressants in general, and anticonvulsants.
- Comorbid conditions, *eg*, depression, anxiety, should be specifically treated.
- Disinhibiting medications (*eg*, benzodiazepines, barbiturates, and opiates), alcohol, and any other substances of abuse should be avoided.

Nonpharmacologic treatments

Psychotherapy

- There is no established treatment of choice.
- Small, uncontrolled series have demonstrated benefit from cognitive, behavioral, and family approaches, as well as psychodynamic therapy; none have used psychodynamic alone.
- Group therapy might benefit, on the basis of affective and interpersonal conflict factors (*see* below).
- Factors seen in reported cases include denial defense mechanisms; object-splitting defense mechanisms; lack of insight; rejection of self-responsibility; difficulty in recognition of feelings in self and others; a propensity to behave, rather than think and feel; situational distress, especially interpersonal; unmet nurturing needs (withheld love); rejection perceptions from parental or love-objects; perceptions of rivalry for parental love; feelings of shame, inadequacy, and helplessness; sexual conflicts; other comorbidities (*eg*, alcoholism).

Behavioral therapy

Behavioral approaches have included the following:

Aversive therapy.

Positive reinforcement with punishment provisions.

Stimulus satiation.

Operant structured fantasies with positive reinforcement.

Treatment aims

To achieve complete cessation of all fire-setting.

Prognosis

Better in those who can identify, verbalize, and work through conflicts in therapy; worse in those with poor capacity for insight or in those with comorbid psychiatric conditions.

- Incidence of relapse during treatment is unknown.
- The chronic and episodic clinical course complicates identification of remission and end of treatment.
- Outcome statistics specific to pyromania are lacking, but reported recidivism rates for treated cases of fire-setting range series from 2%–28%.

Other treatments

Criminal incarceration.

Follow-up and management

Close monitoring and supervision: for public safety and for the patient's clinical progress.

For the acute phase: institutional versus outpatient care.

For the continuation phase: no objective data exist regarding continuation considerations or end point of treatment definition.

General references

Diagnostic and Statistical Manual of Mental Disorders, ed 4. Washington, DC: American Psychiatric Association; 1994.

Kaplan HI, Sadock BJ: *Comprehensive Textbook of Psychiatry*, ed 6. Baltimore: Williams & Wilkins; 1995.

Treatments of Psychiatric Disorders. Washington, DC: American Psychiatric Association; 1989.

Treatments of Psychiatric Disorders, ed 2. Edited by Gabbard GO. Washington, DC: American Psychiatric Press; 1995.

Diagnosis

Definition, signs, and symptoms

• Reactive attachment disorder is a significant disturbance of relatedness beginning prior to 5 years of age. Grossly inadequate or inconsistent care can be either of the inhibited or disinhibited types. In the inhibited type, the child fails to initiate or respond to social interactions and may be excessively guarded, ambivalent, or resistant to comforting. In the disinhibited type, the child is indiscriminate and diffuse in social interactions and relatedness.

• Reactive attachment disorder may be comorbid with developmental delays related to environmental deprivation as well as feeding disorder, rumination disorder, or pica.

Investigations

Careful physical examination: to document concomitant medical problems, growth delay, or physical abuse

Laboratory studies: may show abnormalities related to malnutrition.

Complications

Growth delays.

Malnutrition.

Developmental problems: including language and cognitive delays.

Differential diagnosis

• The disorder is not due to an underlying developmental problem, such as mental retardation or pervasive developmental disorder.
• The developmental type is distinguished from attention deficit–hyperactivity disorder by the child's rapid social attachment.

Etiology

• Disorder is associated with severe emotional or physical neglect.
• There may have been frequent disruptions in primary caretaker or institutionalization.
• "Maltreatment syndrome" may be a more appropriate diagnostic label.

Epidemiology

• Estimated prevalence is 1%, but the syndrome has received little systematic attention.
• Predisposing factors may include severe prematurity with a complicated neonatal course.
• Congenital illness or abnormality, parental poverty, or mental illness.

Treatment

Diet and lifestyle
• Restoration of an adequate caregiver environment, including appropriate nutrition and safe predictable interaction with consistent caregivers, is essential

Pharmacologic treatment
• No pharmacologic treatment is recommended.

Nonpharmacologic treatment
• A multidisciplinary approach to address any medical cognitive or language problems should be instituted.

Individual psychodynamically oriented therapy: may be useful.

Family therapy, close monitoring by a social service agency, and mental health interventions for the parents.

Treatment aims
To achieve developmentally appropriate social interaction.
To improve medical and nutritional status and any cognitive or language delays.

General references
Richters MM, Volkmar F: Reactive attachment disorder of infancy or early childhood. *J Am Acad Child Adolesc Psychiatry* 1994, 33:328–332.

Spitz R: Hospitalism: an inquiry into the genesis of psychiatric conditions in early childhood. *Psychoanal Study Child* 1945, 1:53–74.

Zeanah CH, Mammen OK, Lieberman AF: Disorders of attachment. In *Handbook of Infant Mental Health.* Edited by Zeanah CH. New York: Guilford Press; 1993:332–349.

Diagnosis

General information

• DSM-IV nomenclature and description are not widely accepted. The condition is appropriately termed Rett syndrome.

Symptoms

Stagnation in developmental milestones between 6–18 months: normal pre- and perinatal period and apparently normal early development; thereafter, previously acquired skills are lost, including purposeful hand use, speech, and socialization; if walking has been achieved, gait becomes apraxic and nonpurposeful.

Prominent irritability with periods (often extended) of unprovoked screaming.

Fragmented sleep: may be punctuated by periods of irritability or even laughter without apparent reason.

Bruxism (teeth grinding) and drooling: prominent.

Slow and tedious feeding: with poor chewing skills; constipation may occur.

Cool or cold hands and feet: may even be bluish in color.

Indifference or delayed response to pain: common.

Periodic breathing (breath holding, hyperventilation, or both): may begin between 12–36 months, often preceded by forced expulsion of air or puffing. Air swallowing (bloating) may also occur.

Seizures: consisting of staring spells, complex partial events, or generalized tonic-clonic movements, typically begin after 2 years of age.

Signs

Deceleration in growth rate: head grown may begin decelerating as early as 3 months of age, followed by deceleration in weight gain and linear growth.

Development of stereotypic movements: *eg*, hand washing, wringing, and tapping and apparent in facial musculature and feet; the most prominent sign during the regression phase; alternatively, hand mouthing, picking at clothes, or even tapping the head may be seen; each girl expresses her own repertoire of stereotypies, evolving in type and cadence throughout life.

Hypotonia: typical during infancy, with gradual increasing in tone during childhood and often progressing to rigidity in later years; dystonic posturing is apparent in some and may be progressive.

Truncal ataxia and coarse tremor: may be present to variable degree.

Ambulation: preserved in the majority, although will never occur in ~20% of patients.

Scoliosis: a later sign, usually beginning after 5 years of age.

Investigations

• No specific diagnostic marker is available. It is important to rule out other conditions including inherited metabolic diseases.

Chromosome analysis with high-resolution banding and the FISH probe for Angelman syndrome: should be obtained.

Electroencephalography: preferably with video monitoring; helpful to differentiate seizures from "Rett" behaviors, which lack electrographic accompaniment.

Neuroimaging: *ie*, cranial computed tomograpgy or magnetic resonance imaging; may help exclude a leukodystrophy, neurocutaneous disorder, or metabolic disorder.

Complications

Profound growth deficiency with failure to thrive.

Constipation with impaction.

Progressive scoliosis and other orthopedic deformities.

Differential diagnosis

Autism: girls with Rett syndrome do not fulfill strict criteria for autism. Static encephalopathy (cerebral palsy): the pattern of progression in Rett syndrome would be atypical for a static encephalopathy. Angelman syndrome: acquired deceleration in head growth noted, but happy demeanor, facial features, and often problematic seizures should differentiate from Rett syndrome. Neurocutaneous disorders: mainly tuberous sclerosis, infantile neuronal ceroid lipofuscinosis (especially in Nordic children), fragile X syndrome, and other neurometabolic diseases.

Etiology

• Rett syndrome is most certainly a genetic disorder. The specific mechanism is uncertain, although an X-linked dominant mechanism, lethal in males, is most plausible. Other mechanisms may be operative. Indeed, Rett syndrome may have more than a single etiology.

• The pathogenesis of Rett syndrome is unknown. The pattern of progression; absence of neuropathology seen in progressive disorders; and the combination of reduced brain weight, too small and closely packed cortical neurons, and reduced synaptic connections suggest fundamental interruptions in brain development and maturation. The pecise timing is uncertain, most likely late gestation or early postnatal because deceleration in head (brain) growth is apparent by 3 mo of age.

Epidemiology

• Rett syndrome is generally seen only in females.

• Prevalence rates range from 1:10,000 (in Sweden) to 1:22,000 (in Texas) females. The Swedish data include milder and later onset variants of Rett syndrome, comprising ~20% of the total. Nevertheless, prevalences exceed that for phenylketonuria in females. In the US, ~2500 girls or women are in the International Rett Syndrome Association database.

Treatment

Therapy

Treatment is supportive and symptomatic as no therapy is available to reverse the neurodevelopmental defects in Rett syndrome.

Diet: Feeding is often difficult as chewing and swallowing mechanisms are poorly coordinated. A softened, calorically-supplemented diet may be required. Occasionally, oral intake is so problematic that gastrostomy feeding is required for adequate nutrition. Constipation may be a major concern. Despite various strategies, best results have followed daily milk of magnesia (5-30 ml, usually at bedtime).

Seizures: Carbamazepine, 15 mg/kg/day in two-three doses with meals, has provided effective control with blood levels to 12 (g/ml. Alternatively, sodium valproate, 20-30 mg/kg/day in divided doses with meals (blood levels to 100-120 (g/ml) or Lamotrigine, initial dose of 0.5-1.0 mg/kg/day advancing incrementally every other week to 4-10 mg/kg/day (blood levels 4-20 (g/ml) in divided doses may be employed. Other antiepileptic agents may be considered as well.

Sleep: Occasionally, parents may request medication to assist their daughter's sleep. Chloral hydrate, 20-40 mg/kg, has been helpful. Alternatively, hydroxyzine, 1 mg/kg, or diphenhydramine, 1-2 mg/kg may be effective. Significant tolerance may develop with the last two.

Main side effects

Carbamazepine: lethargy, agitation, leukopenia, skin rash, liver dysfunction, gastric upset.

Sodium valproate: tremor, gastric upset, excessive weight gain, hepatic dysfunction, hyperammonemia, skin rash, thrombocytopenia, agitation.

Lamotrigine: skin rash, especially in combination with sodium valproate.

Sedatives: Excessive sedation.

Main drug interactions

Lamotrigine is associated with significant skin rash and doses should be advanced slowly. In combination with sodium valproate, special caution should be exercised to avoid Stevens-Johnson syndrome. A number of agents elevate carbamazepine levels including erythromycin and related antibiotics, sodium valproate, isoniazid, and cimetidine. Conversely, carbamazepine may lower sodium valproate blood levels.

Nonpharmacologic treatment

Emphasis must be placed on appropriate physical and occupational therapy programs as well as integrated communication therapy to optimize socialization skills and take advantage of eye-pointing which is especially prominent beginning in school age.

Scoliosis may be sufficiently progressive to require surgical intervention. Braces or body jackets appear not to retard development of scoliosis significantly whereas orthotic devices have been effective in preventing deformities at the ankles. Regular assessment by a pediatric orthopedist familiar with Rett syndrome should be initiated by age 5 with periodic evaluations every 6-12 months thereafter. Similarly, a nutritionist should provide semiannual to annual assessments.

Treatment aims

To maintain adequate nutrition and proper bowel function.

To provide effective seizure control and to differentiate seizures from non-seizures so that unnecessary medications are avoided.

To promote appropriate physical, occupational, and educational interventions.

To monitor skeletal development and positioning and provide appropriate orthopedic interventions.

To provide support for the parents and other family members in dealing with this lifelong condition.

Prognosis

Prolonged survival is likely in Rett syndrome. Up to age 10, survival virtually parallels that of the 'normal' female population. By age 35, survival is about 75% versus >97% in 'normal' women. However, girls and women with Rett syndrome will not achieve independent living and up to 40% may not ambulate as adults. Thus, requirements for their care are significant and lifelong.

Long term management

Assessments by experienced physicians and allied health professionals should be conducted on a periodic basis, every 6 months during childhood and adolescence and annually thereafter. This will ensure proper medical management, nutrition, and other therapeutic modalities as well as avoid complications particularly with regard to orthopedic problems.

Key References

Armstrong DD. Review of Rett syndrome. J Neuropath Exp Neurol 1997;56:843-849.

Dure IV LS, Percy AK. The Rett syndrome: An overview. in, Disorders of Movement in Psychiatry and Neurology, Joseph AB, Young RR (eds), Blackwell Scientific Publications, Cambridge, 1998, in press.

Hagberg B. Rett syndrome: clinical peculiarities and biological mysteries. Acta Paediatr 1995;84:971-976.

Percy AK. Neurobiology and neurochemistry of Rett syndrome. Europ Child & Adolesc Psychiatr 1997;6:80-82.

Sekul EA, Percy AK. Rett syndrome: clinical features, genetic considerations, and the search for a biological marker. Current Neurology 1992;12:173-200.

RUMINATION DISORDER

Diagnosis

General information
• Rumination disorder was formerly thought to be a disorder of infancy but is now recognized as being present in all age groups. It is more commonly seen in association with mental retardation, anorexia nervosa, and bulimia nervosa in adolescents and adults. It may also be seen as a reaction to psychosocial stressor in children and adolescents. In such cases, rumination may be self-limited.

Symptoms and signs
Repeated regurgitation and rechewing of food.

Onset after a period of normal functioning (feeding); persists for at least 1 month.

Partially digested food brought into the mouth without apparent nausea, retching, or disgust.

Food either reswallowed following chewing or ejected from the mouth.

In infants
Characteristic posture of straining and arching the back with the head held back, abdominal contractions, and sucking movements of the tongue.

Pleasure from self-stimulating activity.

• Symptoms may occur during or after feeding, often after the child has been put down.

Investigations

History
Careful feeding history: including who feeds the child, positioning, presence of others, levels of stimulation in the environment, and rate of feeding.

Identification of recent physical illnesses or psychosocial stressors.

Length of time between feedings and rumination, frequency of ruminations.

Methods used by the child to initiate ruminations: *eg*, fingers or fist in mouth, rocking, characteristic posturing.

Examination
Physical examination: no pathognomic signs present.

Observation of infants during and after feeding best method of diagnosis.

Attention to maternal–infant interaction during feeding.

Observation of several feedings: may be needed.

Laboratory investigations
• Rule out physiologic causes of vomiting. Consider the following investigations:

Barium esophagraphy (swallow) or upper GI series.

24-hour esophageal pH monitoring.

Esophagascopy.

Complications
Malnutrition.

Dehydration.

Electrolyte disturbances.

Mortality rate of up to 25% in infants with failure to thrive due to rumination.

Maternal aversion: due to disgust over regurgitated food.

Dental decay.

Aspiration pneumonia.

Anemia.

Differential diagnosis
Pyloric stenosis.
Gastroesophageal reflux disease (GERD).
Gastrointestinal infections.
"Normal" vomiting of early infancy.
• Not diagnosed if it occurs exclusively during the course of anorexia or bulimia nervosa.

Etiology
May be precipitated by physical illness or psychosocial stressor.
Understimulation or neglect by caregiver.
Self-soothing/self-stimulating behavior in infants or the mentally retarded.
Habitual behavior.
"Familial ruminators": have been described.

Epidemiology
Prevalence, incidence, and gender distribution not known.
Described as "rare" and "uncommon."
Male-to-female ratios, from 1:1 to as high as 5:1.
Typical age of infant onset, 3–12 months (may be later in mentally retarded).
Childhood onset in reaction to psycho-social stressor.

Treatment

Diet and lifestyle
• Thickened formulas and foods may be of some benefit.

Pharmacologic treatment
• There is no specific pharmacologic treatment.
• If severe and refractory, treat as GERD.

Nonpharmacologic treatment
Maternal–infant interactions enhancement during feedings.

Erect posture during and immediately after feedings.

Distraction reduction during feedings.

Interruption and distraction at onset of rumination.

Modeling of appropriate feeding and interactive behaviors by professional staff (eg, nurses).

Aversive conditioning: lemon juice or tobasco sauce on tongue at onset of rumination.

Maternal and/or family psychotherapy: if indicated.

Social services support: visiting nurse follow-up may be helpful for monitoring and sustaining of progress

Treatment aims
To maintain weight or appropriate weight gain.
To improve maternal–infant bond and family dynamics.
To provide a warm, nurturing environment.

Prognosis
• Psychosocial treatment of infants usually results in improvement in 1–2 wk.

General references
Chartoor et al.: Rumination: etiology and treatment. Pediatr Ann 1984, 13:924–929.

Franco et al.: Rumination: the eating disorder of infancy. Child Psychiatry Hum Dev 1993, 24:91–97.

Mayes et al.: Rumination disorder: differential diagnosis. J Am Acad Child Adolesc Psychiatry 1988, 27:300–302.

Parry-Jones B: Merycism or rumination disorder: a historical investigation and current assessment. Br J Psychiatry 1994, 165:303–314.

Reis S: Rumination in two developmentally normal children: case report and review of the literature. J Fam Pract 1994, 38:521–523.

Diagnosis

Definition

• Schizoaffective disorder is an uninterrupted period of psychotic illness, during which there is a concurrent major depression, manic episode, or mixed episode of depression and mania. Depressed mood must be present during depressive episode.

Symptoms and signs

Delusions or hallucinations: must occur during the episode for at least 2 weeks in the absence of prominent mood symptoms.

Schizophrenia criteria: 6 months of illness and two or more of the following symptoms for 1 month:

1. Delusions
2. Hallucinations
3. Disorganized speech
4. Disorganized or catatonic behavior
5. Negative symptoms

Mood disturbance: should be present for a substantial portion of the illness, including the active and residual phases.

Social and occupational functioning: impaired relative to status prior to onset of illness.

Continuous signs of the illness (for 6 mo) with prominent symptoms (for ≥1 mo or <1 mo if successfully treated).

Investigations

• Clinical assessment in the acute phase should include the following:

Complete psychiatric and general medical histories.

Mental status examination: essential.

Physical and neurologic examinations.

Interviews of collaterals: should be conducted unless the patient objects.

Laboratory studies: not routinely conducted, but when indicated, can include urine screen (for intoxicants or other substances that may induce psychosis or require detoxification), complete blood count, electrolytes and glucose levels, liver enzymes, renal function, thyroid function, and tests for sexually transmitted diseases.

Pregnancy testing (for women) and reproductive health screening.

Neuropsychologic testing: can be beneficial in cases of complicated differential diagnosis and comorbid neurologic disorder.

Neuroimaging and other extensive testing: usually not indicated unless the neurologic examination is abnormal.

Complications

Suicide: suicidal ideation should be evaluated with the focus on the presence of intent or plan, the lethality of the plan, and the presence of command hallucinations (auditory hallucinations [eg, voices urging the patient to harm self or others in cases of homicidal ideation]); a prior history of attempted suicide and coexistent substance abuse are major risk factors; delusions and other positive symptoms are associated with higher incidence of suicide [1]; incidence of completed suicide is 10%–13% over the lifetime for patients with schizophrenic spectrum disorders (50% may attempt).

Comorbid substance abuse: may be seen for nearly 50% of patients.

Homelessness: can be a result of the illness for various reasons for an estimated 12% of chronically ill schizophrenic-spectrum patients; estimates of homeless groups indicate that one third have mental illness, often schizophrenia.

Frequent hospitalizations: common; constitute a major social cost.

Differential diagnosis

• Substance-induced psychosis and contributory medical conditions have been excluded.

• Schizoaffective disorder can be distinguished from mood disorders with psychotic features by a discrete period of psychosis without mood symptoms. In depressive disorder and bipolar mood disorder, psychosis is associated with acute, often severe, mood episodes.

• Disorganized speech and behavior, flat or inappropriate affect, and catatonic behavior (eg, bizarre postures or language patterns, abnormal movements, immobility) may be present at times during the illness but are not prominent in the acute phase. Delusions or hallucinations must be present for at least 2 wk (during which mood symptoms are not prominent) to make the diagnosis.

Etiology

• Risk of developing the disorder is greater when there is a strong family history of the illness, particularly in one or more first-degree relatives. Genetic predisposition is, thus, a major etiologic factor. Prenatal influences (eg, malnutrition, Rh incompatibility) have also been implicated. Stressful life events, physical illnesses, or subclinical disease states have been suggested to function as environmental triggers for schizophrenia spectrum disorders.

Epidemiology

• Estimates of the prevalence of schizoaffective disorder lack agreement, and there remains controversy about this subtype of the psychotic disorders. Overall, schizophrenia lifetime-prevalence rates tend to average 1% of the population for the combined subtypes. Schizoaffective disorder is often associated with a family history of schizophrenia or mood disorder [2].

Treatment

Diet and lifestyle

• Normal diet and exercise levels should be encouraged.

• Alcohol and tobacco use should be discouraged because they may interfere with drug efficacy when prescribing psychoactive medications.

Pharmacologic treatment

• In the acute phase, the goal is to reduce symptoms and the risk of suicide and other dangerous behavior. Antipsychotics and antidepressants (and mood stabilizers for depressed or manic patients) are indicated for most acute patients.

• In the stabilization phase, the goals are to reduce environmental stressors in the patient's life, maintain improved clinical status, and reintegrate the patient into his or her support system and community.

• In the stable phase, the goals are to monitor for adverse medication effects (eg, movement disorders, neuroleptic malignant syndrome), and to improve quality of life and treatment adjuncts that function to avoid relapse.

• Treatment of refractory patients [4] and those with negative symptoms may require the use of atypical neuroleptics (eg, clozapine, quetiapine) or other newer antipsychotics.

Antidepressants

Medications	Dosage, mg/d
Heterocyclics	
Imipramine	150–300
Desipramine	150–300
Amitriptyline	150–300
Nortriptyline	75–125
Protriptyline	15–40
Trimipramine	100–300
Doxepin	150–300
Maprotiline	150–225
Amoxapine	150–400
Trazodone	150–400
Serotonin inhibitors and new drugs	
Fluoxetine	20–80
Bupropion	200–450
Sertraline	50–200
Paroxetine	20–50
Venlafaxine	75–375
Nefazodone	100–500
Fluvoxamine	50–300
Monoamine oxidase inhibitors	
Phenelzine	30–90
Tranylcypromine	20–60

Antipsychotics

Medications	Dosage, mg/d
Low potency	
Chlorpromazine	50–1500
Thioridazine	150–800
Mesoridazine	50–500
High potency	
Molindone	20–225
Perphenazine	8–60
Loxapine	50–250
Trifluoperazine	10–40
Fluphenazine	3–45
Thiothixene	10–60
Haloperidol	2–40
Pimozide	1–10
New antipsychotics	
Clozapine	300–900
Risperidone	4–16
Olanzapine	5–20
Quetiapine	150–750

Mood stabilizers and dosage range

Medication	Dosage, mg/d	Serum level
Lithium Carbonate	600–2400	0.6–1.5 mEq/L
Carbamazepine	600–1600	4–10 µg/mL
Valproic Acid	500–2000	50–1500 µg/mL

Treatment aims

To reduce and stabilize symptoms.
To reintegrate patient into the community.
To educate patient and family.

Nonpharmacologic treatment

Combination therapy: typically involves the use of an antidepressant (when the patient is depressed) and a mood stabilizer (when bipolar symptoms are present) in conjunction with an antipsychotic.

Day treatment programs: can enhance treatment and quality of life for patients with schizoaffective disorder; improvement of daily living skills, social skills, understanding the illness, and need for medication compliance are primary goals; cognitive deficits, if present, need consideration [3].

Psychotherapy: can be beneficial for identifying and minimizing relevant stressors in patient's lives and avoiding relapse and hospitalization.

Group and family therapy: may also be of benefit.

Psychosocial rehabilitation: effective in helping patients identify and pursue long-term life goals.

Electroconvulsive therapy: used in severe mood episodes.

Prognosis

• Schizoaffective disorder is a chronic illness for most patients. Delusions and hallucinations can result in greater risk for suicide. Compliance with treatment is essential to good long-term functioning. Long-term prognosis is intermediate between schizophrenia and mood disorders.

Key references

1. American Psychiatric Association: Practice guidelines for the treatment of patients with schizophrenia. Am J Psychiatry 1997, 154:41–50.

2. Fenton WS, et al.: Symptoms, subtype, and suicidality in patients with schizophrenia spectrum disorders. Am J Psychiatry 1997, 154:2199–2204.

3. Hawkins KA, Sullivan TE, Choi EJ: Memory deficits in schizophrenia: inadequate stimulation or true amnesia? Findings form the Wechsler Memory Scale-revised. J Psychiatry Neurosci 1997, 22:169–179.

4. Brenner HD, Dencker SJ, Goldstein MJ, et al.: Defining treatment refractoriness in schizophrenia. Schizophr Bull 1990, 16:551–561.

SCHIZOID PERSONALITY DISORDER

Diagnosis

Definition
• Schizoid personality disorder is a pervasive pattern of detachment from social relationships and a restricted range of expression of emotions in interpersonal settings, beginning by early adulthood.

Symptoms and signs
Passive responses to adverse difficulties.

Difficulty expressing anger, even when provoked.

Lack of clear goals.

Poor social skills.

Occupational problems: unless work is relatively isolated from social demands.

Sometimes brief psychotic episodes (minutes to hours) in response to stress.

Sometimes predates axis I psychotic disorders.

Can occur together with schizotypal, paranoid, or avoidant personality disorders.

DSM-IV criteria
• Schizoid personality disorder does not occur exclusively during the course of schizophrenia, a mood disorder with psychotic features, another psychotic disorder, or a pervasive developmental disorder, and it is not due to the direct physiologic effects of a general medical condition. (If criteria are met prior to the onset of schizophrenia, add "premorbid," *eg*, "schizoid personality disorder [premorbid].")

• Schizoid personality disorder is indicated by the presence of four (or more) of the following:

1. Neither desires nor enjoys close relationships, including being part of a family.
2. Almost always chooses solitary activities.
3. Has little, if any, interest in having sexual experiences with another person.
4. Takes pleasure in few, if any, activities.
5. Lacks close friends or confidants other than first-degree relatives.
6. Appears indifferent to the praise or criticism of others.
7. Shows emotional coldness, detachment, or flattened affectivity.

Investigations

Psychologic testing
Minnesota Multiphasic Personality Inventory-2: cluster A personality disorders typically are reflected in elevations of scales 6 (paranoia), 8 (schizophrenia), and 0 (social introversion).

Millon Clinical Multiaxial Inventory-III: scale 1 specifically measures for schizoid personality disorders, but some overlap exists between this scale and scale 2A (avoidant), which poses a diagnostic differential issue.

Rorschach: The Exner scoring system is useful in detecting mild thought disorders and emotional trait characteristics.

Laboratory studies
• None are specific.

Complications

Comorbidity
Depression or dysthymia; social phobia; agoraphobia.

Behavioral outcomes
Rejection, sometimes cruelty, from others; isolation and social support deficiencies; employment difficulties (especially in jobs that require social skills).

Differential diagnosis
• Disorders characterized by periods of more persistent psychotic symptoms: delusional disorder, schizophrenia, or mood disorder with psychotic features.
• Disorders of *more severely impaired* social interaction, stereotyped behaviors, and interests (autistic disorder and Asperger's disorder).
• Other personality disorders that are characterized by social isolation and restricted affectivity include the following: Schizotypal personality disorder: has cognitive and perceptual distortions. Paranoid personality disorder: has suspiciousness and paranoid ideations. Avoidant personality disorder: has fear of being embarrassed or inadequate, with excessive anticipation of rejection. Obsessive-compulsive personality disorder: has apparent social detachment that arises from devotion to work and discomfort with emotions (although capacity for intimacy is preserved). Personality change due to a general medical condition, eg, temporal lobe epilepsy. Personality symptoms derived from chronic substance use: premorbid schizoid traits would be absent.

Etiology
• Etiology is not established.
• A close genetic relationship to schizophrenia is doubtful: 1) negative symptoms, more than positive symptoms, have increased heritability in schizophrenia; 2) however, familial relationships between schizoid personality disorder and schizophrenia are not consistently seen; and 3) no neurophysiologic signs (auditory P300 response, smooth pursuit eye tracking) are shared with schizophrenia.
• The dopamine D2 receptor Taq AI allele has a strong association with schizoid and avoidant behavior, as does to a lesser extent the 480-bp VNTR 10/10 allele of the dopamine transporter gene *Dat1*.
• Introversion has been shown to be a highly heritable personality trait.

Epidemiology
Unknown prevalence; wide variance among studies; estimates range from 0.5%–7.0%.
Somewhat more common in men than in women.

Treatment

Pharmacologic treatment
• Controlled pharmacologic treatment studies are lacking.
• Schizoid trait symptoms are not known to benefit from psychotropic medication.
• Low-dose neuroleptics are indicated for frequent or prolonged psychotic states and may prove most effective to diminish anxiety.
• Comorbid conditions, such as depression, should be conventionally treated.

Nonpharmacologic treatment
Supportive psychotherapy
Problem solving.

Social skills training.

Psychoeducation.

Role playing.

Fostering a gratifying, supportive, nonintrusive relationship.

Individual psychodynamic psychotherapy
• Schizoid personality disorder patients rarely seek therapy.
• Treatment usually is sought in response to acute stressors or family influence.
• Psychodynamic therapy usually is a successful benefit if it proceeds slowly, with modest frequency, and respects the patient's discomfort with intimacy, disclosure, and processes of interpersonal interactions.
• If the patient is unable to achieve capacity for interpersonal relationships, then therapy can help better adapt to a life of solitude.

Family therapy
• Schizoid personality disorder patients often live at home and often have first-degree relatives as their sole social support resource.
• Helping family members better understand, accept, and deal with their own emotional issues can foster stronger stability and support for the patient.

Group therapy
• Schizoid personality disorder patients predictably find group work aversive at first.
• If the patient will engage, group therapy offers opportunity for social skills development, insight into social conventions, and possibly a means of strengthening capacity for forming gratifying relationships.

Treatment aims
To maintain stability and support.
To improve social skills and comfort.
To help maximize quality of an isolated lifestyle.

Prognosis
• Insufficient data exist.
• Some schizoid patients can acquire the capacity for comfortable social engagement; substantial improvements have been reported in individual cases.

Follow-up and management
• There is no "acute phase" to the disorder of personality, and its "trait" nature confers long-term perspective.
• Situational decompensations require crisis intervention.
• Psychotherapeutic interventions cited above are intermediate or long-term, with no defined point for termination.

General references
Diagnostic and Statistical Manual of Mental Disorders, ed 4. Washington, DC: American Psychiatric Association; 1994.

Kaplan HI, Sadock BJ: *Comprehensive Textbook of Psychiatry*, ed 6. Baltimore: Williams & Wilkins; 1995.

The Quality Assurace Project: Treatment outlines for paranoid, schizotypal, and schizoid personality disorders. *Aust N Z J Psychiatry* 1990, 24:339–350.

SCHIZOPHRENIA, CATATONIC TYPE

Diagnosis [1,2]

General information

• Presentation must first meet full criteria for schizophrenia and not be better accounted for by another subtype, with essential features marked by psychomotor involvement. Sometimes there is rapid alteration between the extremes of excitement and stupor.

Signs and symptoms

• According to DSM-IV, the clinical picture is dominated by at least two of the following:

1. Motoric immobility as evidenced by cataplexy (including waxy flexibility) or stupor.

2. Excessive motor activity that is apparently purposeless and not influenced by external stimuli.

3. Extreme negativism (an apparently motiveless resistance to all instructions or maintenance of a rigid posturing against attempts to be moved) or mutism.

4. Peculiarities of voluntary movement as evidenced by posturing (voluntary assumption of inappropriate or bizarre posture), stereotyped movements, prominent mannerisms, or prominent grimacing.

• Additional features may include automatic obedience, mimicry, or perseveration.

Investigations [3]

• No definitive lab test is available. Diagnosis is made with comprehensive interview, complete physical examination and detailed history. Because findings of both structural and functional abnormalities have been reported in persons with schizophrenia, neurophysiologic and neuropsychologic assessment may be helpful.

Complications [4]

• During severe catatonic stupor or excitement, patients may need careful supervision to prevent harm to self or others. Other potential risks during catatonia include the following:

Malnutrition.

Exhaustion.

Hyperpyrexia.

Electrolyte disturbance.

Infections.

Neuromalignant syndrome.

Differential diagnosis

• Substance-induced immobility (eg, neuroleptic-induced Parkinsonism). General medical conditions causing immobility.
Manic or major depression episode with severe psychomotor retardation or agitation.

Etiology

• The cause is unknown. The "stress-diathesis model" postulates a person may have a specific vulnerability that, when acted on by stressful environmental influences, allows the symptoms of schizophrenia to develop.

Epidemiology

• The incidence of schizophrenia is estimated to range from 0.030%–0.120% per year for individuals over 15 y of age. Industrialized nations and groups suffering from high levels of cultural disruptions report the greatest numbers. Developing countries tend to have a lower prevalence. Lifetime prevalence of schizophrenia in the US is estimated to be ~1%. Common several decades ago, catatonic schizophrenia is now rare in Europe and North America.

Clinical care

• Course may alternate between active and residual phases.

Treatment

Diet and lifestyle [4]

• As in all illnesses, healthy life habits are recommended, including adequate rest, nourishing diet, abstinence from drugs and alcohol, low stress environment, patient acceptance of healthcare.

Pharmacologic treatment [2,3]

• Conventional neuroleptics as well as the newer (novel) antipsychotics are used to treat all subtypes of schizophrenia. Efficacy varies among patients. No one drug has proved to be more effective.

Conventional neuroleptics

• A wide number of agents are available in pill, injection, and depot injection forms.

• Risperidone and olanzapine are available in pill form only; lorazepam has been shown to be effective during acute phases of catatonic stupor.

Standard dosage	Risperidone, titrated up from 2–6 mg/d; administered on twice daily schedule during acute episodes of psychosis.
	Olanzapine, 5–20 mg/d during acute episode.
	Quetiapine, 300–400 mg/d to a maximum of 750 mg/d.
	Lorazepam, 1–6 mg/d four times daily.
Main side effects	Extrapyramidal symptoms (tremors, restlessness, muscle rigidity), especially with higher doses, drowsiness, orthostatic hypotension, tardive dyskinesia (rare). Enhanced sedation when combined with other CNS depressants.
	Olanzapine: weight gain, orthostatic hypotension; extrapyramidal symptoms including parkinsonism are not common.
	Quetiapine: somnolence, hypotension, lens changes (rare), tardive dyskinesia (rare).
	Lorazepam: drowsiness, rebound insomnia after initial high doses, dry mouth.
Main drug interactions	*Risperidone*: may enhance hypertensive effects when combined with other drugs with same potential.
	Olazapine: may increase effects of antihypertensive agents.
	Quetiapine: potentiates other CNS medications.
	Lorazepam: potentially lethal when combined with alcohol.
Special points	*Lorazepam*: central nervous system (CNS) depressant; caution should be shown in patients with a history of suicide attempts.

Treatment aims

To keep the patient relatively symptom free with the highest functional level on the lowest possible dose of medications with the fewest side effects.

Prognosis

• Patients meeting DSM-IV criteria for schizophrenia generally have poor prognostic features over the short or immediate term. Those with the catatonic subtype of schizophrenia may have a mixed prognosis. Prognosis may be impacted by socioeconomic factors and availability of psychosocial interventions.

Follow-up management

• Psychosocial rehabilitation has become a significant part of the long-term treatment plan of persons with all types of schizophrenia. Goals include medication compliance resulting in reduction of symptoms, patient education, and remediation of disabilities associated with the illness.

Key references

1. *Dignostic and Statistical Manual of Mental Disorders*, ed 4. Washington, DC: American Psychiatric Association; 1994.

2. Bumer D: Catatonia and the neuroleptics: psychobiologic significance of remote and recent findings. *Comp Psychiatry* 1997, 38:193–201.

3. Kaplan HI, Sadock BJ, Grelb JA: *Synopsis of Psychiatry*, ed 7. Baltimore: Williams & Wilkins; 320–342.

4. Northoff G, Wenke J, Demisch L, *et al.*: Catatonic: short-term response to lorazepam and dopaminergic metabolism. *Psychopharmaccology* 1995, 22:182–186.

SCHIZOPHRENIA, DISORGANIZED TYPE

Diagnosis

Symptoms

Disorganized speech and behavior, flat or inappropriate affect.

General schizophrenia criteria: must also be present.

• Patients with this disorder will have two or more of the following symptoms for 1 month: delusions, hallucinations, disorganized speech, disorganized or catatonic behavior, negative symptoms.

Signs

Social and occupational functioning: impaired relative to status prior to onset of illness; cognitive impairment is often present, with a notable decline in functioning relative to premorbid level.

Six months of continuous signs of the illness with at least 1 month of prominent symptoms (< 1 month of symptoms if successfully treated).

Family history of schizophrenia or other mental disorder: occurs in ~25% of the population.

• Illness is chronic in nature and some patients may be treatment refractory.

• Episodic course or periodic worsening may occur.

• Age of onset is usually late teens or early twenties.

Investigations

Clinical assessment in the acute phase: should include a complete psychiatric and general medical history; a mental status examination is essential, and physical and neurologic examination and interviews of collaterals (unless the patient objects) should be conducted.

Laboratory investigations: not routinely conducted; however, when indicated, they can include several components (*eg*, possible urine screen for intoxicants or other substances that may induce psychosis or require detoxification; possible complete blood count, electrolytes and glucose levels, liver enzymes, renal function, thyroid function and tests for sexually transmitted diseases; and possible pregnancy testing and reproductive health screening for females).

Neuropsychologic testing: can be beneficial in cases of differential diagnosis and comorbid neurologic disorder.

Neuroimaging and other extensive testing: usually not indicated unless the neurologic examination is abnormal or unless symptoms and treatment response are atypical.

Complications

Suicidal ideation: should be evaluated with the focus on the presence of intent or plan, the lethality of the plan, and the presence of command hallucinations (auditory hallucinations; voices urging the patient to harm self or others [in cases of homicidal ideation]); a prior history of attempted suicide and coexistent substance abuse are major risk factors.

Suicide: incidence of completed suicide is 10%–13% over the lifetime for patients with schizophrenia, whereas up to 50% may attempt it.

Homelessness: can be a result of the illness for various reasons for an estimated 12% of chronically ill schizophrenic patients; estimates of homeless groups indicate that one third have mental illness, often schizophrenia; patients with disorganized type are vulnerable and require housing aid; frequent hospitalizations are common and a major social cost.

Substance abuse or dependence: reported in 30%–50% of those with schizophrenia.

Differential diagnosis

• Substance-induced psychosis and contributory medical conditions must be excluded.

• Mood disorders with psychotic features (eg, major depressive disorder, bipolar disorder) must be excluded.

• Schizoaffective disorder can be distinguished by discrete periods of mood disturbance and psychosis.

• If there is a history of pervasive developmental disorder, the additional diagnosis of schizophrenia is made only if delusions or hallucinations are present for a month, or less if such symptoms are successfully treated. This would rarely occur in disorganized type schizophrenia.

Etiology

• The risk of developing the disorder is greater when there is a strong family history of the illness, particularly in one or more first-degree relative. Genetic predisposition is thus a major factor. Prenatal influences (eg, influenza, malnutrition, and Rh incompatibility) have also been implicated. Stressful life events, physical illnesses, or subclinical disease states have been suggested to function as environmental triggers for schizophrenia.

Epidemiology

• Estimates vary greater regarding the prevalence of the disorganized subtype of schizophrenia, sometimes referred to as hebephrenia. Studies indicate that 17%–30% of patients may exhibit disorganized type symptoms in the US. In Japan, estimates typically range from 30%–50%. Overall, schizophrenia lifetime-prevalence rates tend to average 1% of the population for the combined subtypes. Disorganized-type schizophrenia is associated with an earlier age of onset, with an insidious development course. Thus, premorbid function is often poor and the disorder often continuous, with a fairly poor prognosis in many individuals.

Treatment

Diet and lifestyle

• Normal diet, rest, and exercise levels should be encouraged.

• Alcohol use and tobacco use should be discouraged because they may interfere with drug efficacy when prescribing neuroleptic medications.

Pharmacologic treatment

Acute phase: the goal is to reduce symptoms and risk of suicide and other dangerous behavior; antipsychotics and antidepressants or mood stabilizers for depressed or manic patients are indicated for most acute patients [1].

Stabilization phase: reduction of environmental stressors in patient's life and efforts to maintain improved clinical status and reintegrate into the community and patient's support system are goals of this phase; attention should be paid to the role of negative symptoms in disorganized–type schizophrenia patients; flat or inappropriate affect and odd behavior and speech may lead to social isolation and depression; antidepressant medication may need to be included in the treatment regimen.

Stable phase: monitor for adverse medication effects such as movement disorders and neuroleptic malignant syndrome; improved quality-of-life and treatment adjuncts that function to avoid relapse are goals of this phase.

• Treatment-refractory patients and those with negative symptoms may require the use of atypical neuroleptics (eg, clozapine) or other newer antipsychotics (eg, olanzapine, risperidone, and quetiapine) [2]. These newer medications are more expensive.

Antipsychotic medications

• The following medications are listed in descending order of extrapyramidal side effects. Chlorpromazine, thioridazine, and mesoridazine are low-potency agents; resperidone, olanzapine, quetiapine, and clozapine are new antipsychotics.

Standard dosage	Haloperidol, 2– 40 mg/d; pimozide, 1– 10 mg/d; fluphenazine, 3–45 mg/d; perphenazine, 8–60 mg/d; trifluperazine, 10–40 mg/d; thiothixene, 10–60 mg/d; molindone, 20–225 mg/d; loxapine, 50–250 mg/d; chlorpromazine, 50–150 mg/d; thioridazine, 150–800 mg/d; mesoridazine, 50–500 mg/d; risperidone, 4–16 mg/d; olanzapine, 5–20 mg/d; quetiapine, 75–750 mg/d; clozapine, 300–900 mg/d.
Main side effects	Sedation (particularly for low-potency agents), orthostatic hypotension. Anticholinergic effects include dry mouth, constipation, blurred vision, tachycardia, urinary retention, memory complaints, confusion and possible delirium. Extrapyramidal effects include dystonia, akithisia, parkinsonism, and neuroleptic malignant syndrome; these may occur for nearly 60% of patients taking antipsychotic medications.

Treatment of extrapyramidal side effects (EPS): options include EPS medications, reduce neuroleptic dosage, change to a newer antipsychotic, or discontinue medication, which is essential in neuroleptic malignant syndrome.

Medications for acute extrapyramidal side effects: Benztropine mesylate (0.5–6.0 mg/d), amantadine (100–300 mg/d), and trihexyphenidyl HCL (1–2 mg/d). Amantadine and trihexyphenidyl HCL may require twice-daily dosages.

Treatment aims
To reduce and stabilize symptoms.
To reintegrate patient into the community.
To educate patient and family.

Prognosis
• Schizophrenia is a chronic illness for most patients. Patients with disorganized-type symptoms tend to have poor social interactions and are prone to isolation and for some depression. Compliance with treatment is essential to good long-term functioning.

Other treatment options
• Day treatment programs can enhance treatment and quality of life for patients with disorganized-type schizophrenia.
• Improvement of daily living skills, social skills, understanding the illness and need for medication compliance are primary goals.
• Psychotherapy can be beneficial for identifying and minimizing relevant stressors in patient's lives and avoiding relapse and hospitalization.
• Group therapy and family therapy may also be of benefit.
• Psychosocial rehabilitation is effective in helping patients identify and pursue long-term life goals.

Key references
1. Practice guidelines for the treatment of patients with schizophrenia. Am J Psychiatry 1997, 154:1–50.
2. Leiberman, JA: Understanding the mechanism of action of atypical antipsychotic drugs: a review of compounds in use and development. Br J Psychiatry 1993, 163–709.

General reference
Fenton WS, et al.: Symptoms, subtype, and suicidality in patients with schizophrenia spectrum disorders. Am J Psychiatry 1997, 154:199–204.

Diagnosis

General information
• Late-onset schizophrenia is a category, not formally classified, for those with first onset of psychosis after 45 years of age.

Symptoms and signs
Focused delusions of persecution: will likely present with beliefs of being followed, watched by others, or being poisoned or gassed; also, ideas of reference.

Auditory hallucinations: visual, olfactory hallucinations.

Often minimal formal thought disorder: thought broadcasting, thought withdrawal, thought insertion, made feelings or behaviors [1,2].

Affect blunted but not flat or bizarre.

• Use criteria for schizophrenia in DSM-IV. Patient most likely will fall under the rubric for paranoid schizophrenia rather than other schizophrenia subtypes.

• Usually presents via family, the police, the court. Patient rarely walks in to complain of symptoms. If patient feels distress, it is likely secondary to others not believing or agreeing with the patient's delusions.

Investigations
Routine laboratory tests: complete blood count, platelets, electrolytes, blood urea nitrogen, creatinine, liver function tests, thyroid function tests (thyroid-stimulating hormone, free thyroxine); measurement of plasma and erythrocytes, folate, and vitamin B_{12} may also be indicated [3].

Magnetic resonance imaging and computed tomography of the head with and without contrast: to rule out tumors, strokes, hemorrhages; likely will show enlarged lateral ventricles without parenchymal atrophy.

Electroencephalography: to evaluate for generalized slowing, consistent with an encephalopathy.

Neuropsychiatric testing: evaluate for preexistent personality traits; evaluate for evidence of a dementing illness; evaluate for personality strengths [3].

Evaluate for coexisting medical illnesses: *eg*, hypertension, diabetes, chronic obstructive pulmonary disease (COPD), cancer, and hearing and visual defects [3].

Complications
Patient often resistant to treatment: due to poor treatment compliance.

Patient dangerous to self or others: if he or she feels threatened by the nature of the delusional material.

Depression: commonly associated intermittently.

• There may be a need for increased social service involvement if family or significant other is not available.

• If patient has other medical illnesses (*eg*, diabetes, COPD), exacerbations can occur secondary to compliance with medications or treatment recommendations that conflict or become incorporated into the delusional material.

Differential diagnosis
Psychosis associated with dementia (cognitive, functional decline).
Delusional disorder (nonbizarre delusions).
Induced psychotic disorder (folie à deux).
Adult-onset schizophrenia (previously unrecognized).
Tumor or neurologic event resulting in symptoms.
Medications resulting in delirium (eg, high-dose prednisone that causes paranoia).
Personality disorder (paranoid, schizoid): function maintained.

Etiology
• Late-onset schizophrenia is presumed to be biologic, but other factors (eg, hearing loss, visual loss, recent immigration) may play a role
• Increased incidence in families with schizoid, paranoid traits or personalities.

Epidemiology
• Late-onset schizophrenia is presumed to be <10% of the total schizophrenia incidence rate.
• Women are affected more than men.
• Single, widow, or widowers are affected more than those who are married.

Treatment

Diet and lifestyle
• Assess for potential harm to self or others.
• Assess home situation that patient finds him or herself in for safety. Residence may require change if involved in the delusional material.
• No special dietary modifications are required; however, do make certain patient is eating and maintaining fluid balance.

Pharmacologic treatment
• General principle can use either conventional antipsychotics (haloperidol, fluphenazine, thiothixene, trifluoperazine) [4] or atypical antipsychotics (olanzapine, risperidone). Doses will generally be higher than those used for psychosis associated with dementia but less than doses for young adult-onset schizophrenia.
• Typical divided doses (morning, bedtime) could include:

Standard dosage	Haloperidol, 0.5–5.0 mg/d.
	Trifluoperazine, 2.0–6.0 mg/d.
	Risperidone, 0.5–3.0 mg/d.
	Olanzapine, 2.5–7.5 mg/d.
Main side effects	Special considerations in the elderly include the development of tardive dyskinesia after 1 month of antipsychotic use, the development of extreme extrapyramidal symptoms (EPS) in those with pyramidal tract strokes, or early Parkinson's disease. The use of anticholinergic agents to decrease the EPS can potentially cause constipation, increase confusion or result in blurry vision, dry mouth, or tremor.

Special considerations
• Clozapine should not be considered until the patient has failed to respond to at least three other antipsychotics, due to risk of bone marrow suppression, especially high with elderly females
• Older persons are likely to be on fixed incomes so cost is a factor in choosing medications, making less expensive conventional neuroleptic agents preferred in some situations.
• Older persons are likely to have multiple medical illnesses, such as Parkinson's disease, wherein the atypical agents might be preferred. Lower doses of conventional/atypical agents might be required in cirrhosis.
• Antipsychotic agent blood levels not part of routine treatment.
• Drug interactions are most likely to occur with seizure medications (phenytoin, phenobarbital, carbamazepine, valproic acid), anticoagulants (warfarin), H_2 blockers (cimetidine), and to a lesser extent with digoxin, rifampin, blood pressure medications, and type I antiarrhythmics.
• Narcotic use may result in need for increased dose of the antipsychotic.
• Alcohol use with antipsychotics is discouraged.
• Tobacco use, especially cigarette smoking, may result in lower drug levels.

Treatment aims
• Late-onset schizophrenia is a serious mental illness, and referral to a psychiatrist is essential to maximize remission potential via compliance with medication.

Prognosis
• Grandiose delusions and delusions associated with sex and jealousy predict a poor outcome over time [5].
• Course is likely chronic but with waxing and waning of symptoms.

Follow-up and management
• The mainstay of treatment is pharmacotherapy (antipsychotics).
• Mood stabilizers (lithium, depakote, antidepressants) are of secondary importance.
• Electroconvulsive therapy is of tertiary importance.
• Supportive psychotherapy is useful to engage patient in the treatment process.
• Insight-oriented psychotherapy contraindicated.

Key references
1. Pearlson OD, Kregor L, Robins PV, et al.: A chart review study of late-onset and early-onset schizophrenia. Am J Psychiatry 1989, 146:1568–1574.
2. Howard R, Cartle D, Wessely S, et al.: A comparative study of 470 cases of early-onset and late-onset schizophrenia. Br J Psychiatry 1994, 163:352–357.
3. Yassa R, Suranyi-Cadotte B: Clinical characteristics of late-onset schizophrenia and delusional disorder. Schizo Bull 1993, 19:701–707.
4. Jeste DV, Lacro JP, Gilbert PL, et al.: Treatment of late life schizophrenia with neuroleptics. Schizo Bull 1993, 19:817–830.
5. Jorgensen P, Munk-Jorgensen P: Paranoid psychosis in the elderly, a follow-up study. Acta Psychiatrica Scand 1985, 72:358–363.

Diagnosis

Signs and symptoms
• There is no pathognomonic sign or symptom for schizophrenia.

DSM-IV diagnostic criteria

General
1. Persistent symptoms related to affect, emotional state, personality, cognition, motor activity, and perception.

2. Persistent symptoms (prodromal/active/residual) for at least 6 months, with two or more symptoms active for at least a month.

3. Symptoms sufficient to cause social or occupational dysfunction.

4. Symptoms not secondary to other psychiatric illness.

5. Schizophrenia is then more discretely diagnosed by subtypes (paranoid, catatonic, disorganized, undifferentiated, and residual).

Explicit
1. Preoccupation with one or more delusions (most frequently of persecution or grandeur).

2. Frequent auditory hallucinations.

3. No prominent symptoms of disorganized speech, disorganized or catatonic behavior, or flat or inappropriate affect.

Investigations [1]
Laboratory screening tests (eg, serum, cerebrospinal fluid, urine): are not diagnostic for schizophrenia; however, they are often necessary to rule out medical causes in the differential for schizophrenia (*see* Differential diagnosis).

Thorough history and physical.

Psychologic testing: can reflect disrupted cognition (*eg*, vigilance, memory, concept formation, attention, retention, and problem-solving ability) and abnormal responses to both projective and objective tests such as the Rorschach and the Minnesota Multiphasic Personality Inventory are common.

Computed tomography and magnetic resonance imaging: have demonstrated lateral and middle ventricle enlargement, and cerebral asymmetry.

Positron emission tomography: may show hypoactive frontal lobes.

Collateral data on the patient's present and premorbid functioning: are often informative.

Complications [1,2]
Increase in incidence of minor physical anomalies.

Soft neurologic signs.

Excessive water intake: can lead to hyponatremia.

Substance abuse: in 30%–50%.

Suicide: 50% attempt, 10% complete.

Difficulties in sustaining work, education, and relationships.

Often victims of crime and homelessness.

Differential diagnosis [1,2]

Substance use
Amphetamines, cocaine, alcohol hallucinosis, Wernicke-Korsakoff syndrome, barbiturate withdrawal, hallucinogens/marijuana, phencyclidine, beta-blockers, buproprion, indomethacin, procainamide, phenytoin, carbamazepine, corticosteroids.

General medical conditions
Central nervous system and other neoplasms; AIDS, herpes, neurosyphilis, and other systemic infections; epilepsy and other brain pathology (normal pressure hydrocephalus, cerebral lipoidosis, Huntington's disease and Wilson's disease, metachromatic leukodystrophy); cardiovascular disease; trauma; toxic exposure (CO, heavy metals); lupus; systemic excesses or deficiencies (acute intermittent porphyria, B_{12} deficiency, homocystinuria, pellagra).

Psychiatric disorders
Autism, schizoaffective disorder, mood disorder with psychotic features, delusional disorder, other brief psychotic disorders, malingering or factitious disorder, obsessive-compulsive disorder with psychotic features, personality disorders.

Etiology [1]
• Excessive dopaminergic activity is postulated, involving numerous dopamine pathways, receptors, and receptor sites.
• Prominent involvement of frontal cortex and the limbic system is implicated.
• Patient may have history of perinatal complications.
• Genetic studies reflect increased (though not complete) concordance in monozygotic versus dizygotic twins.
• Molecular genetic data reflect involvement of chromosomes 5, 6, 11, and 18 in some pedigrees.
• Psychosocial stressors may contribute to the development and evolution of the illness.
• There is no support for the idea that "specific family relation patterns" play a causative role in the development of schizophrenia.

Epidemiology
• The overall incidence of schizophrenia is estimated to be 1.0%–1.5%. Schizophrenia, paranoid subtype may be the most common of all the subtypes.

Treatment

Diet and lifestyle
- Avoid water intoxication and hyponatremia.
- Maintain sobriety (drugs, alcohol, caffeine, nicotine).
- Promote standard medical and dental health maintenance practices (including normal sleep patterns, exercise, and diet), which are often neglected by patient.

Pharmacologic treatment
- Conventional antipsychotic medications treat positive symptoms, and some come in decanoate form, which is useful in noncompliant patients. Conventional antipsychotics (neuroleptics) are less effective with negative symptoms.
- Newer, novel antipsychotic medications have fewer side effects, and treat both positive and negative symptoms.

Conventional antipsychotics

Standard dosage	Haloperidol, 5 mg 1–2 times daily, 2–5 mg i.m. for agitation.
	Polixin decanoate, 25 mg i.m. every 2 weeks.
	Haloperidol decanoate, 50–200 mg i.m. every 4 weeks.
Main side effects	Extrapyramidal symptoms (EPS) or rigidity, akithisia, tremor, hypersalivation, acute dystonic reactions (EPS can be treated with low-dose lorazepam or propranolol).

Novel antipsychotics

Standard dosage	Risperidone, 3 mg twice daily (start with 2–5 mg/d).
	Olanzapine, 5–20 mg at night.
	Quetiapine, 100 mg in morning, 200 mg at night.
	Clozapine, 100 mg once daily (up to 900 mg).
Contraindications	Neuroleptic hypersensitivity; liver dysfunction; for clozapine, history of agranulocytosis or concomitant use with carbamazepine.
Main side effects	Rarely, EPS (increases with higher doses); occasional sedation; occasional dizziness; occasional headache; weight gain; occasional sexual dysfunction; agranulocytosis and seizures with clozapine. Low-potency neuroleptics can cause anticholinergic side effects (eg, dry mouth, urinary retention, delirium, tachycardia, blurred vision), and hypotension. Neuroleptic malignant syndrome (autonomic hyperactivity, lead pipe rigidity, altered mentation, increased creatinine phosphokinase) can be lethal. Tardive dyskinesia is an involuntary choreaform–athetoid movement disorder.
Main drug interactions	Some neuoleptics antagonize anticonvulsants, and may require dosage adjustment; additive with other central nervous system depressants.
Special points	It may take many days or weeks for response; clozapine is associated with agranulocytosis, and requires weekly complete blood counts with differentials. Novel antipsychotics are expensive.

Nonpharmacologic treatment
- Partnership with patient and significant others is critical for long-term management. The philosophy is one of recovery, rehabilitation, and reintegration. Patient and family education about illness and its treatment is essential. Patients should receive education, vocational training, and placement.Enhanced support is available in the community environment (eg, case management, supported housing, day treatment programs, clubhouse settings).

Treatment aims
To reduce or alleviate symptoms to return patient to baseline functioning.

Prognosis
- There is a somewhat later onset (late 20s, early 30s) than other subtypes.
- Majority of untreated patients relapse within 2 y.
- Of those treated with conventional antipsychotics, 30% do not respond.
- More than 50% of patients have poor outcomes, but this is improving with novel antipsychotics.
- Paranoid subtype has a relatively good prognosis, perhaps related to its later onset, relative preservation of personality, cognitive functioning, and affect [2].
- Good prognostic signs include late or acute onset, precipitating stress factors, good premorbid functioning, presence of mood disorder symptoms, family history of mood disorders, married, good support system, presence of positive symptoms.
- Poor prognostic signs include early or insidious onset; lack of precipitating factors; poor premorbid functioning; withdrawn, autistic behavior; family history of schizophrenia; single, divorced, widowed; poor support system; presence of negative symptoms; presence of neurologic signs or symptoms; history of perinatal trauma; no remissions in 3 y; many relapses; history of assaultiveness [3].

Follow-up and management
- Regularly assess the patient's response to medications, monitoring for long-term side effects.
- Regularly assess need for additional community supports.
- Offer routine health maintenance.

Key references
1. Kaplan HI, Sadock BJ (eds): Synopsis of Psychiatry, ed 8. Baltimore: Williams & Wilkins; 1998.
2. Conley R, Merlino J (eds): A Clinician's Approach to Psychotic Disorders. 1988.
3. Diagnostic and Statistical Manual of Mental Disorders, edn 4. Washington, DC: American Psychiatric Association; 1994.

Diagnosis

Symptoms and signs

• This subtype of schizophrenia is characterized by the presence of continuing evidence of schizophrenia-like disturbances, after a fully symptomatic episode but without a full set of active symptoms or sufficient symptoms to meet diagnostic criteria for another subtype of the illness. Critical features include the following:

Absence of prominent delusions.

Absence of hallucinations.

Absence of disorganized speech.

Absence of grossly disorganized or catatonic behavior.

• Continuing evidence of the disturbance is indicated by the following:

Presence of "negative" symptoms: affective flattening or blunting, poverty of speech or speech content, thought blocking, poor grooming, lack of motivation, social withdrawal, anhedonia, attention defects, cognitive defects.

• If delusions or hallucinations are present they are in a milder form and not accompanied by strong affect. Examples include odd beliefs, strange behaviors, unusual perceptual experiences.

Investigations

• There are no laboratory tests that are indicative of residual schizophrenia. The disorder has no single clinical sign or symptom that is pathognomonic. The diagnosis is made via a comprehensive interview, physical examination, and detailed history. It is important, however, to rule out any physical condition that may mimic the symptoms of the illness. Possible physical causes of similar syndromes might include the following:

Infections.

Brain tumors or other neurologic diseases.

Metabolic disorders.

Endocrine disorders.

Vascular disorders.

Toxicity (including substance abuse and dependence).

Nutritional deficiencies.

Autoimmune deficiencies.

Complications

Death: a higher mortality rate from accidents and natural causes due to other conditions being misdiagnosed.

Suicide: attempted by 50% of all patients with schizophrenia; 10% ultimately "completed."

Depression: occurs intermittently in a majority of cases.

Substance abuse: 30%–50% may meet diagnostic criteria for alcohol abuse or dependence.

Differential diagnosis

Substance-induced psychosis.
Delirium or dementia.
Affective disorders.
Medical conditions.
Personality disorders.
Malingering or factitious disorder.

Etiology

• The cause of residual schizophrenia is not known. It most likely is the result of a number of factors, including genetic, neurologic, and environmental. It includes patients whose clinical presentations, treatment responses, and courses of illness are varied.

Epidemiology

• Precise data on residual schizophrenia have been difficult to obtain.
• The lifetime prevalence of schizophrenia in the US is estimated to be 1.0%.
• Peak ages of onset are 15–25 for men and 25–35 for women.

Clinical course

• Prodromal syndrome may last ≥1 y before psychosis.
• Function >5 y from initial diagnosis is predictive of later course of disorder.
• Positive symptoms often lead to hospitalization. As time progresses, positive symptoms become less severe. Negative or deficit symptoms may increase in severity over time.
• Resolution of negative symptoms, especially the chronic residual syndrome, continues to be a perplexing challenge [1].
• May be time limited and represent a transition between a full-blown episode of schizophrenia and compete remission. However, it may also be continuously present for many years, with or without acute exacerbations [2].

Treatment

Diet and lifestyle
• Balanced diet and adequate rest are recommended.
• Reduction of stressful situations and abstinence from substance abuse are essential.

Pharmacologic treatment
• Regarding symptom reduction and relapse prevention, therapy with antipsychotic drugs plays the most important role [1]. For both acute and maintenance treatment, antipsychotic medications are usually necessary.

Haloperidol
• Available in pill, concentrate, injectable and decanoate (long-acting) forms.

Standard dosage	2–20 mg/d orally for acute psychosis and maintenance; 2–5 mg i.m. for acute agitation.
Contraindications	History of neuroleptic malignant syndrome (NMS).
Main side effects	Extrapyramidal symptoms (tremor, akithisia [benztropine, 1–2 mg daily, is useful in the control of extrapyramidal disorders]), restlessness, muscle stiffness, sedation, tardive dyskinesia, NMS (rarely).
Main drug interactions	Potentiating effects of other central nervous system (CNS) depressants.
Special points	Antipsychotic drugs should be given in a manner that will minimize side effects.

Risperidone

Standard dosage	2–10 mg twice daily (usually 4–6 mg four times daily)
Main side effects	Hypotension, insomnia, agitation, restlessness, tremors, muscle stiffness, headache, anxiety.
Main drug interactions	Patients should avoid using alcohol.
Special points	High cost; available only in tablet form.

Olanzapine

Standard dosage	5–20 mg daily (usually 10 mg daily).
Main side effects	Sedation, weight gain, dizziness.
Main drug interactions	Enhanced sedation with other CNS depressants.
Special points	High cost, available only in oral form.

Quetiapine

Standard dose	300–400 mg/d up to a maximum of 750 mg/d.
Main side effects	Somnolence, hypotension, lens changes (rare), tardive dyskinesia (rare).
Main drug interactions	Potentiates other CNS medications.
Special points	High cost, available only in oral form.

Clozapine
• Useful in patients who are nonresponsive to conventional antipsychotics.

Standard dose	300–600 mg/d (up to 900 mg).
Main side effects	Agranulocytosis (1%–2%); requires weekly complete blood count monitoring; seizures.
Main drug interactions	Do not use with carbamazepine.

Nonpharmacologic treatment
• Hospitalization may be necessary to provide intense support and structure when patients decompensate.
• Group therapies focused on real-life plans, problems, and relationships; reduces social isolation, increases cohesiveness, and improves reality testing.
• Individual psychotherapy, including supportive focus on building relationships and acceptance.
• Social skills training produces improvement in specific behaviors but less in symptoms and community functioning.
• Family-oriented therapies or education with focus on problem-solving strategies.
• Vocational rehabilitation can promote development of prevocational and vocational skills, and job placement and maintenance.

Other treatment options
• Fluphenazine decanoate and haloperidol decanoate are available for i.m. injection every 1–4 weeks. Good for noncompliant patients.
• Lithium may be effective in reducing psychotic symptoms in up to 50% of patients with schizophrenia; usually used with concomitant neuroleptic.

Key references
1. Moller HJ: Treatment of schizophrenia: state of the art [review]. Eur Arch Psychiatry Clin Neurosci 1996:229–234.
2. Diagnostic and Statistical Manual of Mental Disorders, ed 4. Washington, DC: American Psychiatric Society; 1994.

General references
Kaplan H, Sadock B: Synopsis of Psychiatry, ed 7. Williams and Wilkins: 1994.

Pen DL, Meuser KT: Research update on the psychosocial treatment of schizophrenia. Am J Psychiatry 1996, 607–617.

Diagnosis

Definition
Undifferentiated schizophrenia is diagnosed when the patient meets the primary criteria for Schizophrenia but no one type of symptom is prominent (as in the paranoid, disorganized or catatonic types).

Signs and symptoms

Positive symptoms
• Positive symptoms need to be present for a significant portion of time during a 1-month period, and there needs to be continuous signs of the disturbance for a continuous 6-month period.

Delusions.

Hallucinations.

Disorganized speech.

Grossly disorganized behavior.

Negative symptoms
Flat or blunted emotions.

Lack of interest.

Limited speech.

Lack of motivation or energy.

Investigations
• Because no sign or symptom is pathognomic, schizophrenia cannot be diagnosed without a complete personal and family history. Neurologic causes and substance abuse should be ruled out.

• Tests that may determine a diagnosis of schizophrenia include drug screen, electrocardiogram, general chemistry screen, complete blood count, magnetic resonance imaging or computed tomography scan, urinalysis, electroencephalogram, neuropsychologic and general psychologic testing.

Complications
Suicide: ~10% of patients are at risk for completed suicides.

Depression: 25% of all patients with schizophrenia experience clinical depression.

Substance abuse: 30%–50% of all patients with schizophrenia use alcohol or drugs at some point in their illness.

Differential diagnosis
Substance-induced disorders.
Physical or neurological conditions (eg, vascular disorders, metabolic disturbances, autoimmune deficiencies, endocrine disorders, nutritional deficiencies, infections, brain trauma, temporal lobe epilepsy or psychotic disorder due to a general medical disorder).
Delirium or dementia.
Mood disorders.
Other psychotic disorders (eg, schizoaffective, schizophreniform, brief psychotic, delusional).
Personality disorders (eg, schizotypal, schizoid, paranoid personality).
Factitious disorder or malingering.

Etiology
• The cause of schizophrenia is unknown. It may comprise a group of disorders with multiple causes including genetic, neuropathologic, viral, and environmental.

Epidemiology
• The prevalence of schizophrenia (all types) in the general population ranges from 1%–1.5%.
• Men tend to have an earlier onset than women. Peak ages are 15–25 y of age for men and 25–35 y for women. Undifferentiated schizophrenia tends to have an earlier onset than other types.

Clinical course
• Prodromal signs and symptoms may occur weeks or years before an active phase, usually develop slowly, and include social withdrawal, loss of interest in usual activities, deterioration in functioning in various areas, and unusual behavior.
• Undifferentiated type is associated with an early history of behavioral difficulties.
• Active phase of schizophrenia is characterized by acute psychotic symptoms that are fairly responsive to treatment.
• Within 2 y of an active phase, between 70%–80% of nonmedicated patients will "relapse" into another active phase, and 30%–40% will relapse even when medication compliant.
• The active phase is followed by a period during which patients often continue to experience negative symptoms. Baseline functioning may deteriorate following each successive active phase.

Treatment

Diet and lifestyle

Balanced diet.

Low stress and structured environment.

Abstinence from alcohol and illegal drugs.

Adequate rest.

Pharmacologic treatment

• There are two main classes of drugs used to treat schizophrenia: conventional antipsychotics and the novel antipsychotics.

Conventional antipsychotics

• Neuroleptic antipsychotics (eg, chlorpromazine, fluphenazine, haloperidol, thiothixene, trifluoperazine, perphenazine, and thioridazine) have been considered the conventional methods for treating schizophrenia. They are most effective in treating the positive symptoms of schizophrenia but have less impact on negative symptoms. In addition, they are associated with serious adverse side effects (eg, tardive dyskinesia and neuroleptic malignant syndrome [NMS]).

Standard dosage	Haloperidol, 2–5 mg i.m. (for acute agitation); 5–20 mg/d orally or decanoate (long-lasting), 50–200 mg i.m every 2–4 weeks (for maintenance).
Contraindications	History of tardive dyskinesia or NMS.
Main side effects	Extrapyramidal symptoms, including acute dystonic reactions, akithisia, parkinsonism, tardive dyskinesia, NMS (rare but of concern).
Main drug interactions	Enhanced sedative effect with other CNS depressants.

Novel antipsychotics

• Atypical antipsychotic drugs (eg, risperidone, quetiapine, clozapine, and olanzapine) are relatively new on the market and can be costly. However, they are effective in treating both the positive and negative symptoms of schizophrenia and are associated with fewer and less severe adverse side effects.

Standard dosage	Risperidone, 4–6 mg daily is usual but can range from 2–10 mg/d.
	Olanzapine, 5–20 mg/d; usual dosage is 10 mg daily.
	Quetiapine, 300–400 mg/d (up to a maximum of 750 mg/d).
	Clozapine (useful in patients who do not respond to other antipsychotics), 300–600 mg/d up to 900 mg.
Main side effects	*Risperidone*: orthostatic hypotension, tachycardia, extrapyramidal symptoms at higher doses, tardive dyskinesia, insomnia, agitation, anxiety, and headache.
	Olanzapine: sedation, weight gain, dizziness.
	Quetiapine: somnolence, hypotension, lens changes (rare), tardive dyskinesia (rare).
	Clozapine: agranulocytosis, seizures.
Main drug interactions	*Risperidone*: enhanced sedative effect with other CNS depressants.
	Olanzapine: enhanced sedative effect with other CNS depressants.
	Quetiapine: potentiates other CNS medications.
	Clozapine: do not use with carbamazepine.

Treatment aims

• During the active phase, treatment is focused on ending the current acute psychotic episode.
Following a psychotic episode, treatment should continue in order to improve functioning and prevent future psychotic episodes.

Prognosis

• 20%–30% of patients have a good recovery.
• Good prognosis has been linked to late or acute onset, good premorbid adjustment, mood disorder symptoms, good support systems, and positive symptoms.

Follow-up and management

• Medication compliance is essential to relapse prevention and can be enhanced by the following:
Careful titration of antipsychotics to minimize side effects.
Ensuring continuity from inpatient to outpatient care.
Family and patient education about the nature of the illness and the need for medication.
Concurrent treatment of potential substance abuse problems.
Assuring the patient has a stable living situation.

Nonpharmacologic treatment

Hospitalization (may be necessary during the active phases of schizophrenia).
Psychosocial rehabilitation.
Vocational rehabilitation.
Family education.
Individual and group therapy.

General references

Kaplan HI, Sadock BJ, Grebb JA: *Kaplan and Sadock's Synopsis of Psychiatry: Behavioral Sciences Clinical Psychiatry*, ed 7. Baltimore: Williams & Wilkins; 1994.

Fenton WS, McGlashan TH: Natural history of schizophrenic subtypes. *Arch Gen Psychiatry* 1991, 48:969–977.

McGlashan TH, Fenton WS: Classical subtypes for schizophrenia: literature review for DSM-IV. *Schizophrenia Bull* 1991, 17:609–632.

Diagnosis

Signs and symptoms

• The symptoms of the disorder are identical to schizophrenia except the illness lasts for >1 month but <6 months, and impaired social functioning is not a requirement for the diagnosis. The essential features of the illness are:

1. Good premorbid functioning.

2. Sudden onset of psychotic symptoms.

3. Symptoms last >1 month but <6 months.

4. Predominance of positive symptoms with negligible negative symptoms.

5. Symptoms are not related to substance abuse or any medical condition.

6. Symptoms are not related to schizoaffective or mood disorder.

Positive symptoms
Hallucinations.

Delusions.

Confusion.

Perplexity.

Grossly disorganized speech and behavior.

Negative symptoms
Inappropriate affect.

Social withdrawal.

Poor personal hygiene.

Anhedonia.

Investigations

• There is no laboratory test available that is indicative of schizophreniform disorder. The diagnosis is made by interviewing the patient and by obtaining a comprehensive history and a complete physical examination. Particularly with an initial episode, it is important to rule out any physical condition that might mimic the symptoms of the disorder. Some possible physical causes might be vascular disorders, toxicity, metabolic disturbances, autoimmune deficiencies, endocrine disorders, nutritional deficiencies, infections, brain trauma, temporal lobe epilepsy. Laboratory screening tests might include toxicology screen, chemistry panel, thyroid function tests, and complete blood count.

Complications

Suicide: there is a significant risk of suicide; in one study, there was an 8% rate of completed suicide (death) among those with schizophreniform disorder.

Depression: periods of depression after the psychotic symptoms abate are common.

Change in diagnosis to one with poorer prognosis: if symptoms persist for >6 months.

Treatment

Diet and lifestyle
• As in all conditions, it is important to maintain a healthy lifestyle with a balanced and nutritious diet, adequate rest, exercise, avoidance of alcohol and drugs, and a decrease in the level of stress.

Pharmacologic treatment
• Neuroleptics (conventional antipsychotics) or the newer atypical antipsychotics are used to treat the symptoms of schizophreniform disorder. There is no evidence that any particular neuroleptic is better at treating the disorder than another, although an individual patient might respond better and have fewer side effects to a particular drug.

Risperidone
• One of the newer atypical antipsychotic medications useful in treating acute psychotic symptoms. Available only in pill form.

Standard dosage	Titrated up to 4–6 mg/d to a maximum of 6–12 mg/d administered on a twice-per-day schedule for an acute psychotic episode.
Main side effects	Orthostatic hypotension, drowsiness, extrapyramidal symptoms at higher doses (eg, dystonic reactions, restlessness, tremor, muscle rigidity), tardive dyskinesia.
Main drug interactions	Should be used with caution in combination with drugs or alcohol that effect the central nervous system (CNS). May enhance the hypertensive effects of other drugs with this potential.

Olanzapine
• An atypical antipsychotic for control of psychotic disorders, it is generally well tolerated and has fewer side effects than the conventional antipsychotic agents.

Standard dosage	10 mg/d orally for acute psychotic symptoms; the dosage may be adjusted within a range of 5–20 mg/d, depending on the clinical status of the patient.
Main side effects	Sedation, weight gain, orthostatic hypotension, extrapyramidal symptoms (eg, akathesia and parkinsonism) are common.
Main drug interactions	Enhanced sedation with other CNS depressants.

Quetiapine
Standard dose	300–400 mg/d up to a maximum of 750 mg/d.
Main side effects	Somnolence, hypotension, lens changes (rare), TD (rare).
Main drug interactions	Potentiates other CNS medications.
Special points	High cost; available only in oral form.

Clozapine
• Useful in patients who don't respond to other antipsychotics.

Standard dose	300–600 mg/d (can go up to 900 mg/d).
Main side effects	Agranulocytosis, seizures.
Main drug interactions	Do not use with tegretol.

Haloperidol and other conventional neuroleptics
• Wide number of agents, available in pill, injection and depot injection forms.

Standard dosage	2–20 mg/d (average 10 mg/d) orally during acute episodes.
Main side effects	Extrapyramidal symptoms (eg, parkinsonian tremor, stiffness, dystonia, akathisia), sedation, neuroleptic malignant syndrome (rare, but of concern).
Main drug interactions	Many potentiate other CNS drugs.

Prognosis
• According to DSM-IV, the following are good prognostic features:
Onset of prominent psychotic symptoms within 4 wk of the first noticeable change in usual behavior or functioning
Confusion or perplexity at the height of the psychotic episode
Good premorbid social and occupational functioning
Absence of blunted or flat affect
• If the illness lasts only a short period of time, the prognosis is likely to be better.

Nonpharmacologic treatment
Hospitalization: often indicated for a first episode of psychosis in order to keep the patient safe, and to rule out medical conditions that might be responsible for symptoms.
Individual therapy: helpful to deal with issues surrounding the illness after psychotic symptoms are under control.
Patient and family education: particularly important for monitoring the symptoms and increasing participation in treatment.
Electroconvulsive therapy: may be indicated for those patients with marked catatonic or severe depression.

Special considerations and other drugs
• The newer atypical antipsychotic medications are much more expensive than the conventional antipsychotic medications, although they are generally better tolerated.
• It usually requires a 3–6-month course of antipsychotic drugs to treat psychotic symptoms fully
• 75% of patients with Schizophreniform disorder usually respond with noticeable reductions in symptoms with antipsychotic medication treatment within 8 days.
• Anticholinergic drugs are used to treat the extrapyramidal side effects, eg, Cogentin (0.5–6.0 mg/d), Artane (1–15 mg/d), Symmetrel (100–300) mg/d.
• Neuroleptic malignant syndrome is rare (1%–2% of patients treated with antipsychotic medications) but is a potentially fatal complication.

SCHIZOTYPAL PERSONALITY DISORDER

Diagnosis

Definition
• Schizotypal personality disorder is a pervasive pattern of deficits and discomforts in social and interpersonal relationships, with perceptual distortions and eccentricities of behavior, appearance, and speech.

Symptoms and signs
Unusual phrasing or construction of speech; unconventional use of words; no significant looseness of associations; distress and decreased desire for close relationships: in contrast with schizoid personality disorder, (no distress and no desire for close relationships); **transient psychotic episodes:** lasting minutes to hours; in response to stress.

DSM-IV criteria
• Schizotypal personality disorder does not occur exclusively during the course of schizophrenia, a mood disorder with psychotic features, another psychotic disorder, or a pervasive developmental disorder.

• The disorder is indicated by the presence of five or more of the following:

1. Ideas of reference.

2. Odd beliefs or magical thinking that influences behavior and is inconsistent with subcultural norms.

3. Unusual perceptual experiences, including bodily illusions.

4. Odd thinking and speech.

5. Suspiciousness or paranoid ideation.

6. Inappropriate or constricted affect.

7. Behavior or appearance that is odd, eccentric, or peculiar.

8. Lack of close friends or confidants other than first-degree relatives.

9. Excessive social anxiety that does not diminish with familiarity and tends to be associated with paranoid fears rather than negative judgments about self.

Investigations
Psychologic testing
Minnesota Multiphasic Personality Inventory-2: possible elevations of scales 6 (paranoia), 8 (schizophrenia), and 0 (social introversion); **Millon Clinical Multiaxial Inventory-III:** scale 5 specifically measures for schizotypal personality disorder; **Rorschach:** The Exner scoring system is useful in detecting mild thought disorders and emotional trait characteristics.

Neuropsychologic testing
Impaired performance on the following tests of perceptual gating and orientation: auditory P300 responses between chronic schizophrenia and controls; prolonged reaction times in switching attention between auditory and visual modalities; deficits in sensorimotor gating; impaired auditory selective attention during interference tests; abnormal galvanic skin orienting responses; Wisconsin Card Sorting Test perseveration errors; California Verbal Learning Test impairment; Trail-making Test, Part B performance problems; facial expression recognition deficits; attention deficits.

Complications
Comorbidity: depressive disorders (50% incidence); anxiety disorders; concurrent personality disorder of another type (eg, schizoid, paranoid, avoidant, borderline).

Behavioral outcomes: isolation and social support deficiencies; employment difficulties (especially in jobs that require social skills); less likely to attempt suicide than those with other personality disorders; misinterpretations, paranoia, and ideas of reference complicate marriage and close relationships; reduced frequency of marriages and close relationships.

Differential diagnosis
• Psychotic disorders (delusional disorder, schizophrenia, mood disorders with psychotic features) have longer and more severe psychotic episodes.
• Autistic disorder or Asperger's disorder have more severe deficits in social awareness, emotional reciprocity, and stereotyped behaviors.
• Expressive language disorders have more primary language disturbances, with attempts to compensate by other means of communication.
• Other personality disorders include the following:
Paranoid and schizoid: do not have the same fashion of cognitive and perceptual distortions or the extent of eccentricity and oddness.
Avoidant: desire relationships but feel constrained by fear of rejection.
Narcissistic: may have fears of imperfections or flaws being revealed that "look" suspicious or socially withdrawn.
Borderline: have manipulative behaviors, with any reactive psychotic episodes usually linked to pronounced mood symptoms; those with borderline personality disorder usually desire intimacy but may be socially isolated as a consequence of anger episodes or mood instability.

Etiology
• Schizotypal personality disorder is a characterologic phenotypic variant of a schizophrenic genotype (a "schizophrenia spectrum" disorder).
• Biologic markers in common with schizophrenia include lateral ventricular enlargement, reduced prefrontal cortical mass, increased cerebrospinal fluid and plasma homovanillic acid levels, and impaired smooth-pursuit eye-tracking movement.
• There are prefrontal and left hemispheric neuropsychologic performance deficits (see Neuropsychologic testing).
• Adoptive and family studies find higher prevalence among first-degree relatives of those with schizophrenia; schizophrenia and other psychotic disorders are more prevalent among the relatives of schizotypal patients.

Epidemiology
• The prevalence in the general population is ~2%–5%.
• It is possibly more common in men than in women.

Treatment

Pharmacologic treatment

- Low-dose neuroleptics are helpful for paranoia, reactive thought disorganization, and periods of escalated anxiety; whether treatment is episodic or continuous depends on individual case determination.
- Comorbid conditions (*eg*, depression, insomnia, panic or anxiety) should be specifically treated.
- Incidence of medication-related adverse effects is typically high
- Very low doses of neuroleptics or anxiolytics often are effective.
- Medication compliance is often difficult.
- Discuss tardive dyskinesia and other neuroleptic-related risks.

Nonpharmacologic treatment

Schizotypal characteristics influencing psychotherapy

Sense of discontinuity with time and other people.

Anhedonia: a common schizotypal trait.

Tendency to misinterpret social situations.

Concrete and humorless interpersonal style.

Problems with ego boundaries, distortions of the sense of self.

Need for education and accurate interpretations of reality: especially in respect to interpersonal situations.

Hypochondriacal tendencies: in one third of cases.

Supportive therapy

- Maintain a "safe" emotional distance.
- Caution is necessary regarding sensitivity and tendencies for shame perception.
- Keep the pace slow.
- Useful supportive interventions include gradual therapeutic alliance and relationship via nonjudgmental acceptance and session regularity; sympathetic listening, empathetic interest; education, advice, assistance with problem solving; encouragement, exhortation; the therapist as "reality organ" (auxiliary ego).

Cognitive-behavioral therapy

- The first priority is establishing a solid therapeutic relationship.
- Discover underlying beliefs.
- Discover dysfunctional assumptions and cognitive errors that lead to unhappiness and distress.
- Explore automatic thoughts.
- Active therapist involvement through the Socratic method, with the ultimate treatment goal begin to replace negative beliefs, assumptions, and automatic thoughts with more realistic and positive ones.

Behavioral therapy

- Behavioral therapies include social skills training, role playing and rehearsal, and formal educational and training resources.

Group therapy

- Group therapy has positive potential on diminished social anxieties, interpersonal insights and skills, and the capacity and confidence for developing friendships.
- There is negative potential for rejection by other members and threatening material in group dialogue (excessive dynamic or insight orientation).

Family therapy

- Family therapy should be educational and supportive.

Treatment aims

Short-term: to achieve crisis stabilization and situational support.
Long-term: to achieve stability of reality orientation, maximal psychosocial functioning.

Other treatments

- Self-help groups: usually too threatening.
- Day treatment programs: beneficial for some.
- Vocational rehabilitation services.
- Partial hospital programs: useful as intensive psychosocial therapy resources.
- Acute inpatient treatment: only for crisis decompensation.
- Long-term inpatient treatment is virtually never needed.

Prognosis

- Relatively stable course.
- Approximately 10%–20% later develop schizophrenia or another psychotic disorder.

Follow-up and management

For the acute phase

Crisis stabilization.
Close monitoring of medication effectiveness and side effects.
Active, directive therapist intervention.

For the continuation phase

Often indefinite for the long term.
Agenda shifts to gradual insights, belief reorientation capacities, confidence, and comforts.
For some, expanded interpersonal relationships; for others, expanded solitary activities and interests.

General references

Kaplan HI, Sadock BJ: *Comprehensive Textbook of Psychiatry*, ed 6. Baltimore: Williams & Wilkins; 1995.

Task Force on Treatments of Psychiatric Disorders: *Treatments of Psychiatric Disorders*. Washington, DC: American Psychiatric Association; 1989.

Treatments of Psychiatric Disorders, ed 2. Edited by Gabbard GO. Washington, DC: American Psychiatric Press; 1995.

Diagnosis

Definition

• The substances in this category include the benzodiazepines, the carbamates (eg, meprobramate), the barbiturates (eg, secobarbital), and the barbiturate-like hypnotics (eg, glutethimide, methaqualone). This class of substances includes almost all of the prescription sleeping medications and almost all prescription antianxiety medications, except for the nonbenzodiazepine antianxiety agents.

• Sedative hypnotic problems may be classified into three distinct categories:

Sedative hypnotic dependence: dependence is characterized by physiologic dependence and withdrawal symptoms; the substance taken in larger amounts or over a longer period then intended; significant drug-seeking behavior; and continued use despite social, psychologic, occupational, or physical consequences.

Sedative hypnotic abuse: abuse may occur alone or, more commonly, in conjunction with other substances; abuse is marked by recurrent use in situations in which use is physically hazardous and by continued use despite knowledge of having persistent or recurrent social, occupational, psychologic, or physical problems caused or exacerbated by the substances; when these behaviors are accompanied by evidence of tolerance, withdrawal, or compulsive using behaviors, a diagnosis of dependence should be made.

Physical dependence: marked by tolerance of and withdrawal from the substances in this class; current research shows that physiologic dependence may set in after as little as 2–4 weeks of continued use; this is differentiated from addiction by the lack of significant drug-seeking behaviors and psychosocial impairment.

Symptoms and signs

• Substances in this class are central nervous system depressants and, therefore, elicit effects similar to alcohol in their action. Common signs of sedative hypnotic intoxication include impaired psychomotor functioning, slurred speech, difficulty with concentration, impairment in ability to recall information, behavioral disinhibition, respiratory depression, impaired reflex eye movements, cardiovascular depression.

• A withdrawal syndrome emerges on cessation or decreased dosage of these substances. The most frequent symptoms of withdrawal tend to be indistinguishable from the typical manifestations of anxiety.

• Common symptoms of withdrawal include anxiety, insomnia, restlessness, agitation, irritability, muscle tension, nausea, coryza, diaphoresis, lethargy, hyperacusis, aches and pains, blurred vision, depression, nightmares, hyperreflexia, ataxia. Less common withdrawal symptoms include psychosis, seizures, persistent tinnitus, confusion, paranoia, paranoid delusions, hallucinations.

• Overdose can be reached quickly with this class of drugs due to their synergistic effect with other central nervous system depressants. Common signs of sedative-hypnotic overdose include stupor, coma, periods of silence on electroencephalogram, pupillary constriction, diminished or absent pupillary and corneal reflexes, slow or rapid and shallow breathing, Cheyne-Stokes breathing, delayed gastric emptying, shock, and hypothermia.

Investigations

• A detailed chemical use history is recommended. Important factors to include in this history are as follows:

Family history of chemical use; amount, frequency, and duration of sedative-hypnotic use; concurrent substance use and abuse: particularly alcohol, other sedative-hypnotic agents, opiates, and cocaine; **prior abuse of sedative hypnotics; prior history of substance abuse or dependency; problems associated or concurrent with sedative-hypnotic:** eg, familial, occupational, marital, social, physical, and psychological; **toxicology screen, complete blood count, and blood chemistry:** may be helpful in delineating a diagnosis.

Differential diagnosis

• Complications or consequences of sedative hypnotic abuse are often mistaken for secondary rather than primary problems (eg, seizure disorders, alcohol dependence, head trauma from motor vehicle accidents).

• Patients may present with complaints that, if investigated, are seen as consequences of sedative-hypnotic problems (eg, social, familial, marital, occupational impairments).

• Psychiatric complaints often mistaken for sedative hypnotic problems include anxiety, panic attacks, insomnia, restlessness, agitation, irritability, and generalized aches and pains.

• Comorbid diagnoses include:
Anxiety disorders (eg, generalized anxiety disorder, panic attacks), depressive disorders, adjustment disorder, somatoform disorder, personality (axis II) disorders (eg, borderline, histrionic), dementia, head trauma, anorexia or bulimia.

Etiology

• Risk factors for sedative hypnotic abuse include the following:
Family history of substance or alcohol problems; past history of substance or alcohol problems; female gender; middle-aged and elderly patients (>40 y of age); concurrent psychiatric illness, particularly the anxiety-related diagnoses.

Complications

Physical: substances in this class work synergistically with each other, and toxicity may be reached quickly; toxicity may be fatal if not managed; patients may present with hypertension, liver disease, seizures, tremors, and physical symptoms of withdrawal.

Social: disruption in familial, social, and occupational functioning may be evident in the addicted patient; individuals may exhibit behavioral disinhibition when intoxicated; patients may report to a physician with physical trauma associated with behavioral disinhibition or psychomotor retardation.

Psychologic: patients may present with symptoms of anxiety, panic attacks, insomnia, depression, and other stress-related complaints (eg, restlessness, irritability).

Treatment

Diet and lifestyle

• Patients are encouraged to resume regular eating habits and sleep patterns. Additionally, patients are encouraged to develop prosocial stress-management activities, along with maintaining a more balanced schedule of activities.

Nonpharmacologic treatments

• Referrals to substance-abuse treatment centers or self-help groups (eg, Narcotics Anonymous) is the most common form of treatment. Practitioners should cultivate a contact within the substance-abuse treatment community to recommend facilities that match patient needs and preferences.

Pharmacologic treatment

Withdrawal

• Hospital admission requirements for detoxification depend on the quantity, frequency, and duration of sedative-hypnotic use. Discontinuation of sedative-hypnotic use can be facilitated by informing patients of the possible withdrawal symptoms prior to treatment. A method of gradual dose reduction is most effective in easing patients out of both withdrawal and physical dependence. In general, two methods of tapering exist: 1) a gradual dose reduction of the abused medication, and 2) a tapering schedule designed to substitute longer-acting for shorter-acting sedative hypnotics, with the gradual tapering off of the medication. A dose equivalency of 30 mg of phenobarbital per daily dose of sedative hypnotic (or 70% of the estimated daily dose if the patient has a poor history) is used in tapering. Alternatively, substitution of a longer acting benzodiazepine (eg, chlordiazepoxide or clonazepam) for a shorter-acting drug (eg, alprazolam) can be achieved using a taper schedule based on the drug half-life from which the patient is being withdrawn. Carbamazepine (up to 800 mg/d total) and flumazenil have shown some success in ameliorating the physical and some of the anxiety-related symptoms of sedative-hypnotic withdrawal.

Overdose

• Hospital admission to monitor vital signs is recommended. Gastric lavage, activated charcoal, and magnesium citrate may be helpful. Additionally, general respiratory and cardiovascular support may be required. Flumazenil has been shown effective in reversing the effects of sedative hypnotic overdose.

• Flumazenil is indicated for management of benzodiazepine withdrawal and overdose.

Standard dosage	Initial dose, 0.2–0.4 mg i.v. for 30 seconds, then every 30 seconds to a maximum dosage of 3 mg (for i.v. use only).
Main drug interactions	Neuromuscular blockade; effects must be fully reversed; reversal of benzodiazepine effects may be associated with the onset of seizures in high-risk populations (eg, concurrent sedative-hypnotic withdrawal, recent therapy with cyclic antidepressants or parenteral benzodiazepine, and seizure activity prior to administration of flumazenil); not recommended in cases of serious cyclic antidepressant poisonings, as manifested by motor abnormalities, dysrhythmias, anticholinergic signs, and cardiovascular collapse at presentation.
Special points	Patient should be monitored carefully; not recommended in children; use with caution in head-injury patients, drug and alcohol patients, and psychiatric patients because drug may provoke panic attacks; may precipitate convulsions or restrict cerebral blood flow.

Treatment aims

To achieve and adhere to abstinence from mood- and mind-altering drugs.

To educate on alternative methods of coping with concurrent presenting psychiatric problems.

To educate and facilitate family and peer support.

For physical dependence: to facilitate the discontinuance of sedative-hypnotic use.

Follow-up and management

• Primary goal of follow-up is to prevent and identify signs of relapse.

• Family and peer support is essential for continued abstinence.

• Management of concurrent psychiatric diagnosis, if applicable, by therapeutic or psychiatric interventions is essential. Referrals for anxiety and sleep-related disorders are often beneficial in helping patients maintain abstinence. Buspirone and selective serotonin reuptake inhibitors have shown success in treating many of the concurrent psychiatric complaints of patients.

• Management by primary care physician of concurrent physical problems associated with or caused by sedative-hypnotic use.

General references

Diagnostic and Statistical Manual of Mental Disorders, ed 4. Washington, DC: American Psychiatric Association; 1995:261–270.

Hayner G, Galloway G, Wiehl WO: Haight Ashbury free clinic's drug detoxification protocols: Part 3: benzodiazapines and other sedative-hypnotics. *J Psychoactive Drugs* 1993, 25:331–335.

Milhorn TH Jr: *Chemical Dependence: Diagnosis, Treatment and Prevention.* New York: Springer-Verlag; 1990:149–166.

Parran T: Prescription drug abuse: a question of balance. *Med Clin North Am* 1997, 81:967–978.

Sussman N: Treating anxiety while minimizing abuse and dependence. *J Clin Psychiatry* 1993, 54(suppl):44–51.

Woods JH, Winger G: Current benzodiazapine issues. *Psychopharmacology* 1995, 118:107–115.

Diagnosis

Symptoms and signs

Absence of speech in at least one social situation: despite the ability to speak in other situations; absence of speech must be persistent for at least 1 month but, if in the classroom, not limited to the first month of the school year; must significantly interfere with social or academic functioning.

Communication using gestures, monosyllabic utterance, or by pulling or pushing others.

Extreme shyness, clingy behavior, withdrawal, negativity, or temper outbursts.

Compulsive behaviors: may occasionally be seen.

• This disorder may begin prior to 5 years of age but not come to medical attention until school age. The disorder may persist for several months or years.

Investigations

Careful parent and child interviews.

Physical examination: including a neurologic assessment and evaluation of oral, sensory, and motor functioning.

Speech and language evaluation: essential; audiometry should be included in the speech assessment.

Complications

Significant social and academic impairments.

Low self-esteem.

Differential diagnosis
• An underlying communication disorder must be ruled out.
• Lack of knowledge of the local language must also be eliminated as a causal factor.
• The presence of pervasive developmental disorder, a psychotic disorder, or severe mental retardation.
may preclude the diagnosis of selective mutism.
• If criteria are met, a diagnosis of social phobia may be made concomitantly.

Etiology
• An anxious, shy, or inhibited temperament has been shown to be associated with the disorder. Occasionally psychodynamic factors related to the sudden loss of a caretaker or to a traumatic event may be indicated.

Epidemiology
• The prevalence is less than 1% in school-age children, with females more commonly affected than males.

Treatment

Pharmacologic treatment
• Treatment of a comorbid condition (*eg*, an anxiety disorder) may be beneficial.
• Fluoxetine has been helpful in single-case and small, controlled trials.

Nonpharmacologic treatment
• Integrated treatment approach involving multidisciplinary team of parents, educators, and a speech therapist may hold the greatest possibility of success.
• Cognitive-behavioral and psychodynamic therapies may be included based on specific needs and circumstances.

Treatment aims
To achieve a decrease in anxiety, with appropriate speech production in social situations and consequent improvement in social and academic functioning.

General references
Dow SP, Sonies BC, Scheib D, et al.: Practical guidelines for the assessment and treatment of selective mutism. *J Am Acad Child Adolesc Psychiatry* 1995, 34:836–846.

Diagnosis

Definition
• Separation and anxiety disorder is defined as developmentally inappropriate and excessive anxiety in response to separation from home, parents, or loved ones.

Symptoms and signs
• Anxiety symptoms range from anticipatory uneasiness to panic to tantrums and pleading.

• They must be present for at least 4 weeks and present before 18 years of age.

• Anxiety may manifest as a variety of somatic symptoms, such as recurrent abdominal pain or palpitations. • Other symptoms include recurrent unrealistic worries about harm befalling loved ones or an untoward event causing separation, refusal to go to school or elsewhere due to these fears, sleep difficulties, reluctance of refusal to fall asleep without the loved one near, nightmares with separation themes, and the child making frequent contact with and communicating desire to return to the loved one.

Investigations
Thorough psychosocial and family history.

Physical examination.

Somatic complaints in relation to episodes of separation: may preclude investigative procedures.

Differential diagnosis
Depression.
Pervasive developmental delay.
Early stages of a psychotic illness.
Panic disorder or generalized anxiety disorder.
Truancy.
Phobic avoidance.
Medical causes for somatic symptoms.

Etiology
Recent experiences of loss or change.
Illness or death of a family member.
Disruptive change of home or school.
Positive family history of anxiety disorders, depression, somatization disorder, or alcoholism.
Anxiety within the family communicated to the child, particularly regarding separation.

Epidemiology
Prevalence, 3.5% to 5.4%.
Peak incidence, ~11 y of age and equal between boys and girls.
Slightly lower socioeconomic class.

Treatment

Pharmacologic treatment

Antidepressants.

Imipramine: up to 3-5 mg/kg/d with baseline and follow-up electrocardiography.

Selective serotonin-reuptake inhibitors: *eg,* fluoxetine up to 1 mg/kg (usually 0.5 mg/kg).

Nonpharmacologic treatment

Hospitalization with enforced separation and a progressive reunification schedule: when patient's illness is severe and refractory to outpatient intervention efforts.

Behavioral therapy.

Parent guidance.

Enforced separation at natural and usual times: encourage extrafamilial activities and relationships.

Praise for successful separation attempts and behavioral reinforcement of success.

Systematic desensitization.

Family intervention: to address how anxiety is transmissible in a family; family therapy.

SEXUAL AROUSAL DISORDER, FEMALE

Diagnosis

Symptoms and signs [1]

Little or no sexual pleasure with partner during physical intimacy or intercourse.

Concomitant failure to achieve or maintain vaginal lubrication and engorgement: despite normal sexual stimulation.

Feeling "dead" or numb when with partner: but no physical signs, eg, pain, panic, or aversion.

• To be considered a disorder, the disturbance must cause significant subjective distress or relationship problems. Symptoms may be lifelong or acquired, generalized, or situation-specific. Normal excitement from self-stimulation may be present.

• Symptoms may go undetected or underreported by many females.

• Individuals may have tried home remedies, eg, lubricants.

Investigations

History: diagnosis is made from history.

Physical evaluation: to rule out possible contributory or causative medical factors (eg, abnormal genital anatomy, endocrinopathy [including diabetes], neuropathy, and medication use).

Psychologic assessment and testing: may reveal characteristics, behaviors, or disorders that may be contributing to the intensity, duration, or frequency of orgasmic difficulties; screening for depression, anxiety, and relational problems is particularly important.

Assessment of the patient's (and partner's) understanding of normal sexual anatomy and function.

Complications

Sexual inadequacy: affected females may feel that they are sexually inadequate; the patient's partner, similarly, may feel that he or she is at fault for failing to provide adequate sexual stimulation or satisfaction.

Avoidance of sexual relationships, decreased sexual desire, painful intercourse, serious marital dysfunction, and other psychiatric disorders: may result.

Negative effects of home remedies: for the vaginal area or contraceptive effectiveness, eg, petroleum-based jellies can cause irritation and bacteria growth.

Differential diagnosis

• This disorder is very difficult to differentiate from hypoactive sexual desire disorder.

Etiology

• The degree to which "normal" females can and do experience sexual arousal probably varies considerably. Cases in which there is virtually no arousal or pleasurable response to sexual thoughts or stimulation usually have significant psychologic contributors, which may include unhealthy attitudes towards sex (especially inappropriate guilt or belief that sex is unnatural or unclean), conflict or dissatisfaction with one's partner, history of sexual abuse or trauma, history of prostitution, fear of intimacy, and fear of pregnancy. Conflicts over sexual identity or preference may occasionally give rise to this disorder.

• Medical concerns (eg, hormonal changes, vascular problems, and neurologic concerns) may result in decreased physiologic sexual arousal. These concerns may then interact with psychologic concerns to create a combined etiology.

Epidemiology

• Prevalence of the disorder is unknown. Sexual arousal (and, previously, frigidity) is a vague term that has made systematic research into this disorder difficult. Additionally, females are often reluctant to report this problem or are sometimes unaware that a problem exists.

Treatment

Diet and lifestyle

• Body image and self-esteem are important to feeling "sexual" and deserving of receiving pleasure from a partner. Appropriate interventions, such as weight loss and exercise, may be beneficial.

Pharmacologic treatment

• Treatment with short-acting benzodiazepines on an as-needed basis may be helpful in cases accompanied by anxiety over sexuality or sexual performance.

• Bupropion is being studied as a drug to increase arousal but is unproven for this indication.

• Associated (or causative) depression should be treated with antidepressants, but only bupropion, mirtazepine, and nefazodone appear to be relatively free of adverse sexual side effects.

Nonpharmacologic treatments

• Treatment will most likely include the following components:

1. Education for female and her partner regarding sexual anatomy and normal sexual function.

2. Enlistment of the partner's cooperation, understanding, and patience.

3. Increasing patient's ability to feel comfortable with her body in the presence of a partner.

4. Sex therapy: may include sensate focus exercises, relaxation therapy, increased awareness that orgasmic capacity should not be used as a measure of "success" for a sexual encounter, that a very satisfactory sexual relationship can exist in the absence or orgasms for one or both of the partners, guided/directed masturbation, sharing of pleasure points with her partner, and discovering variations of stimulation to enhance sexual experiences.

5. Addressing relationship problems and conflicts over intimacy and sexuality.

6. Addressing sexual abuse or sexual trauma. Treatment of individuals who have been sexually traumatized or abused is difficult and best undertaken by a clinician who has the experience and time necessary to help the patient safely and successfully resolve these traumatic experiences.

7. Bibliotherapy: many helpful books (see General references) are available to help the woman become more comfortable with and knowledgeable about her sexuality.

8. Psychotherapy: generally assumes that all females are biologically capable of attaining orgasm; treatment goals include becoming comfortable with nudity and genitalia, feeling safe in her relationship, and focussing on the receipt of pleasure that is free of guilt or expectations.

Treatment aims

To address medical problems that may contribute to decreased sexual arousal. To increase sexual satisfaction by means of enhancing and accepting one's sexuality.

Prognosis

• Prognosis is variable. Patient motivation is essential. Treatment sought only to please the partner has a lower success rate than that which is sought to understand and explore the patient's own sexual difficulties. Lifelong cases have a poorer prognosis than those cases that are acquired.

Key reference

1. Rosen RC, Beck JG: *Patterns of Sexual Arousal*. New York: The Guilford Press; 1988.

General references

• *See* General references for Orgasmic disorder, female.

Diagnosis

Definition [1]
• Sexual aversion disorder is defined as a fear of or intense aversion to genital contact with a partner or to nongenital aspects of sex (*eg*, kissing or breast touching), with a compelling urge to avoid the feared or repulsive activity. The aversion causes significant distress or interpersonal difficulty. Resistance to behavioral "homework" assignments is common.

Symptoms and signs [1]
• Sexual activities may be associated with panic attacks and/or flashbacks from a previous sexual trauma.

• Fear and aversion may result from specific sexual acts (*eg*, penetration) or they may result from overall sexual behaviors and feelings

• To avoid sexual activities, individuals may engage in various behaviors including decreasing their attractiveness by wearing baggy clothing, not eating, or overeating; going to bed early or late; becoming overinvolved in work, family, or social activities; or traveling frequently.

Investigations
History: inquire regarding underlying anxiety disorders (*eg*, obsessive-compulsive fear of touching or germs); relationship problems; fear or dislike of one's partner; sexual identity disturbances; and history of sexual, physical, and emotional abuse.

Psychologic testing: may offer information concerning other psychopathology that exacerbates or contributes to the sexual aversion.

Complications
Hypoactive sexual arousal.

Inhibited orgasm.

Dyspareunia or vaginismus.

Abnormal intimacy and romantic relationships.

Partners feeling rejected, undesirable, or inadequate.

• Demanding genital contact as a therapeutic approach may actually exacerbate the severity of the patient's symptoms.

• Individuals may have attempted self-medication through the use of alcohol or other intoxicating substances.

Differential diagnosis
Hypoactive sexual desire disorders (HSDs): involve simple loss of sexual desire in the absence of a phobic component; there is no appetite for erotic interchange with a partner, and the patient is not actively repelled or afraid as with sexual aversion [1].

Occasional sexual aversion that is not persistent or recurrent, or sexual aversion that does not cause marked distress or relationship problems: not considered to be a sexual aversion disorder.

Relationship problems: may result in decreased sexual activity and repulsion of one partner for the other; the aversion in this circumstance is to the other partner rather than sexual activity per se.

Etiology
• Early indoctrination that sex or the body is unnatural, sinful, or "dirty" is common.

• A history of sexual abuse as well as fear of germs (especially HIV), touching, intimacy, and pregnancy may cause or contribute to the disorder.

Epidemiology
• Sexual aversion disorder occurs in both sexes but is more common in females.

• Prevalence is unknown but is estimated to occur in 1%–2% of the general population, and it commonly occurs with other anxiety disorders.

Treatment

Pharmacologic treatment

• Use of antianxiety medications, such as the benzodiazepines (usually on an "as needed" basis), as an adjunct to treatment can reduce the patient's anxiety to manageable levels, but alone does not cure these patients [2].

Nonpharmacologic treatment

• Treatment is frequently multifaceted. Depending upon the etiologic nature of the disorder for a particular individual, the treatment may be patterned after treatment for phobias and posttraumatic stress disorder (PTSD) or as a severe case of hypoactive sexual desire disorder. Generally, the same techniques are utilized with varying emphasis upon each technique. Both approaches often include the following:

Education regarding normal sexual function and relationships.

Psychotherapy: may be necessary to help the patient understand and resolve the contributory components to the sexual aversion.

Sensate focus exercises: designed to decrease performance anxiety and increase enjoyment of sensual experiences; for some individuals with sexual aversion, sensate focus is not effective and may actually aggravate the severity of the symptoms [3]; therefore, it is indicated only after complete assessment of the individual's needs.

Exposure therapy: extinguishing the sexual phobic response by means of gradually exposing the individual to the feared situation and allowing the anxiety to habituate; the sexual exposure prescribed for sexual aversions should be individualized and controlled so that the patient's anxiety remains tolerable during the duration of these therapeutic exercises; the patient must be desensitized slowly, with very small increments of exposure to the previously avoided sexual situation until the phobic response is extinguished [4].

Relaxation therapy: may be helpful in decreasing anxiety and increasing motivation to engage in exposure therapy.

Treatment aims

To reduce aversion or fear associated with sexual activity.
To address additional concerns that may have been related to the occurrence of this disorder (eg, relationship difficulties, past sexual trauma).

Prognosis

• Without treatment, the expected course is similar to that of simple phobias and PTSD.
• With treatment, prognosis is largely dependent upon identification and correction of underlying causative or contributory psychologic factors.

Key references

1. Kaplan HS: The Sexual Desire Disorders: Dysfunctional Regulation of Sexual Motivation. New York: Brunner/Mazel; 1995
2. Masters WH, Johnson VE: Human sexual inadequacy. Boston: Little, Brown; 1970.
3. Kaplan HS: Sexual aversion disorder. In Case Studies in Sex Therapy. Edited by Rosen RC, Leiblum SR: New York: The Guilford Press; 1995.
4. Kaplan HS: Sexual Aversions, Sexual Phobias, and Panic Disorders. New York: Brunner/Mazel; 1986.

General references

• See General references for Orgasmic disorder, female.

Diagnosis

Definitions [1–4]

• According to the DSM-IV, hypoactive sexual desire disorder (HSD) is characterized by persistently or recurrently low or absent sexual fantasies and desire for sexual activity, which causes marked distress or interpersonal difficulty and is not due a medical condition, a substance (drug of abuse or medication), or another major psychiatric disorder (*eg*, major depressive disorder).

• The judgment of deficiency or absence is made by the clinician, taking into account factors that affect sexual functioning (*eg*, age and the context of the person's life). Although desire does tend to decline with age, in the absence of illness, the sex drive should continue to function well into advanced old age. Although frequency of sexual activity does not equate with desire, one of the most widely accepted definitions of low frequency is any sexual activity occurring less than once every 2 weeks for persons ≤55 years of age.

Lifelong versus acquired HSD

• One should determine whether the condition is lifelong or developed after a period of normal functioning. Majority of cases are acquired. Lifelong type is more common in women than men.

Global versus situational HSD

• Some people may only have difficulty with a certain partner, type of partner, or specific sort of sexual activity, yet they may remain interested in masturbating, fantasy, and other partners. Others may have no interest in any and all sexual activities and are devoid of sexual fantasies. Situational HSD may be more likely to have psychologic etiologies, but organic processes can still be contributing factors. Global dysfunction may result from either psychogenic or organic processes.

HSD due to psychologic factors versus combined factors

• This is a difficult distinction to make and undoubtedly most cases are due to combined factors to some degree.

Investigations

Assessment for depression: decreased desire is a common symptom of depression and a side effect of many antidepressants; lifetime prevalence of mood disorders is increased in patients with HSD.

Assessment for other sexual disorders: ~40% of patients with HSD present with another sexual dysfunction; in males, erectile dysfunction is most common [3]; if present, urologic or gynecologic referral may be indicated.

Assessment for possible medication side effects: numerous medications (*see* Differential diagnosis) can decrease desire; patients are often unaware of the potential for such effects.

Assessment of the couple: the complaint of low desire may actually represent an excessive level of desire in the other partner; partners may merely have levels of desire on opposing ends of the normal continuum; the complaint may also be a manifestation of more generalized relationship discord.

Laboratory investigations: generally do not indicate abnormalities; common levels checked include testosterone level, prolactin level, thyroid-stimulating hormone, estrogen level, follicle-stimulating hormone, and luteinizing hormone.

Complications

Relationship stress.

Impairment of procreation.

Exacerbation of comorbid psychiatric conditions.

Differential diagnosis [1,5]

Sexual aversion disorder.

Substance abuse.

Side effects of medications (eg, antihypertensives, antidepressants, antipsychotics, antiandrogens).

Decreased desire as a component of another Axis I disorder (eg, major depressive or anxiety disorders).

Hypogonadal states.

Decreased desire secondary to another sexual dysfunction (eg, organic impotence or dyspareunia) Hyper- and hypothyroidism.

Hyperprolactinemia.

Any medical conditions causing chronic pain, fatigue, or malaise.

Etiology [1]

Low testosterone: more consistent finding in men not as clear in women [2].

Relationship factors: lack of trust and intimacy, conflicts over power and control, lack of physical attraction, and interpersonal dependency (emotional reliance on others); these factors may be more important for women than for men [3].

Sexual inactivity: prolonged inactivity sometimes results in suppression of desire.

Intrapsychic anxiety and anger: both emotions have been postulated to act as a "turn off" in some cases [2].

Other sexual dysfunction: low desire may be a response to another condition that is interfering with sexual functioning (eg, erectile dysfunction or dyspareunia) [3].

• Risk factors include history of major depressive disorder, sexual abuse, relationship distress, low testosterone, chronic substance abuse. For males, the degree of emotional reliance on others is associated with risk for HSD. Female professionals have a higher risk than female nonprofessionals [1–3].

Epidemiology

Overall population rate, 20% [5].

Female-to-male ratio, 2:1 (but incidence of males is increasing) [5].

Percentage of couples presenting to sex therapy clinics and diagnosed with HSD, 40%–55% [3].

Typical presentation in women, early 30s; in men, mid- to late 40s [3].

Treatment

Pharmacologic treatment [1,5]

• Results of pharmacologic treatment have been disappointing. Several agents have been touted as aphrodisiacs, but as yet, none have been proven effective for the majority of cases.

• Hormone augmentation in patients with normal levels has been shown to be ineffective.

Hormone replacement (testosterone)

• Hormone replacement is indicated only if level of testosterone is low (<300 µg/dL for men; <25 µg/dL for women).

Standard dosage	In men, long-acting testosterone ester, ethanoate, or propionate in aqueous solution, 150–300 cm3 i.m. every 2–3 weeks until patient reports return of normal libido.
	In women, long-acting testosterone ester, ethanoate, or propionate in aqueous solution, 10–30 cm^3 (10% of male dose),
	Oral methyl testosterone, 5 mg 2–4 times per week, or
	Combination of estrogen, 0.65 mg, and methyl testosterone, 1.25 mg.
Contraindications	Prostatic carcinoma or hypertrophy; male breast cancer; severe cardiac, hepatic, or renal disease; pregnancy class X; hypercalcemia; diabetes mellitus.
Main side effects	In males: feminization, priapism, oligospermia, alopecia, prostatic hypertrophy, carcinoma.
	In females: amenorrhea or oligomenorrhea, virilization.
	In both sexes: edema, acne, suppression of hypodensity lipoprotein cholesterol.
Main drug interactions	Increases plasma concentrations of cyclosporine and the anticoagulant action of warfarin.
Special points	Increased risk of hepatotoxicity: patients should be monitored closely for signs of liver damage, especially those with a history of liver disease.
	Polycythemia: periodic hemoglobin and hematocrit determinations should be considered in patients receiving long-term therapy.

Bupropion

• Bupropion has been shown to increase desire in HSD populations, but conclusive replication of these results has not yet been obtained.

Standard dosage	150–300 mg/d or twice daily.
Contraindications	Pregnancy rating B, anorexia or bulimia nervosa, seizure disorder, hepatic disease.
Main side effects	Agitation, anxiety, restlessness, insomnia, weight loss, headache, tremor.
Main drug interactions	Potentially fatal interaction with monoamine oxidase inhibitors.
	Hepatic enzyme induction yields a large number of potential drug interactions.

Follow-up and management

• Psychotherapy usually requires more sessions than for other sexual disorders. Continued vigilance for other psychiatric conditions (which are increased in this population and more amenable to treatment) is recommended.

Treatment aims

To increase capacity for and enjoyment of sexual functioning.
To improve interpersonal relationships.
To identify and treat other secondary conditions that may be contributing to the problem.

Nonpharmacologic treatment [1,5]

Psychotherapy

• Despite the lack of controlled data supporting the efficacy of therapy, most experts in the field agree that some form of therapy is useful. Traditional sex therapy techniques, although still employed in most treatment programs, are less useful for HSD than for other sexual disorders. More global forms of therapy utilizing cognitive-behavioral and psychodynamic principles are recommended.

• Couples therapy appears to be superior to individual therapy. For women, focusing on psychologic symptoms and relationship stress is generally more helpful. For men, assessment for other sexual dysfunction is primary [3].

Prognosis [5]

• HSD is generally regarded as the most difficult sexual disorder to treat, with successful outcomes in <50% of patients. Markers of poorer prognosis in HSD include younger age of couple, shorter duration of problem, and lifelong and global types. Motivation of male partner may be the most predictive factor in heterosexual females with HSD.

Key references

1. Kaplan HS: *The Sexual Desire Disorders* New York: Brunner/Mazel, Inc.; 1995.

2. Beck JG: Hypoactive sexual desire disorder: an overview. *J Consult Clin Psychol* 1995, 63:979–927.

3. Donahey KM, Carroll RA: Gender differences in factors associated with hypoactive sexual desire. *J Sex Marital Ther* 1993, 19:25–39.

4. *DSM-IV* Washington, DC: American Psychiatric Association; 1995.

5. Rosen RC, Leiblum SR: Hypoactive sexual desire. *Psychiatr Clin North Am* 1995, 78:707–727.

Diagnosis

Symptoms and signs
• This paraphilia involves sexual excitement derived from receiving psychologic or physical pain, humiliation, and/or suffering.

• There is significant distress or impairment in functioning due to fantasies, urges, or actual masochistic behaviors.

• Symptoms are present for >6 months.

• Submission of the sexual masochist is usually demonstrated by various means: flagellation (*eg*, spanking, whipping); bondage (*eg* ropes, gags, handcuffs, blindfolds, chains); pain, relatively safe (*eg*, ice, hot wax, biting, face slapping); pain, potentially dangerous (*eg* burns, piercing, pins, tattoos, branding, fisting); and humiliation (*eg*, psychologic degradation, role-playing an animal or baby, urination or defecation rituals).

• The term *sadomasochism* refers to consensual sadistic and masochistic sexual behavior (bondage/discipline or dominance/submission) and is considered a questionable diagnosis. The ethics of "treating" this behavior is currently under debate.

• Many individuals who engage in sadomasochism will "play" either dominant or submissive roles. These individuals are referred to as switchables, duals, or middles.

• Sadomasochists usually follow stereotypical scripts of role-playing such as master–slave, teacher–student, and guardian–child.

• Most masochists enjoy but are not reliant on these behaviors for sexual satisfaction. Some individuals are incapable of sexual satisfaction without masochistic rituals.

Investigations
Laboratory investigations: none are indicated.

Psychologic testing: may identify additional psychiatric disorders and paraphilias contributing to the severity of the masochistic behavior.

Penile plethysmography: may offer additional information to establish arousal associated with this behavior; the reliability of this measure is questionable, however, and may result in false-negative information.

Complications
Legal implications of behavior: some masochistic individuals may become sexual offenders and commit sex crimes due to cognitive distortions that excuse offensive behavior (further paraphilias may develop as masochism loses its novelty).

Impaired social or sexual functioning: the individual may only be able to achieve sexual arousal through masochistic activities; this behavior may strain social and sexual relationships resulting in emotional loneliness; however, many individuals report that their sadomasochism behavior does not interfere with their functioning in other areas of their life.

Infection and other medical problems, including death: may arise from the activities engaged in such as fisting, anal intercourse, exposure to fecal matter, and hypoxyphilic behavior (*eg*, autoerotic asphyxiation); although most sadomasochists follow carefully designed scripts and allow a previously agreed on "safe word" it is possible that the activity may progress too far or that the sadistic partner may not adhere to the agreed guidelines.

Other information
• Related paraphilias include urophilia (sexual arousal associated with urinating on someone or being urinated on), coprophilia (sexual arousal associated with defecating on someone or being defecated on), hypoxyphilia (sexual arousal associated with oxygen deprivation; may result in injury or death, usually by accident; has been associated with other masochistic behaviors, transvestitism, and self-observation; reported deaths include individuals ranging from 10–60 years of age, usually males).

Differential diagnosis
Normal sexual arousal: sadomasochistic individuals typically do not engage in dangerous pain, but rather simulated or less dangerous pain. When consensual, this sexual behavior is not necessarily considered a disorder.
Self-defeating behavior: individuals may engage in behavior that is self-defeating or self-mutilating, but not for sexual arousal.

Etiology
• No single theory is accepted to explain the heterogeneity of masochistic behavior and there appear to be subtle differences in male and female masochistic desires as well as individual differences.
Biologic theory: evidence not available.
Behavioral theory: suggests that masochistic behavior is paired with sexual arousal (classic conditioning), which is inherently positive (operant conditioning); the masochistic behavior is further reinforced by masturbatory fantasies and may be associated with increased autonomic nervous system arousal (from danger, risk, and so on).
Escape theory: suggests that individuals are drawn to sadomasochistic behavior to escape their identity and act out a new, sometimes, opposite persona.
Opponent-process theory: this learning theory suggests that fear, discomforting, and painful, experiences initiate an opponent process of pleasure (eg, skydiving, rock climbing).
Psychodynamic theory: suggests that the individual wants to dominate but is psychologically conflicted and therefore submits to be dominated; other theories have been posited with little or no supportive data.

Epidemiology
• In the United States, sadomasochism between consenting partners is not considered rare and is possibly common.
• In sadomasochism, more individuals describe themselves as masochistic than sadistic.
• Age of onset is early adulthood.
• Prevalence is slightly more male than female.
• Some comorbidity exists with other paraphilias or sexual dysfunction.
• There is conflicted evidence of the psychiatric comorbidity of masochists.

Treatment

General information

• The ethical implications of "treating" someone for masochism are heavily debated. Most agree, however, that if the individual is uncomfortable with their arousal pattern and have been given information about its acceptance or if the individual is engaging in dangerous activities and risk-taking behavior (eg, hypoxyphilic behaviors or not screening their partners), treatment is appropriate. Unfortunately, the effectiveness of treatment is questionable.

Pharmacologic treatment

Psychotropic medication

• These medications are thought to work by treating the "obsessional" nature of the disorder and by taking advantage of their sexual side effect profiles.

• Dosage has not been well documented. Dosing is hypothesized to be similar to dosing for obsessive-compulsive disorder and titrate until symptoms are controlled or side effects are intolerable.

Standard dosage	Fluoxetine, 20–80 mg/d.
	Paroxetine, 20–60 mg/d.
	Sertraline, 50–200 mg/d.
	Clomipramine, 150–300 mg/d.
	Fluvoxamine.
Main side effects	*All agents*: gastrointestinal upset, diarrhea, vomiting, anorexia, agitation, insomnia, sexual dysfunction.
Main drug interactions	*All agents*: potentially fatal interaction with monoamine oxidase inhibitors; potentially fatal interaction with antiarrythmic medications; serotonergic crisis (hypertension, hyperpyrexia, seizures) is possible in patients on other serotonergic medications.
	Clomipramine: may also be associated with dry mouth, orthostasis, constipation, weight gain, urinary retention, cardiac dysrhythmias, and lowered seizure threshold.

Hormonal agents

• Hormonal agents been shown to be effective in suppressing sexual urges, but they may truncate the individual's sexual life and result in decreased compliance with medication.

Standard dosage	Medroxyprogesterone acetate, 500 mg/wk i.m. or 80 mg/d orally.
	Leuprolide acetate, 7.5 mg/mo i.m. or 1 mg/d s.c.
Contraindications	*Medroxyprogesterone acetate:* use cautiously in patients with hyperlipidemia (serum lipoproteins [high-density lipoprotein and low-density lipoprotein] should be monitored during therapy), thrombophlebitis, thromboemboloic disease, asthma, congestive heart failure, nephrotic syndrome or other renal disease, or cardiac disease; may exacerbate major depression, migraine, or seizure disorder; should not be used with bromocriptine (the combination would be counterproductive).
	Leuprolide acetate: patients with urinary tract obstruction may have worsening of symptoms during the first weeks of treatment; flutamide (250 mg orally 3 times daily) should be given concurrently during the first 2 weeks of therapy to prevent a possible transient increase in sex drive; androgens and estrogens are relatively contraindicated and would defeat the purpose of leuprolide therapy.
Main side effects	*All agents*: weight gain, hypertension, lethargy, hot flashes, mood lability (during early treatment), phlebitis (rare), and gynecomastia (rare).

Treatment aims

To reduce masochistic behavior or reduce dangerous masochistic behavior.

Prognosis

• Without treatment, masochism tends to remain a preference in sexual behavior, fantasies, and urges.

• A reasonable goal may be to reduce the frequency and intensity of masochistic behavior, fantasies, and urges and decrease the dangerousness of the activities.

Follow-up and management

• Some individuals benefit from locating their state's network of individuals interested in sadomasochism.

• Patient may need counseling to improve skills relating to sexual partners in a nonmasochistic manner.

• Assess need for counseling regarding paraphilias or other psychopathology.

• Monitor for likelihood of engaging in sexual offenses or sex crimes.

Nonpharmacologic treatment

• Cognitive-behavioral therapy may include the following:

• Behavior therapy to reduce inappropriate sexual arousal and increase appropriate sexual arousal.

• Challenging distorted thinking and beliefs, especially those concerning justification for the paraphilic behavior.

• Social skills training, assertiveness training, communication skills training.

• Relapse prevention to help identify vulnerable thoughts and situations and intervene to prevent or stop the behavior by using various cognitive and behavioral skills.

General references

Laws DR, O'Donohue W: *Sexual Deviance*. New York: Guilford Press; 1997.

Levitt EE, *et al.*: The prevalence and some attributes of females in the sadomasochistic subculture: a second report. *Arch Sex Behavior* 1994, 23:465–473.

Blanchard R, Hucker S: Age, transvestism, bondage, and concurrent paraphilic activities in 117 fatal cases of autoerotic asphyxia. *Br J Psychiatry* 1991, 159:371–377.

Diagnosis

Symptoms and signs

- This paraphilia involves sexual excitement derived from administering psychologic or physical pain, humiliation, and/or suffering.
- There is significant distress or impairment in functioning due to fantasies, urges, or actual sadistic behaviors.
- Symptoms are present for >6 months.
- The "victim" of the sexual sadist may be nonconsenting or consenting (sexual masochist). When engaging in these activities with a consenting individual, the activity is typically referred to as sadomasochism.
- Dominance of the sexual sadist is usually demonstrated by various means: flagellation eg, spanking, whipping); bondage (eg, ropes, gags, handcuffs, blindfolds, chains); pain, relatively safe (eg, ice, hot wax, biting, face slapping); pain, potentially dangerous (eg, burns, piercing, pins, tattoos, branding, fisting); humiliation (eg, psychologic degradation, forcing into the role of an animal or baby, urinating or defecating on the other person's body).

Sexual sadists with nonconsenting partners

- Sexual sadists with nonconsenting partners may engage in torture to the point of serious injury or death, may engage in sexual activity with corpses, and frequently increase in sadistic intensity until they are caught.

Sadomasochism

- Sadomasochism refers to the consensual sadistic and masochistic sexual behavior (also known as "bondage and discipline" and "dominance and submission").
- Many individuals who engage in sadomasochism will "play" either dominant or submissive roles. These individuals are referred to as switchables, duals, or middles.
- Sadomasochists usually follow stereotypical scripts of role-playing such as master–slave, teacher–student, and guardian–child.
- Most sadomasochists enjoy but are not reliant on these behaviors for sexual satisfaction. Some individuals are incapable of sexual satisfaction without sadomasochistic rituals.

Investigations

Laboratory investigations: none are indicated.

Psychologic testing: may suggest additional psychiatric disorders contributing to the severity of the sadistic behavior.

Penile plethysmography: may offer additional information to establish arousal associated with this behavior and assess for arousal associated with other paraphilias; the reliability of this measure is questionable, however, and may result in false-negative information.

Complications

Legal implications of behavior: sexual sadism may result in sadistic murder, rape, and injury to others, as well as a variety of other illegal activities.

Impaired social or sexual functioning: the individual may only be able to achieve sexual arousal through sadistic activities; some sadistic individuals are also sadistic toward living beings in a nonsexual context that may additionally hinder relationships; in contrast, many individuals engaging in sadomasochism report that their sexual behavior does not interfere with their functioning in other areas of their life.

Infection and other medical problems: may arise from the activities engaged in, such as fisting, anal intercourse, exposure to fecal matter, drinking blood, and eating body parts or organs (as in the case of some sadistic killers); some of these medical issues are examined under Sexual masochism.

Differential diagnosis

Normal sexual arousal: sadomasochistic individuals typically do not engage in dangerous pain but rather simulated, less dangerous pain. When consensual, this sexual behavior is not necessarily considered a disorder.
Psychosis: psychotic individuals may engage in sadistic behavior for reasons other than sexual excitement, and the behavior exists only during the course of the illness.

Etiology

- No single theory is accepted to explain the complexities and range of sexually sadistic behavior.

Epidemiology

- In the United States, sadomasochism between consenting partners is not considered rare.
- Sexual sadism with nonconsenting partners is considered rare.
- Age of onset for sexual sadists/ sadomasochism is in early adulthood with a chronic course.
- Sexual sadists with nonconsenting adults are almost exclusively male, whereas participants in sadomasochism are both male and female.
- High comorbidity exists with other paraphilias or sexual dysfunction.
- Patients may have antisocial and/or narcissistic personality disorders.

Other information

- Sadistic murder may occur as a means of increasing arousal, or may be necessary for arousal, or could result from an escalation of sadistic behavior into a "frenzy."
- Anorectal fatalities generally result from perforation of the rectal walls, as in "fisting" (the insertion of a fist into the anus or vagina).
- Related paraphilias include the following: urophilia (sexual arousal associated with urinating on someone or being urinated on); coprophilia (sexual arousal associated with defecating on someone or being defecated on); vampirism (sexual arousal associated with drawing or drinking blood); piqueurism (the act of stabbing the victim in the breasts or buttocks before escaping); necrophilia (sexual arousal associated with corpses or mutilating corpses; some cases result from extreme aggression following a murder; other cases involve individuals deceased for a period of time).

Treatment

General information

• Very little data have been collected regarding treatment modalities or treatment efficacy for sexual sadism. Frequently these individuals do not seek treatment themselves but rather are forced into treatment due to legal difficulties. Sadomasochists may not be distressed by their behavior and therefore only seek treatment under certain circumstances. Treatment for sexual sadists and sadomasochists tends to be similar.

Pharmacologic treatment

Psychotropic medication

• These medications are thought to work by treating the obsessional nature of the disorder and by taking advantage of their sexual side effect profiles.

• Dosage has not been well documented. Dosing is hypothesized to be similar to dosing for obsessive-compulsive disorder, titrating until symptoms are controlled or side effects are intolerable.

Standard dosage	Fluoxetine, 20–80 mg/d.
	Paroxetine, 20–60 mg/d.
	Sertraline, 50–200 mg/d.
	Clomipramine, 150–300 mg/d.
	Fluvoxamine.
Main side effects	*All agents*: gastrointestinal upset, diarrhea, vomiting, anorexia, agitation, insomnia, sexual dysfunction.
	Clomipramine: may also be associated with dry mouth, orthostasis, constipation, weight gain, urinary retention, cardiac dysrhythmias, and lowered seizure threshold.
Main drug interactions	*All agents*: potentially fatal interaction with monoamine oxidase inhibitors, potentially fatal interaction with antiarrythmic medications, serotonergic crisis (hypertension, hyperpyrexia, seizures) possible in patients on other serotonergic medications.

Hormonal agents

• These have been shown to be effective in suppressing sexual urges, but they may truncate the individual's sexual life, resulting in decreased compliance with medication.

Standard dosage	Medroxyprogesterone acetate, 500 mg/wk i.m. or 80 mg/d orally.
	Leuprolide acetate, 7.5 mg/mo i.m. or 1 mg/d s.c.
Contraindications	*Medroxyprogesterone acetate*: use cautiously in patients with hyperlipidemia (serum lipoproteins [high-density lipoprotein and low-density lipoprotein]) should be monitored during therapy), thrombophlebitis, thromboemboloic disease, asthma, congestive heart failure, nephrotic syndrome or other renal disease, or cardiac disease; may exacerbate major depression, migraine, or seizure disorder; should not be used with bromocriptine (the combination would be counterproductive).
	Leuprolide acetate: patients with urinary tract obstruction may have worsening of symptoms during the first weeks of treatment; flutamide (250 mg orally 3 times daily) should be given concurrently during the first 2 weeks of therapy to prevent a possible transient increase in sex drive ;androgens and estrogens are relatively contraindicated and would defeat the purpose of leuprolide therapy.
Main side effects	*All agents*: Weight gain, hypertension, lethargy, hot flashes, mood lability (during early treatment), phlebitis (rare), and gynecomastia (rare).

Treatment aims

To reduce voyeuristic behavior.
To improve sexual functioning with consenting individuals and to prevent relapse.

Prognosis

• Without treatment, the course of this disorder tends to be chronic; although the actual behavior may decrease as the patient ages, his fantasies may remain voyeuristic in content.

• Indicators of poor prognosis include the following:
Early age of onset.
No guilt for the behavior.
High frequency of engaging in the behavior.
Poor sexual and social relationships.

Follow-up and management

• Identify vulnerable situation to prevent relapse.

• Encourage consensual sexual activities.

• Assess need for counseling regarding paraphilias or other psychopathology.

Nonpharmacologic treatment

• Cognitive-behavioral therapy seeks to identify antecedent thoughts, situations, and behaviors that lead to the paraphilic behavior. This therapy also seeks to increase the patient's ability to identify these vulnerable situations and intervene to prevent or stop the behavior by using various cognitive skills and behavioral skills.

General references

Laws DR, O'Donohue W: *Sexual Deviance*. New York: Guilford Press; 1997.

Levitt EE, et al.: The prevalence and some attributes of females in the sadomasochistic subculture: a second report. *Arch Sex Behavior* 1994, 23:465–473.

Diagnosis

Definition

• Delusional disorders are a group of disorders of unknown etiology, the principal feature being the presence of a nonbizarre delusion (ie, situations that can occur in real life). In shared psychotic disorder (SPD), also called folie à deux, a delusion develops in an individual in the context of a close relationship with another person who has an already established delusion and requires that the delusion be similar in content to that of the person who already has the delusion. The disturbance cannot be accounted for by schizophrenia or a mood disorder or be due to the effects of drugs or a medical condition.

• Jules Baillarger first described the syndrome, calling it folie à communiquè in 1860. Later in 1877, Laseque and Fabret termed it folie à deux.

Symptoms and signs

Length of association: duration of the association between primary and secondary in SPD is relatively long and measurable in years; range varied between 1–79 years.

Length of exposure to primary's psychosis: inconsistently reported; the length of exposure ranged from a matter of hours to 11 years; the majority of cases reported the onset to have occurred in <1 year.

Majority of relationships within the nuclear family: couples (married or living together) accounted for ~30% of SPD patients; siblings accounted for another 30%; parents and children accounted for 31%, of which the child was the secondary ~74% of the time.

Diagnosis of the primary: schizophrenia (~45% of cases), mood disorders (13%), and delusional disorders (11%).

Social isolation: the pair's obvious and extreme physical and social isolation is evident in approximately two thirds of cases; in all cases, the nature of communication and interaction with others is impaired.

Type of delusion shared by content: persecutory (~75% of cases) and grandiose.

Comorbidity: in 62% of secondaries (depression, dementia, and mental retardation).

Family history: in 55% of secondaries; in only 35% of patients was there a positive family history of Axis I psychiatric illnesses in primary relatives other than the primary.

• Coleman and Last [1] listed the following as prerequisites:

1. The primary must be in the early stages of his or her illness (ie, he or she has to take positive steps to influence the partner).

2. The primary and secondary must be in close proximity for a long time.

3. Sharing the dominant person's delusion must be of some advantage to the secondary person.

4. The primary must represent authority in the eyes of the secondary.

5. Most commonly, the psychosis develops when both are living in poverty.

• The role of hereditary factors in the etiology has been suggested because of the significant number of blood relatives affected, but confounding variables (eg, closeness of relationships within the family, their duration, a dominant–submissive factor that is operative to some degree, relative isolation of the family from the community) are conductive to the production of this phenomenon.

• Predisposing factors include isolation, rigid authoritarian family structure, physical handicap, poverty, ambivalence in relationship, dependency or submissiveness, female sex (?), young age, passive or low self-esteem, sensory impairment, cerebrovascular disease, low intelligence, and genetic predisposition to psychotic disorders.

Differential diagnosis

• Diagnosis of SPD is made only when delusion is not due to a substance or a general medical condition.

• Differential diagnosis is rarely a problem.

• SPD can be distinguished from a phenomenon explicable on the basis of a transient belief induced by powerful suggestion (eg, superstitious practices).

• Consider affective or mood disorder with psychotic features if no close relationship with a dominant person with a psychotic disorder or if psychotic symptoms precede onset of shared delusions.

• Consider factitious disorder and malingering with predominantly psychologic signs and symptoms.

Etiology

• SPD may evolve because both partners share some psychologic benefits from it. The secondary accepts the dominant partner's delusion rather than risk the deterioration of the close, gratifying relationship. For the primary, the transfer of delusion may be a final attempt to keep in touch with reality by maintaining a meaningful relationship with at least one other person.

• Psychodynamically, the secondary may have repressed oedipal fantasies in which the primary becomes identified with a parent.

• According to learning theory, the recipient learns the abnormal behavior from the more dominant, driving primary.

• Brill first introduced psychoanalytic interpretation, emphasizing the importance of identification. The essential relationship between the two partners is one of ambivalence—a compound of love and hate.

• Pulver and Brunt stressed the role of hostility. The dominant partner provokes the submissive one into accepting delusions rather than provoking a break-up of the relationship.

Epidemiology

• The disease is probably rare; incidence and prevalence figures are lacking. Literature is mostly case reports.

• Mean age of primaries is ~48 y, with a range of 9–81 y; secondaries is 43 y, with a range of 10–81 y.

• Sex of the secondary is female in ~62% of cases; male, ~38%. Both female and male secondaries are more likely to be affected by a female primary, which occurs in >70% of cases. Patient unit was the same sex more often than mixed.

Treatment

General information

• The majority of treatment modalities reported mention only the short-term effects of pharmacologic treatment policies and physical separation on the recipient. Long-term treatment has seldom been studied.

• In most cases, separation of the dependent patient is achieved by admitting the primary to a psychiatric center.

• In children who are secondaries, separations from the inducer usually leads to the disappearance of psychotic symptoms (in 12 of 14 cases), but this is far less often the case with adult recipients (16 of 29).

• It is also possible that the secondary suffers from a serious mental disorder. It may be necessary to admit him or her to a psychiatric center as well.

• Often, both the primary and secondary require treatment with antipsychotic drugs.

• Psychotherapy with nondelusional members of patient's family should be undertaken. Psychotherapy with both submissive and dominant partners may be undertaken later. To prevent recurrence, family therapy and social interventions to modify family dynamics are useful.

Characteristics of the partners in a *folie à deux*

• The primary may have (in order of frequency) schizophrenia, delusional disorder, affective illness, dementia, dominant and forceful personality, or better education and higher IQ than secondary.

• The secondary usually has a submissive and dependent personality, physical disability, or sensory impairment and may be reclusive, suspicious, or depressed.

Subtypes

Folie imposè: delusions of a psychotic person are transferred to an intimately associated and mentally sound one; the delusions of the secondary disappear after separation.

Folie simultanè: The simultaneous appearance of an identical psychosis occurs in two intimately associated morbidly predisposed individuals; there is no change with separation.

Folie communiquè: Both individuals have a true psychotic illness, but the onset of symptoms in the secondary patient is after the primary; they may share delusional ideas that have originated from either; symptoms are maintained even after separation.

Folie induitè: New delusions are adopted by a psychotic individual under the influence of another psychotic individual.

Course

• Little is known about the age of onset (usually middle to late adulthood, but it appears to be quite variable). Without intervention, the course is usually chronic because the disorder most commonly occurs in relationships that are long-standing and resistant to change. With separation from the primary, the secondary's delusional beliefs disappear (either quickly or slowly). However, sometimes the beliefs may be sustained, at times becoming so extended that other psychotic symptoms may be superimposed.

General references

Diagnostic and Statistical Manual of Mental Disorders, ed 4. Washington, DC: American Psychiatric Association; 1994.

Enoch MD, Trethowan WH: Uncommon Psychiatric Syndromes, ed 2. Bristol, England: John Wright & Sons; 1979.

Manschreck TC: Delusional disorder and shared psychotic disorder. In Comprehensive Textbook of Psychiatry, ed 6. Edited by Kaplan BJ, Sadock Baltimore, MD: Williams and Wilkins; 1995.

Mentjox R, Van Houten CA, Kooinan CG: Induced psychotic disorder: clinical aspects, theoretical considerations, and some guidelines for treatment. Compr Psychiatry 1993, 34:120–126.

Silveira JV, Seeman MV: Shared psychotic disorder: a critical review of the literature. Can J Psychiatry 1995, 40:389–395.

Diagnosis

Definitions
• There are three types of sleep disorders—nightmare disorder, sleepwalking disorder, and night terror disorder.

• Nightmares are dreams that waken the child, leaving him or her feeling scared and anxious and with a sense of dread. The dreamer awakens completely and becomes alert (in contrast to night terror disorder, in which the child remains confused and disoriented and typically returns to sleep). Nightmares occur during rapid eye movement (REM) sleep, a sleep phase in which there can be no body movement and, therefore, is not associated with sleepwalking.

• Sleepwalking is one of the parasomnias and is considered a disorder of arousal. Sleepwalking occurs during non-REM sleep (sleep stages 3 and 4) rather than during dreaming or REM sleep. Sleepwalking is a sleep-state transition disorder.

• Night terror is defined as an incomplete awakening during stages 3 or 4 non-REM sleep, with intense fear and panic. There may be an initial scream. The child doesn't recognize parents or other familiar persons and will typically fight off attempts to hold and console him. Night terrors occur during the first third of the night, and the child has no memory of the event the next morning.

Symptoms and signs
Nightmare disorder
• *See* Definitions

Sleepwalking disorder
• During sleepwalking, the somnambulist makes repetitive movements, typically sitting up in bed. Most children do not actually walk, but when they do, they typically walk around their room without a goal or may walk to their parents or to the bathroom. They have a blank stare and are relatively unresponsive. Movements are clumsy. On awakening, the child has no memory or only a vague awareness that something happened during the night. Daytime functioning is typically normal. There are no diagnoses consistently associated with sleepwalking in children. MMPI profiles of adults do not support sleepwalking as a "hysterical dissociation."

Night terror disorder
• Night terrors are characterized by a sudden partial arousal from non-REM sleep with a loud cry and autonomic and behavioral manifestations of fear. The child may appear to be awake but is not. He or she may thrash around in the bed, eyes open with a blank look. Autonomic activity may include racing heartbeat, rapid breathing, diaphoresis, and flushing. The child typically does not calm when you walk into the room and will not meaningfully interact with the environment or anyone in it. Instead of being comforted by being held, he may thrash even more wildly in an attempt to get loose. Attempts to waken the child are usually unsuccessful. He will not recall the event if awakened at the time or if questioned about it the next morning.

Differential diagnosis
Nightmares and night terrors
• Night terrors should be differentiated from nightmares. In nightmares, the child is awake and is comforted by the presence of his parents; he or she can recall a dream or dream fragment. In night terrors, the child is not fully awake, is not comforted by familiar people, and often has no recall of the event upon awakening the next day. Night terrors should also be differentiated from nocturnal seizures.

Sleepwalking
• Automatism, such as chewing and swallowing, may occur during either seizures or sleepwalking. Seizures can occur any time during the day or night, whereas sleepwalking occurs only at night. Patients with seizures do not typically have a family history of sleepwalking or night terrors. Electroencephalography can be helpful. Malingering should be suspected when a patient demonstrates complicated and goal-directed behavior during an episode. In malingering, the episodes usually last more than 15 minutes and may occur at any time during the night.

Etiology
Nightmares
• High fevers can increase the frequency of nightmares, as can emotional upset and sexual abuse.

Sleepwalking
• Sleepwalking is concordant six times more frequently in monozygotic twins than in dizygotic twins. The child of a parent with a history of sleepwalking is six times more likely to sleepwalk than a child of parents without this history.

• Central nervous system immaturity is a causative factor in childhood sleepwalking as suggested by the presence of sudden rhythmic high-voltage bursts of delta-frequency during sleep in sleepwalkers up to 17 y of age.

• Fever and certain medications can precipitate sleepwalking episodes. Elevated body temperature suppresses stages 3 and 4 of non-REM sleep and is sometimes followed by a rebound.

Night terrors
• Episodes can be precipitated by fever, recovery from sleep deprivation (rebound effect on stage 3 and 4 sleep), and some medications. Although there is no increase in comorbid diagnoses in children, adults with sleep terrors often have another psychiatric diagnosis.

Treatment

General information

Nightmare disorder

• A child aged 2 years may not know that what happened during his dream was not real. When the child awakens frightened, he or she will need help separating dream from reality in order to return to sleep. If the child is too frightened to return to sleep, the parent should remain with him or her in the room but should not make a habit of taking the child into parent's bed.

• Provide the child with comforts suitable to age and stage of development.

• Enter into the child's fantasy by suggesting that his teddy bear will stay awake and chase the monsters so that he can return to sleep without worry.

• Offer him a flashlight for reassurance if he fears the dark.

• If a child has frequent nightmares, the underlying cause should be evaluated. If separation issues precipitate nightmares, games like peek-a-boo and hide-and-seek can help the child to tolerate separation and anticipate the parent's return.

• If toilet training leads to increased nightmares, it may be necessary to back off for awhile.

• Children can be helped to understand their dreams with books on the subject (*see* General references).

• Avoiding frightening TV shows, movies, and videos can decrease the frequency of nightmares in susceptible children.

Sleepwalking disorder

• Parents may need to be reassured and instructed to lead their children back to bed without waking them.

• Insufficient sleep or irregular sleep schedules can trigger sleepwalking and should be avoided.

• Because a child can injure himself while sleepwalking, dangerous objects should be removed and stairways gated.

• Diazepam, cloncypum and imipramine may be used to treat episodes of sleepwalking when medication is indicated.

Night terror disorder

• The child should not be wakened, but rather the episode should be allowed to run its course, and the child should be settled back in bed without waking.

• Night terrors occur more frequently with emotional stress and exhaustion.

• Adequate sleep on a regular schedule can less the frequency of episodes as can stress reduction.

Prognosis

Nightmares

• Nightmares are developmental and will abate with maturity, unless maintained by specific traumatic events.

Sleepwalking and night terrors.

• Most children simply outgrow sleepwalking and require no special treatment.

Epidemiology

Nightmares

• Nightmares are part of normal development and occur in nearly all children.

• Infants have REM sleep in which there may be smiles suggestive of dreams, but it is not until 2 y of age that the child develops the intense fear that will awaken him or her.

Sleepwalking

• Sleepwalking is much more common in children than in adults. Between 10–15% of children aged 5–12 y have at least one episode of sleepwalking.

• The prevalence of somnambulism is 1%–6% in the general population.

• Incidence is 4–6 times more common in patients with Tourette syndrome and migraine headaches. Between 25%–33% of sleepwalkers have nocturnal enuresis. Ten percent of children and 50% of adults who sleepwalk also have night terrors. Somnambulism affects both sexes equally.

• Sleepwalking typically occurs during sleep stages 3 and 4 and is most prevalent between 4–8 y of age.

Night terrors

• Sleep terrors occur most commonly in children between ages 4–12 y of age, diminishing during adolescence, but can occur in adults as well. Sleep terrors are somewhat more common in boys than in girls and may occur in more than one family member. Overall prevalence is 3% in childhood. Family history of partial arousals may be as high as 60%.

General references

Adair R, Bauchner H: Sleep Problems in Childhood. *Curr Probl Pediatr* 1993.

Ferber R: *Solve Your Child's Sleep Problems.* New York: Simon & Schuster; 1985.

Masand P: Sleepwalking. *Am Family Phys*, 1995, 51.

Wise M: Parasomnias in children. *Pediatr Ann* 1997, 26:7.

Diagnosis

Symptoms

Strong and persistent fear of social or performance situations in which embarrassment or humiliation may occur: specific social or performance situations almost always provoke an immediate anxiety response, which may take the form of a panic attack; social or performance situations are avoided or endured with intense anxiety; the fear is seen as excessive and unreasonable (except in children); the fear causes significant interference with functioning or marked distress; the condition persists for at least 6 months in children <18 years of age.

Typical fears: *eg*, evaluation (negative or positive) by others; social interaction; and speaking, eating, drinking, and writing in public.

Associated phenomena: hypersensitivity to criticism or rejection, difficulty with assertiveness, low self-esteem.

• The "general" subtype is reserved for those patients whose fears are related to all or almost all social situations.

Signs

Any of the following, when confronted with or anticipating feared social situations:

Blushing.

Gastrointestinal discomfort, nausea, diarrhea.

Cold and clammy hands, sweating.

Palpitations.

Shaky voice, tremors, muscle tension.

Confusion.

Urgency to urinate.

Investigations

Laboratory studies: none are routine.

Instruments: symptom severity can be measured by the Hamilton Anxiety Scale, Social Phobia and Anxiety Inventory, Fear of Negative Evaluation Scale, or the Brief Social Phobia Scale.

Complications

Underachievement: underachievement in school or work due to test anxiety, avoidance of public speaking, or fear of situations involving authority figures or colleagues.

Limited social support: difficulty building social support networks, lower likelihood of marriage.

Comorbidity: other psychiatric disorders occur in 70% of people with social phobia, which is associated with and often precedes other anxiety, substance-related (particularly alcohol), mood, and somatization disorders.

Suicidal ideation: increased rate of suicide attempts mostly accounted for by comorbidity.

Avoidant personality disorder: often diagnosed in addition to generalized social phobia; may be an alternate conceptualization of the condition.

Differential diagnosis

Generalized anxiety disorder, specific phobia: anxiety or fear *not* focused mainly on embarrassment or humiliation.

Panic disorder: unexpected panic attacks and subsequent avoidance of multiple situations are thought to trigger the attacks.

Agoraphobia: fear and avoidance of characteristic situations (eg, the market-place), which may or may not involve embarrassment or humiliation; when in a feared situation, people with agoraphobia tend to prefer having the company of a trusted companion, but those with social phobia may not.

Avoidant personality disorder: pervasive social avoidance, feelings of inadequacy, and fear of negative evaluation; extensively overlaps with generalized social phobia.

Schizoid personality disorder, pervasive developmental disorder: avoidance of social situations due to lack of interest in relating to other people.

Depression: social avoidance due to depressed state (resolves when depression remits).

Separation anxiety disorder in children: avoidance of social situations due to fear of separation from caretaker.

Performance anxiety, shyness: anxiety or avoidance without clinically significant impairment or marked distress.

• Social phobia is not diagnosed if social anxiety and avoidance are related only to potentially embarrassing symptoms of a medical or mental disorder (eg, obesity, tremor). Anxiety disorder not otherwise specified may be diagnosed if social avoidance is clinically significant in these cases.

Etiology

• Chemical (eg, dopaminergic, serotonergic, noradrenergic dysregulation), genetic, and environmental (conditioning, modeling) contributions are likely.

• Behavioral inhibition in childhood may be a precursor in some cases.

Epidemiology

• Lifetime prevalence is 3%–13%.

• Onset typically is in mid-adolescence, although it may start in childhood. Onset >25 y of age is not common.

• Prevalence is greater for women than for men in community samples. Men predominate in clinical settings.

• Course is often continuous and lifelong, although attenuation in severity in adulthood is common.

Treatment

Diet and lifestyle
- Use of alcohol to self-medicate social phobia may complicate treatment.
- Successful treatment may facilitate positive lifestyle changes.

Pharmacologic treatment [2,3]

Standard dosage	Monoamine oxidase inhibitors (MAOIs), *eg*, phenelzine (30–90 mg/d in 3 divided doses).
	Benzodiazepines, *eg*, clonazepam (1–6 mg/d) or alprazolam (0.5–4.0 mg/d) in 3 divided doses.
	Beta-blockers, *eg*, propranolol (10–20 mg 1 h before performance).
	Selective serotonin-reuptake inhibitors (SSRIs), *eg*, fluoxetine (20–80 mg/d), fluvoxamine (50–300 mg/d), paroxetine (20–60 mg/d), or sertraline (50–200 mg/d).
Contraindications	*MAOIs*: difficulty managing dietary restriction.
	Benzodiazepines: addiction potential; caution with dependent personality disorder or alcohol or drug abuse.
	All drugs: patients with hepatic impairment.
Main side effects	*MAOIs*: orthostatic hypotension, weight gain, edema, sexual dysfunction, insomnia, sedation.
	Benzodiazepines: sedation, fatigue, memory impairment, ataxia, dysarthria, incoordination, confusion, paradoxical excitement/aggression.
	Beta-blockers: bradycardia, hypotension, depression, insomnia, decreased sexual ability.
	SSRIs: sexual dysfunction, nervousness, gastrointestinal problems, insomnia, dizziness.
Main drug interactions	*Benzodiazepines*: additive effects with alcohol and other central nervous system (CNS) depressants.
	MAOIs: potential hypertensive crisis with tyramine containing foods; increased effects and toxicity with SSRIs, tricyclics, barbiturates, and CNS depressants.
	SSRIs: should not be used within 14 days of MAOI use.
Special points	*MAOIs*: most effective pharmacologic treatment, especially for generalized social phobia.
	Beta-blockers: effective for performance anxiety on as-needed basis but not for generalized social phobia.
	All drugs: Relapse associated with discontinuation.
	Tricyclics are not effective for social phobia.

Nonpharmacologic treatment [2,4]

Behavioral or cognitive-behavioral therapy: cognitive retraining to change dysfunctional interpersonal thinking; desensitization (via rehearsal, exposure, and/or relaxation); social skills training; treatment outcome similar for behavioral and cognitive-behavioral treatments; exposure to feared stimuli generally involved in effective treatments; group treatment format frequently used; lower relapse rates after treatment discontinuation than with drugs is probably due to development of active coping skills; symptom improvement may even increase after treatment is complete; no current evidence of synergistic effects combining drug and psychologic treatment.

Treatment aims
To alleviate both fear and avoidance.
To develop anxiety-management skills.
To modify thinking and behavior.

Prognosis
- Often appears to lead to depression, alcohol abuse, and other psychiatric illness if untreated (vast majority of cases are untreated).
- Best demonstrated short-term treatment efficacy is with MAOIs; ~66% of patients respond, although 8 wk of treatment required for full therapeutic effects.
- Pharmacologic treatment often works faster, but therapy is as effective in the long term and more effective at relapse prevention.
- Comorbidity and generalized subtype are associated with poorer prognosis.

Follow-up and management
- Long-term treatment should be psychologic. Treatment effects of therapy have been found to be more durable than effects of drugs after treatment discontinuation. "Booster" sessions may be helpful in solidifying improvement in some cases.

Treatment strategy
- Although efficacy of the SSRIs may be less than that of the MAOIs, SSRIs have become first-line treatment because of their greater safety and tolerability.
- MAOIs and benzodiazepines are second-line treatments unless contraindicated.
- In nongeneralized cases, beta-blockers should be tried before commitment to continuous treatment with MAOIs or benzodiazepines.

Key references
1. Schneider F, *et al.*: Social phobics: comorbidity and morbidity in an epidemiological sample. *Arch Gen Psychiatry* 1992, 49:282.1
2. Turner S, *et al.*: Behavioral and pharmacological treatment for social phobia. In *Long-term Treatments of Anxiety Disorders.* Edited by Mavissakalian M, Prien R. Washington, DC: American Psychiatric Press; 1996.
3. Jefferson W: Social phobia: a pharmacologic treatment overview. *J Clin Psychiatry* 1995, 56(suppl 5):18–24.
4. Juster H, Heimberg R: Social phobia: longitudinal course and long-term outcome of cognitive-behavioral treatment. *Psychiatric Clin North Am* 1995, 18:821–842.

SOMATIZATION DISORDER

Diagnosis

Definition
• Somatization disorder (formerly Briquet's syndrome) is characterized by a history of multiple physical complaints (beginning before 30 years of age and occurring over several years) that cannot be explained adequately based on physical and laboratory examinations and that result in treatment being sought or significant impairment in functioning.

Symptoms and signs
• The following four symptom criteria must be met over the course of the illness (although not all criteria need have occurred simultaneously):

1. Four pain symptoms related to at least four different sites or functions.

2. Two gastrointestinal symptoms (other than pain), including nausea, bloating, diarrhea, food intolerance, and vomiting (when not pregnant).

3. One sexual symptom (other than pain), including sexual indifference, erectile or ejaculatory dysfunction, irregular menses, menorrhagia, and vomiting throughout pregnancy.

4. One pseudoneurologic symptom (other than pain), including at least one symptom or deficit that suggests a neurologic condition (eg, conversion symptoms [hysterical paralysis, aphonia, or blindness, difficulty swallowing or a lump in throat, pseudoseizures, etc.], dissociative amnesia, or loss of consciousness other than fainting).

• These symptoms cannot be fully explained after appropriate investigations by a general medical condition or the direct effects of a substance, and they are not intentionally produced or feigned (see Differential diagnosis).

• Those who fail to meet stringent DSMñIV criteria for somatization disorder yet demonstrate a tendency to seek medical attention for somatic symptoms that have no pathophysiologic basis may meet criteria for undifferentiated somatoform disorder, pain disorder, or conversion disorder.

• Somatization may also be conceptualized as "the expression of emotional discomfort and psychosocial stress in the physical language of bodily symptoms" [1]. As such, somatization is a universal process (eg, "butterflies in the stomach" as an expression of anxiety) that becomes pathologic only when symptoms are misattributed to disease and medical attention sought.

Investigations
Diagnostic strategy for detecting somatization [2]
• Carefully elicit psychosocial information from the start of the encounter.

• Avoid changing diagnostic strategy midstream (sudden switch from biomedical to psychosocial inquiry is often perceived as a prelude to rejection: "it's all in your head").

• Somatization is not a diagnosis of exclusion. Look for positive indicators of somatization, including history of parental illness or disability; childhood neglect or abuse; childhood obligation to care for sick parents (or siblings); patient has received much medical attention but with limited results; history of polysurgery with limited results; illness onset in psychologically meaningful setting (significant life transitions); histrionic personality style; illness has an idiosyncratic or symbolic meaning for patient; description of symptoms is vague, inconsistent, or bizarre; symptoms persist despite allegedly specific medical therapy; patient denies possible psychological role of symptoms; comorbid psychiatric illness (especially depression, anxiety, substance abuse); analgesic misuse or abuse; unexplained gross disability; denial or minimizing of life problems; symptoms function to communicate distress to physician and family.

Further investigations
• Further investigations should be limited once 1) the appropriate work-up of presenting physical complaints has established the absence of pathophysiology sufficient to explain presenting symptoms, and 2) the diagnosis of Somatization Disorder has been established.

Differential diagnosis
• Must rule out general medical conditions that present with sometimes confusing symptom pictures (eg, multiple sclerosis, systemic lupus erythematosus or other collagen-vascular diseases, acute intermittent porphyria, endocrinopathies). Anxiety disorders, mood disorders, schizophrenia with somatic delusions, undifferentiated somatoform disorder, pain disorder associated with psychologic factors, conversion disorder, dissociative disorder, hypochondriasis, factitious disorder with predominantly physical signs and symptoms, malingering.

Etiology
Multifactorial etiology: truly a biopsychosocial phenomenon. Neurobiologic factors: decreased corticofugal inhibition may allow increased nociceptive input; brain hemispheric asymmetry with impaired interhemispheric communication may impair translation of affective distress into appropriate language. Psychodynamic factors: somatized symptoms act as defensive compromise formations, resolving intrapsychic conflicts. Behavioral factors: abnormal adoption of the "sick role" is a learned behavior with many secondary rewards; some family and medical systems act to perpetuate illness behaviors. Sociocultural factors: family-of-origin illness beliefs shape how somatic experiences are interpreted; subcultural and cultural illness beliefs also shape attribution of somatic symptoms.

Epidemiology
Strictly defined DSM-IV somatization disorder
General population: 0.2%–0.5% lifetime. Primary care outpatients: 5%–10%. Specialty clinics (eg, pain clinics): ~40%. Female-to-Male ratio: 5:1.

Somatization as a process
Primary care outpatients: 25%–60%.
• Approximately 10% of medical services are provided to patients with no evidence of organic illness (this excludes patients with known psychiatric syndromes).

Complications [3]
Iatrogenic injury.
Functional impairment..

Treatment [2,4,5]

Diet and lifestyle management
- Reduce external stressors to the greatest extent possible.
- Get adequate exercise.
- Avoid substances of abuse, especially excessive alcohol use.

Pharmacologic treatment
- Pharmacologic treatment is not indicated for somatization disorder, except to treat comorbid depression, anxiety, or objectively verified comorbid physical disorders.

Nonpharmacologic treatment
Clinical management strategy for chronic somatization
- Assure adequate (not heroic) medical evaluation.
- Centralize care under a single physician to discourage doctor-shopping and polypharmacy.
- Agree upon mutually acceptable language and labels for symptoms.
- Don't dispute the reality of the patient's complaints.
- Discuss appropriate goals. Emphasize coping rather than cure.
- Reassure continued physician involvement. Schedule regular follow-up visits independent of symptom status.
- Perform regular physical exams. Limit tests and procedures (especially invasive ones) to those indicated by objective findings rather than subjective complaints.
- Use medications only when indicated.
- Refer for psychiatric care if the patient is agreeable or if there are major comorbid psychiatric disorders. Emphasize that referral is not dismissal.

Other treatment options
Concurrent psychiatric management: physician consultation with a psychiatrist or ongoing comanagement with a psychiatrist can help the somatizing patient understand the nature of mind–body links while providing treatment of comorbid psychiatric disorders and support for the primary care physician.

Psychotherapy: some type of psychosocial therapeutic management is strongly recommended in all cases for optimal response.

Follow-up and management
- Regularly scheduled follow-up visits (eg, monthly) with the primary care provider, independent of symptom status, are the keystone of ongoing management. As the somatizing patient accepts that the physician will be available predictably, the frequency and severity of somatized complaints often decreases.
- Remain vigilant for concurrent physical illnesses. Somatizing patients have the same rates of common physical ailments as any other patient. Regular physical exams and appropriate work-up of objective physical findings will prevent errors of omission.

Treatment aims
To maintain a collaborative working alliance with a type of patient often experienced as difficult or frustrating. To identify flare-ups of somatization and address the underlying life stressors appropriately.
To reduce inappropriate use of medical resources and, thus, reduce risk of iatrogenic injury.
To monitor somatizing patients for patterns of symptoms indicative of authentic physical illness.

Prognosis
- Somatization disorder has a chronic course over the individual's lifetime, with waxing and waning of symptoms in response to life stressors.
- Be alert for "symptom substitution" (ie, when one symptom resolves, another equally mysterious symptom takes its place, prompting further work-up).

Key references
1. Barsky AJ, Klerman GL: Overview: hypochondriasis, bodily complaints, and somatic styles. Am J Psychiatry 1983, 140:273–283.
2. Kaplin C, Lipkin M Jr, Gordon G: Somatization in primary care: patients with unexplained and vexing medical complaints. J Gen Intern Med 1988, 3:177–190.
3. Gureje O, Simon GE, Ustun TB, Goldberg DP: Somatization in cross-cultural perspective: a World Health Organization study in primary care. Am J Psychiatry 1997, 154:989–995.
4. Bass C: Somatization: Physical Symptoms and Psychological Illness. Oxford, England: Blackwell Scientific Publications; 1990.
5. Bass C, Benjamin S: The management of chronic somatisation. Br J Psychiatry 1993, 162:472–480.

General reference
American Psychiatric Association: Diagnostic and Statistical Manual of Mental Disorders ed 4. Washington, DC: American Psychiatric Press; 1994.

SPECIFIC PHOBIA

Diagnosis

Definition
• A specific phobia is an exaggerated fear of a stimulus that a patient can clearly identify as anxiogenic.

• Common examples of specific phobias include fears of driving, flying, snakes, rats, insects, and people with AIDS.

• Phobias are currently classified into one of five types:

1. Animal (*eg*, snakes, roaches, mosquitos, dogs, cats).

2. Natural environment (*eg*, tornadoes, lightning, cliffs).

3. Blood, injection, or injury (*eg*, seeing blood drawn by venipuncture or by trauma, receiving a shot)

4. Situational (*eg*, elevators, tunnels, bridges, boats).

5. Miscellaneous (*eg*, phobia of exposure to others with an illness and risk of acquiring the illness; phobia of situations leading to choking, vomiting, incontinence).

General information
• Ironically, a phobia is often incongruent with a patient's overall lifestyle. For example, a zoologist who works effortlessly with terrestrial animals may have a phobia only of eels; or a person who has a phobia of bridges because of possible collapse on the way to work may routinely speed to work along alternate routes, accepting the speeding risk as necessary.

• People who have exaggerated fears of certain stimuli, but who never encounter the stimulus and are not distressed, have a subclinical, nondiagnosed specific phobia that may evolve into a diagnosable phobia if a change in circumstances forces exposure to the stimulus.

Diagnostic variations in children
• In children, exposure to the phobic stimulus may be manifested behaviorally (*eg*, crying, running, hiding) more often than verbally.

• Children may not recognize the fear as exaggerated, irrational, or inconsistent with peer norms.

• Symptoms must be present at least 6 months to give a diagnosis of specific phobias in children because minor, fluctuating, magnified fears are common in childhood.

Symptoms and signs
• The stimulus may lead to any of the following responses:

Intense anxiety: if directly exposed to the stimulus.

Panic attack: if directly exposed to the stimulus.

Avoidance of future exposure to the stimulus: with possible constriction of activities.

Painful suffering and anxiety: if the stimulus, because of occupational or societal demands, must be encountered and cannot be avoided.

Worrying and anticipatory distress: between exposures to the stimulus.

Shame, self-condemnation, or other negative self-evaluations: over having the exaggerated fear.

Investigations
Psychiatric rating scales: phobias (especially milder ones accompanying other psychiatric conditions) may be incidentally uncovered in the Hamilton Rating Scale for Anxiety or other anxiety rating scales; the Fear Survey Schedule and Anxiety Sensitivity Index Catalog exaggerate fears more completely and may reveal phobias.

Laboratory work-up: no specific tests are available for this condition.

Differential diagnosis
Other anxiety disorders (eg, generalized panic with or without agoraphobia, pure agoraphobia, social phobia; less commonly, obsessive-compulsive or posttraumatic stress); psychoses with fearful delusions; hypochondriacal fears of one's own disease; anorexia and bulimia nervosa food fears.

Etiology
Psychologic factors: thought to be predominant in most phobias and include traumatic events that persist as phobia; observation of traumatic events in others; unexpected panic attack in a previously benign, tolerated situation, then subsequent association of the fear of the panic experience with that situation; persistent, calamitous warnings from significant others (eg, parents) about the dangers of some situations, then subsequent adoption of that view as natural.

Biologic factors: blood injection or injury phobia shows the greatest evidence of possible biologic substrate, with patients showing a high frequency of vasovagal fainting and characteristic cardiovascular response of a drop in heart rate after a transient rise in heart rate upon stimulus exposure.

Epidemiology
• Specific phobia was the most common psychiatric diagnosis in women by the Epidemiologic Catchment Area study in the early 1980s.

• Most phobias develop in childhood or the mid-20s.

Complications
• Phobic patients are generally able to adjust to their condition and develop few complications. Possible complications in those who could not compensate for their magnified fears include job loss, change in living arrangements (eg, a person with a dog phobia living in a neighborhood into which newcomers with dogs move), marital tension, or school problems. Some medical complications could arise. If forced into exposure to a phobic stimulus, a patient with a preexisting heart arrhythmia may develop symptoms resulting from a panic attack. Patients with blood, injection, or injury phobia may avoid medical or dental care for years and neglect needed diagnosis or treatment of easily identified problems.

Treatment

Diet and lifestyle

• No diet accommodations are necessary or helpful.

• If possible, lifestyle changes may completely eradicate a specific phobia (if the evoking stimulus can be reliably avoided).

• With blood, injection, or injury phobia, letting the patient recline is a simple maneuver that may prevent dangers arising from fainting.

Pharmacologic treatment

Benzodiazepines

Standard dose	Lorazepam, 0.5–2.0 mg (1–3 h preexposure), Clonazepam, 0.5–2.0 mg (1–3 h preexposure), Clorazepate, 3.75–7.50 mg (2–4 h preexposure), or Diazepam, 2–10 mg (1–3 h preexposure).
Contraindications	History of substance dependence with high risk of relapse; poorly compensated respiratory disease. Because of side effects, a job that requires supreme mental alertness could be disastrous. Benzodiazepines may decrease reaction time and mental acuity. Use caution while driving and in other situations requiring full mental capacity.
Main side effects	Drowsiness, amnesia, ataxia.
Main drug interactions	Synergism with alcohol may cause central nervous system depression and, infrequently, death.

Nonpharmacologic treatment

Behavioral treatment

• Behavioral treatment is considered the best treatment for simple phobias.

Exposure therapy: patients challenge their phobia by exposing themselves to the phobic stimulus, generally in gradations but sometimes totally (flooding); the stimulus may be confronted by only the imagination or by direct contact; a therapist guides the patient and titrate as well as discusses the stereotyped phobic responses as the patient proceeds; the patient is not asked to relax during exposure but rather is encouraged to face the stimulus boldly and to gradually see that it is not to be feared as much as formerly believed.

Systematic desensitization: patients are helped to couple willful relaxation with a mental image of the phobic stimulus; a therapist asks the patient to learn a relaxation technique, then asks the patient to exercise this technique while imagining the stimulus; eventually, the feeling tone of relaxation replaces the old phobic response of fear.

Participant modeling: a therapist helps model contact with the phobic stimulus without fear; the therapist personally faces the stimulus to demonstrate that it is indeed possible not to have fear of the stimulus; with this behavioral leadership in place, the patient then confronts the feared stimulus (with successively less and less direct therapist help) until it is neutral.

Treatment aims

To reduce symptoms and life impairment.

Prognosis

Usually good when patient accepts treatment and pursues it with dedication. Poorer when specific phobia accompanies other significant psychiatric problems or patient is unmotivated.

Follow-up and management

Generally at patient's discretion, depending on recurrence of symptoms or emergence of new ones.

Other treatment options

• For some patients, supportive or insight-oriented psychotherapy may be helpful.

General references

Chapman TF, Fyer AJ, Mannuzza S, Klein DF: A comparison of treated and untreated simple phobia. *Am J Psychiatry* 1993, 150:816–818.

Diagnostic and Statistical Manual of Mental Disorders ed 4. Washington, DC: American Psychiatric Association; 1994:405–411.

Gabbard G: *Treatment of Psychiatric Disorders*, vol 2. Washington, DC: American Psychiatric Press; 1995:1453–1475.

Himle JA, Crystal D, Curtis GC, Fluent E: Mode of onset of simple phobia subtypes: further evidence of heterogeneity. *Psychiatry Res* 1991, 36:37–43.

Diagnosis

DSM-IV diagnostic criteria

1. Repetitive, seemingly driven, and nonfunctional motor behavior (*eg*, hand shaking or waving, body rocking, head banging, mouthing of objects, self-biting, picking at skin or bodily orifices, hitting own body).

2. The behavior markedly interferes with normal activities or results in self-inflicted bodily injury that requires medical treatment (or would result in an injury if preventive measures were not used). Specify "with self-injurious behavior."

3. If mental retardation is present, the stereotypic or self-injurious behavior is of sufficient severity to become a focus of treatment.

4. The behavior is not better accounted for by a compulsion (as in Obsessive–compulsive disorder), a tic (as in tic disorder), a stereotypy that is part of a pervasive developmental disorder, or hair pulling (as in trichotillomaina).

5. The behavior is not due to the direct physiological effects of a substance or a general medical condition.

6. The behavior persists for 4 weeks or longer.

Symptoms

• As described in diagnostic criterion 1, a stereotypy can be any type of repetitive, nonfunctional movement. Stereotypies may involve specific external objects, and they may also be related to particular times of day or other activities. Occasionally, interruption of performance of stereotypies may result in significant stress or discomfort. In the presence of mental retardation, historical features (*eg*, the association of anxiety, the need to perform, or relief upon performance) may be inferred.

Signs

• In the absence of self-injurious features, there may be no physical findings. Self-injurious or self-mutilatory behaviors will be apparent in the form of bleeding skin lesions secondary to picking, biting, or chewing or secondary to misshapen skull and face from chronic head banging.

Investigations

• Investigations should focus on the sequelae of stereotypies, especially if injurious. Bone and skull radiographs and investigation of anemia should be considered if behaviors are severe.

Complications

Head banging: if severe, can result in fracture and/or intracranial trauma.

Infection, sepsis: caused by open wounds or maceration.

Differential diagnosis

Tics and Tourette syndrome.
Obsessive–compulsive disorder.
Rett syndrome.
Lesch–Nyhan syndrome.
Neuroacanthocytosis.
Autism.
Pervasive developmental disorder.

Etiology

• Stereotypic behavior may occur as part of normal development, but it is typically mild and transient. The pathogenesis of stereotypies is not known. The association of stereotypies with mental retardation, autism, and stroke argue for a central nervous system cause. Stereotypies may also be associated with sensory deprivation or confinement, suggesting a role for sensorimotor integration.

Epidemiology

• The epidemiology of this disorder is unknown, but stereotypic movement is considered relatively frequent in the mentally retarded population, especially among the institutionalized and the visually handicapped.

Treatment

Lifestyle management

• The only effective treatment programs typically involve behavioral modification programs. Even so, these methods are not always of benefit to the patient. Physical restraints or protective clothing (*eg*, helmets) may be required to prevent injury to self or others.

Pharmacologic treatment

• Although treatment with sedative hypnotics, tricyclics, and benzodiazepines has been tried, there is no proven method of ameliorating stereotypies. Recently, it has been suggested that stereotypic movements may have an obsessive–compulsive component, and serotonin-reuptake inhibitors have been used, but benefits remain anecdotal.

Treatment aims

• Stereotypies may demand attention if they interfere with activities or if they bring unwanted attention to an individual. However, in the case of retarded persons, such a consideration may not be of significance. On the other hand, in patients with self-injurious behaviors, it is of the utmost importance that protective measures be taken (eg, helmets, face masks, gloves, etc.).

Prognosis

• In the retarded population, no long-term data exist regarding the natural history of stereotypies. However, recent reports of stereotypic movements in the nonretarded population suggest a much milder course, with some ability to suppress these movements. The prevalence of these movements with advancing age is not known.

General reference

Tan A, Salgado M, Fahn S. The characterization and outcome of stereotypic movements in nonautistic children. *Movement Disorders.* 1997, 12:47–52.

Diagnosis

Definition

• Acute stress disorder (ASD) is a typical pattern of dissociation, anxiety, and behavioral symptoms developing after direct or indirect exposure to severe or life-threatening trauma. Traumatic stressors may be natural or man-made disasters or physical or psychologic injuries to self or others [1]. The onset of ASD may be immediate or delayed up to 1 month after exposure to the traumatic stress. The duration is usually 2 days to 4 weeks (longer duration may signify posttraumatic stress disorder [PTSD]).

• ASD is classified into acute, subacute, and chronic phases, which facilitates in the selection of treatment modality. The chronic phase usually fulfills qualifications for PTSD.

Signs and symptoms [2]

Acute phase (lasts minutes to hours)

Emotional shock.

Paradoxical calm.

Psychic numbing.

Denial: including denial of or amnesia for the traumatic event and/or of physical injury.

Motor "freezing" or restlessness.

Insomnia.

Hypervigilance increasing to panic and flight.

Irritability.

Pervasive anxiety.

Unprovoked aggression.

Impaired cognition.

Subacute phase (lasts hours to weeks)

Marked behavioral change.

Somatization.

Dissociation.

Delirium.

Intrusive memories, "reliving" the traumatic event, flashbacks (which may presage PTSD).

Avoidance of reminders of traumatic event.

Guilt and shame: often accompanied by depression.

Dissociation.

Investigations

Careful history of traumatic event: discuss its meaning to the patient and clarification of patient's role.

Thorough psychiatric history (including family and social history): to uncover preexisting psychiatric disorders or special vulnerabilities.

Physical and neurologic examinations, including brain imaging when indicated: to delineate confounding injuries.

Mental status examination: to rule out clinical symptoms of psychiatric disturbance.

Laboratory tests: for substances and medical illnesses that mimic or provoke symptoms of stress and anxiety (eg, urine drug screen, toxic screen, blood sugar)

Psychologic tests: to clarify diagnosis, assess depth of mood disorder, etc.

Differential diagnosis

PTSD and other anxiety disorders. Exacerbation of other, preexisting mental disorders.

Direct effects of traumatic injuries.

Confounding medical illnesses or injuries.

Delirium: in 20% of emergency room patients; prominent among the elderly, substance abusers, the severely injured (100% of those on ventilators or with >30% burns), and those with preexisting Axis I and II disorders (33% and 20% of accident patients in emergency rooms, respectively).

Etiology

• ASD is caused by an identifiable, major traumatic stressor.

• 45% of injured adults display marked emotional and/or behavioral change in subacute phase, but only 33% warrant psychiatric diagnosis.

• Among injured civilians, 1% show "freezing," 5% panic or blind flight, 10%–20% strong anxiety without behavioral symptoms (acute phase).

• 44% of severely burned adults (16% of those burned less severely) suffer psychiatric disorders. Behavioral dysfunction is found in 75% of accidentally injured civilians.

• Residual, nonorganic psychiatric disorder is found in 17% of accidentally injured adults at 1 y after trauma, in 9% at 2 y; 6% have organic mental disorder [3].

• Physical injury and unfamiliarity with stressors often intensify severity; temporal, spatial, or emotional proximity to the stressors also increases severity [4].

Complications

Suicide.

Social or occupational disability: both in victims and in their families [3].

Decompensation leading to major depression or anxiety disorder.

Delayed wound healing: disturbed behavior from ASD may complicate recovery from physical injuries; injured patients are more vulnerable to all complications of ASD.

Chronic physical disability.

Psychotic decompensation.

Symptoms persisting beyond 6 months: may indicate PTSD.

Treatment

Diet and lifestyle

• Stabilize physical injury or illness by 1) establishing a recovery environment (*eg*, rest, respite, safety, someone to talk with [especially in disasters]), 2) repairing social organization (*eg*, provide media director, outreach programs, self-help groups), 3) stabilizing individual patient, and 4) locating and mobilizing family and social support system.

Nonpharmacologic treatment

Psychotherapy

• Assess patient's mental status.

• Gather information about patient's family, residence, employment, nature of traumatic stress and role in it.

• In the acute phase, use the crisis intervention model [5] and a structured but flexible approach. Provide ego support.

• In the subacute phase, use a dynamic approach to explore the patient's vulnerabilities and unique reactions to the traumatic event. Reconcile any misunderstandings.

• Support groups, biofeedback, hypnosis, family therapy, and occupational rehabilitation may also be of benefit.

Pharmacologic treatment

• Treat symptoms of severe anxiety, insomnia with benzodiazepines (zolpidem also may be used for insomnia).

• Depression (usually delayed) may not require antidepressant medication unless severe or protracted.

• Treat psychotic decompensation with antipsychotic medication (*eg*, olanzapine, risperidone, haloperidol, loxapine).

Treatment aims

To counter regression, retraumatization (by stigmatization and victimization), and chronicity.

To restore psychosocial functioning, family, occupational, and sociopolitical structures when possible.

Prognosis

• Prognosis is variable, depending upon proximity to traumatic event, presence and severity of injuries, and preexisting psychopathology (which worsen prognosis) and robustness of psychosocial support, intact social structure, and vigorous and appropriate treatment (which improve prognosis).

• Early intervention is crucial to a favorable outcome.

• Psychosocial setting of injury, preexisting personality, and level of mental stability strongly affect morbidity and response to treatment.

• Victims familiar with disasters fare better than those without such experience.

Key references

1. Krystal H: *Massive psychic trauma.* New York: International Universities Press; 1968.

2. Malt UF, Weisaeth L: Traumatic stress: empirical studies from Norway. *Acta Psychiatrica Scandanavia* 1989, 80:11–137.

3. Rosenbaum A, Hoge SK: Head injury and marital aggression. *Am J Psychiatry* 1989, 146:1048–1051.

4. Goldberg J, True WR, Eisen SA, Henderson WG: A twin study of the effects of the Vietnam War on PTSD. *JAMA* 1990, 263:1227–1232.

5. Doyle BB: Crisis management of the suicidal patient. In *Suicide Over the Life Cycle.* Edited by Blumenthal S, Kupfers D. Washington, DC: American Psychiatric Press; 1990.

General reference

Malt UF: The traumatic effects of accidents. In *Individual and Community Responses to Trauma and Disaster.* Edited by Ursano, McCaughey, Fullerton. New York: Cambridge University Press; 1997.

Diagnosis

Signs and symptoms

Alcohol-induced persisting dementia

Decline in functional abilities: due to memory loss, especially capacity for new learning and retention.

Impairment in at least one other cognitive function: aphasia, apraxia, agnosia, executive.

• The decline in function is not temporary but is permanent even with a period of abstinence and stable nutrition of 1 year.

Other substance-induced persisting dementia

Decline in functional abilities: same as with alcohol-induced persisting dementia.

Changes in cognitive and memory function leading to deficits in functional skills: associated with the use of marijuana, barbiturates, benzodiazepines, cocaine, and solvents; little information is available regarding the development of dementia due to the these drugs.

General information

• The information that follows applies largely to alcohol abusers; however, treatment recommendations may be equally applicable to any substance-induced dementia.

Investigations

History

Careful assessment of substance use history: to establish association with cognitive decline and functional deficits.

Corroboration of substance use and functional capacity by family.

Laboratory tests

Liver function tests: several are consistently elevated in the chronic alcoholic (eg, γ-glutamyltransferase, serum glutamic-oxaloacetic transaminase, serum glutamate pyruvate transaminase).

Carbohydrate-deficient transferrin: may be more sensitive and specific than liver function tests.

Screening questionnaires

Michigan Alcohol Screening Test (Selzer, 1971)

Alcohol Use Inventory (Wanberg et al., 1977)

Drinking Profile (Marlatt, 1976)

• The instruments listed may be valuable aids in diagnosing dementia associated with alcohol abuse.

Neuropsychologic tests

• Documenting memory and cognitive impairments is an essential component of diagnosis. Formal cognitive and memory tests provide measures of current functioning that can be compared with expected premorbid abilities to estimate the presence and extent of impairment.

Neuroimaging studies

• Recent neuroimaging studies have consistently found increased cerebrospinal fluid volume in the ventricular system of older, nutritionally impaired alcoholics. Bilateral atrophy involving frontal and frontal-temporal-parietal-cortical areas has been noted in alcoholics regardless of age and nutritional state. Assessment of cerebral blood flow has also indicated that frontal and parietal-cortical areas are susceptible to alcohol damage.

Differential diagnosis

Dementia due to the following:
Alzheimer's disease.
Vascular disease.

Delirium due to the following:
Substance withdrawal.
Medical illness.
Intoxication.

Etiology

• Risk factors include the following:
Length of substance abuse history.
Chronic, regular, and heavy substance use.
Poor nutritional status.

Epidemiology

• Approximately 10% of chronic alcoholics develop dementia due to alcohol abuse, placing an estimated 1% of the population at risk. An additional 5%–15% of alcoholics will have mild cognitive impairments that do not meet the criteria for dementia.

Complications

Comorbid psychiatric illness: a large percentage of chronic substance users also have serious mental disorders (eg, major depression, bipolar affective disorder, obsessive-compulsive disorder, or psychosis); in addition, personality disorders (eg, dependent, antisocial, narcissistic, and borderline) are evident. Poor social support: the chronic substance abuser often has few family ties or friends to assist with treatment; unemployment and homelessness are consequences that undermine effective treatment. Medical illness: liver disease (cirrhosis), heart disease, malnutrition (eg, thiamine deficiency), and pancreatitis are potential physical consequences of prolonged alcohol abuse.

Treatment

Diet and lifestyle

• Ensuring consistent, healthy nutrition may benefit in moderating the progression of the dementia. In many instances, thiamine supplementation may be necessary, but it rarely reverses established dementia.

• As with other individuals suffering from dementia, the alcoholic requires placement in a structured-living setting to maintain safety and sobriety. Often, family members are not able or available to care for the individual.

Pharmacologic treatment

• Medications are not now available to enhance the cognitive functioning of people with alcohol-related dementia; however, consideration might be given to drugs used to manage other forms of dementia (*eg*, Aricept).

• If patients have comorbid depressive illness, standard pharmacologic approaches are indicated. Tricyclic antidepressants (TCAs), selective seritonin-reuptake inhibitors, and monoamine oxidase inhibitors (MAOIs) could benefit individuals with affective illness. However, the anticholinergic effects of TCAs may worsen memory, and patients may be too cognitively impaired to manage MAOI medications.

• If evidence of mania due to bipolar disorder is observed or derived from the history, lithium, Tegretol, or Depakote are among the options to consider.

• As in other dementias, combative behavior may be seen with the confusion common in these demented patients. Haloperidol 0.5–5.0 g orally or i.m. may be indicated.

Nonpharmacologic treatment

Alcoholics Anonymous (AA): once the chronic alcoholic has become severely impaired cognitively, AA is no longer an effective treatment alternative; in cases of less severe impairment, involvement with AA may be helpful after recovery of abilities has occurred.

General references

Jernigan TL, *et al.*: Reduced cerebral grey matter observed in alcoholics using magnetic resonance imaging. *Alcoholism: Clinical and Experimental Research* 1991, 15:418–427.

Rourke SB, Loberg T: The neurobehavioral correlates of alcoholism. In *Neuropsychological Assessment of Neuropsychiatric Disorders.* Edited by Grant I, Adams KM. New York: Oxford University Press; 1996.

Volkow ND, *et al.*: Recovery of brain glucose metabolism in detoxified alcoholics. *Am J Psychiatry* 1994, 151:178–183.

Diagnosis

Definition
• Suicide attempt can be defined as a voluntary act intended to end the life of the actor. Although not a mental disorder itself, suicide attempt can be a fatal complication of mental disorder and can result from the self-destructive impulses that accompany mood, substance use, thought, or personality disorders [1]. Common means of attempted suicide include intentional overdoses, jumping from a height, self-induced gunshot or knife wounds, self-induced lacerations, hanging, and self-immolation.

Signs and symptoms
• Patients who have attempted suicide usually present for treatment of the physical consequences of the attempt (eg, traumatic injuries, toxic overdoses, burns) or the psychologic source of despair that leads to the attempt (eg, depression, substance intoxication). Physical signs and symptoms depend on the selected mode of attempted suicide. Similarly, psychologic symptoms largely depend on the underlying psychiatric disorder.

Investigations
• The best and most effective investigation is a careful and empathic patient interview.

• No reliable screening instruments or tests for suicide risk are available.

• After careful examination for injury sustained in the attempt and therapeutic attention to such injuries as indicated, all survivors of a suicide attempt should be examined to screen for the presence of mental disorder and to estimate the risk of a recurrent suicide attempt.

• All attempts at suicide should be taken seriously and evaluated. Evaluation should include history from the patient and collateral sources, a full mental status examination, elaboration of the details of the attempt and any persistent suicidal ideation, and assessment of any risk factors for repeated suicide attempts.

Complications
Death: from injuries sustained in the current attempt.

Subsequent successful suicide attempt.

Residual physical injury and disability: as a consequence of the attempt.

Differential diagnosis
Accidents.
Victimization by violent acts of others.
Idiopathic toxic drug reactions.
Extreme intoxication without suicidal intent.

Etiology
• Approximately 95% of patients who complete suicide suffer from a mental disorder.
• Completed suicide is associated with depression in ~50% of cases, with substance abuse or intoxication in ~25% of cases, with psychotic illnesses in ~10% of cases, and with character disorders in ~5% of cases.
• Depressive disorders carry the highest sustained risk of suicide (15%–25% lifetime risk).
• Alcohol and other substance use disorders also markedly increase the risk of suicide attempts; 21% of those who commit suicide are intoxicated at the time.
• Other factors that elevate the risk for suicide include male gender, past history of suicide attempts, family history of mental disorder or suicide, chronic illness, being single, unemployed, and socially isolated.
• Unsuccessful suicide attempts are more likely to be impulsive acts performed by a person who is ambivalent about a desire to die and who chooses a relatively low-risk method of suicide (eg, witnessed overdose). Such attempts are more common in females and younger persons, in the setting of acute life stresses, and in patients who are intoxicated or who suffer from personality disorders.

Epidemiology
• Suicide is the eighth leading cause of death in America; the third leading cause of death in those <25 y of age. Suicide rates appear to be declining in adults (except in the elderly) but increasing among adolescents and children.
• The overall incidence of suicide in the US is 10–12:100,000 deaths.

Treatment

General information

• The first and most important aspect of treating those who have survived a suicide attempt is the maintenance of patient safety. Most suicidal ideation will resolve; proper treatment will hasten this process. Those who make decisions about management and disposition (*eg*, whether to use restraints or one-to-one supervision, whether to transfer the patient for inpatient psychiatric care) of suicide attempt survivors should err on the side of patient safety. For a patient experiencing a depth of despair sufficient to trigger a suicide attempt, contact with a concerned and empathic clinician can be lifesaving.

Pharmacologic treatment

• Pharmacologic treatment should be directed to the underlying cause of the suicide attempt (*eg*, antidepressants for depression, antipsychotics for psychosis, etc.).

Treatment Aims:
To ensure patient safety.
To resolve suicidal ideation and reduce the risk of repeated suicide attempt.
To resolve the underlying disorder(s) that precipitated suicide attempt.

Prognosis
• If the acute precipitant of an unsuccessful suicide attempt is detected and treated, the majority of those who attempt suicide recover and do well; however, 6%–8% of those who survive a suicide attempt will die by suicide within 5 y. Patients with a history of repeated suicide attempts are at high risk of more attempts in the future.
• The low base rate of suicide combined with the relatively low rate of recurrent suicide attempt makes accurate prediction of future suicide risk very difficult. Attempts to refine prognostic accuracy in suicide-risk prediction have not been successful [2]. Suicide risk evaluation is best viewed as a short-term assessment of suicide risk, valid for a period of ~24–48 hours.

Follow-up and management
• Follow-up care should be directed to the underlying cause of the suicide attempt. Serial assessment of suicidal ideation or behavior is indicated, especially at times of increased symptomatology.

Key references
1. Blumenthal SJ, Kupfer DJ (eds): *Suicide Over the Life Cycle: Risk Factors, Assessment, and Treatment of Suicidal Patients.* Washington, DC: American Psychiatric Press; 1990.
2. Pokorny AD: Prediction of suicide in psychiatric patients: report of a prospective study. *Arch Gen Psychiatry.* 1983, 40:249–257.

General references
Hirschfeld RM, Russell JM: Assessment and treatment of suicidal patients. *N Engl J Med* 1997, 337:910–955.

Shuster JL, Stern T: Suicide. In *Intensive Care Medicine,* ed 3. Edited by Rippe JM, Irwin RS, Alpert JW, Fink MD. Boston: Little, Brown & Co.; 1996:2521–2525.

Stern TA, Mulley AG, Thibault GE: Life-threatening drug overdose: precipitants and prognosis. *JAMA* 1984, 251:1983–1985.

Diagnosis

Symptoms and signs

• The classic triad consists of chorea, hypotonia, and emotional lability. Affective changes have received the most attention recently, and patients may complain of restlessness, anxiety, "twitchiness," and/or impulsivity. Motor complaints range from mild clumsiness to impaired gross motor skills such as dressing or eating with utensils.

Chorea: Patients demonstrate distal adventitious movements that are more pronounced with distraction; they may sit on their hands and cross their legs to minimize movement.

Motor impersistence: difficulty with maintaining a forceful contraction results in "milkmaid's grip"; impersistence is typically also present with forced eye closure or tongue protrusion.

Abnormal gait: the classic choreic "dancing" gait is best appreciated while ambulating normally; patients also have significant problems with tandem gait and postural instability.

Dysarthria and dysphagia: may occur secondary to involvement of bulbar musculature; findings are asymmetric in ~20% of patients.

Investigations

Mental status examination and behavioral history: should be performed to document any symptoms of obsessive-compulsive disorder (OCD), other anxiety disorders, or other psychologic problems; an effort should be made to ascertain pertinent family, psychosocial, and medical history to determine if there is any familial tendency toward OCD or if a tic disorder is present.

Antistreptolysin (ASO) and anti-DNase B (ADB) titers: serum should be obtained to assess the presence of group A β-hemolytic streptococcal (GABHS) infection.

Complications

Rather sudden or subacute onset of motor abnormalities: may contribute to patients suffering significant loss of self-esteem; this may be further exacerbated by comorbid anxiety disorders.

School and/or employment issues: often of major importance, depending on the degree of abnormal movements and psychologic problems.

Differential diagnosis

Drug-induced chorea: neuroleptics, anticonvulsants, oral contraceptives.
Metabolic causes: hyperthyroidism, hypoparathyroidism, pseudohypoparathyroidism.
Pregnancy: chorea gravidarum.
Familial choreas: benign hereditary chorea, Huntington's disease, paroxysmal movement disorders.
Collagen-vascular disease: systemic lupus erythematosus, periarteritis nodosa.
Other: Wilson's disease, Tourette syndrome, cerebrovascular accident.

Etiology

• Sydenham's chorea is a major manifestation of acute rheumatic fever (ARF) and is sufficient to make a diagnosis of a first attack. To make the diagnosis secure, however, it is necessary to document evidence of a recent GABHS. A history of a positive throat culture accompanied by signs of an infection and/or elevated ASO or ADB titers is considered sufficient to demonstrate GABHS infection. Antistreptococcal titers may not become elevated for 2–3 mo after an infection and may remain elevated for 4–6 mo. The documentation of infections in GABHS carriers remains controversial.
• Demonstration of a temporal association is not proof of causality. Nevertheless, the association is so well characterized that it is sufficient to make the diagnosis if no other cause for chorea can be determined.

Epidemiology

• ARF is relatively uncommon, although regional outbreaks have occurred in the US over the past 15–20 y. Among patients with ARF, 10%–20% will develop Sydenham's chorea.

Treatment

Diet and lifestyle
• No particular dietary modifications are recommended.

• Patients need to modify their daily activities to accommodate to abnormal motor function. During the course of Sydenham's chorea, they may need to suspend driving or activities requiring manual dexterity and/or hand-eye coordination.

Pharmacologic treatment
• Sydenham's chorea is typically self-limited, with a course of 2–6 months. Treatment is usually aimed a motor symptoms only when severe enough to significantly impact on the patient. Behavioral symptoms may respond to traditional agents for anxiety, OCD, or impulsivity.

For chorea
• Neuroleptics may be beneficial, with efficacy related to the degree of D2 blockade.

Standard dosage	Neuroleptics, eg, haloperidol, pimozide, fluphenazine, and thiothixene (dosage must be individually titrated in children, and in all patients, it is advisable to start at a low dose).
Contraindications	Previous sensitivity (eg, neuroleptic malignant syndrome), history of tardive dyskinesia. Pimozide may prolong QT interval on electrocardiography and is not recommended in patients with arrhythmogenic conditions.
Main side effects	Lethargy, dysphoria, dystonic reactions, akathisia, tardive dyskinesia.
Special points	Degree of side effects must be weighed against the severity of symptoms. The risk of developing tardive dyskinesia in children is felt to be remote but must be discussed with patients and their families.

For target symptoms
Standard dosage	Anxiolytics (eg, benzodiazepines).
Main side effects	Somnolence, paradoxical agitation, occasionally dependence.
Special points	The transience of symptoms in most patients will obviate the need for pharmacologic intervention.

For OCD symptoms
Standard dosage	Selective serotonin-reuptake inhibitors (SSRIs).
Main side effects	Somnolence, anticholinergic effects, impotence.
Special points	The transience of symptoms in most patients will obviate the need for pharmacologic intervention.

Treatment aims
To adjust to what is typically a transient alteration in motor function; occasionally, evaluation by an occupational therapist is more beneficial in this regard than pharmacologic means.

Prognosis
• Well over 90% of patients have resolution of their symptoms within 6 mo of presentation.

Follow-up and management
• Patients should be monitored closely to assess the degree of motor and psychologic adaptation. If medications are used, efficacy and side effects should be assessed periodically.

Other treatment options
• Refractory cases of Sydenham's chorea are rare. Clinical investigations are ongoing to evaluate the role of auto-immune processes, and treatment trials are ongoing to assess plasmapheresis and immunosuppression for the treatment of Sydenham's chorea.

Diagnosis

Symptoms and signs [1–3]

Abnormal, purposeless, involuntary movements: most commonly consisting of orolingual dyskinesias (lip smacking, chewing, tongue thrusting, lateral jaw movement, grimacing), dystonias, or choreiform movements of the extremities, associated with chronic antipsychotic use.

Athetosis; pelvic thrusting; disorders of speech, swallowing, or breathing: in more severe cases.

Tongue fasciculations: often an early sign.

• These movements worsen with stress and disappear with sleep and, temporarily, with voluntary suppression. Patients are often unaware of them.

Investigations

Standardized rating scales: *eg*, the Abnormal Involuntary Movement Scale, used to screen for tardive dyskinesia (TD) and to follow severity over time.

Complications [2–4]

Cosmetic disfigurement: including dental and denture problems.

Speech impairment and difficulty eating (including involuntary retching and vomiting).

Respiratory distress: characterized by gasping, grunting, dyspnea and cyanosis, can be life-threatening.

Abnormal gait: causing falls and injuries.

Differential diagnosis [1,2]

Withdrawal dyskinesia.
Dyskinesias due to other drugs (eg, L-dopa, metoclopramide, amphetamines, anticholinergics, phenytoin, lithium).
Basal ganglia disorders (Huntington's disease, Wilson's disease, Sydenham's chorea).
Hypoparathyroidism.
Tourette's syndrome.
Movements associated with schizophrenia, advanced age, or ill-fitting dentures.

Etiology [2–4]

• Risk factors include the following:
Age (increased incidence, severity, and persistence in elderly; also greater chronicity in those with nonorofacial TD at baseline).
Female gender, particularly in elderly.
History of a mood disorder or brain surgery.
African-American race.
Diabetes mellitus.
Alcohol abuse.
• More controversial risk factors include the following:
Dose of and time on antipsychotic.
Smoking.

Epidemiology [2–4]

• Prevalence is 10%–20% in patients treated with antipsychotics for >1 y; greater in high-risk groups (up to 50%).
• Disease rarely appears <6 mo of treatment.
• Spontaneous remissions are relatively common (18%–30%).

Treatment

Pharmacologic treatment [2–5]

• Assess need for continued antipsychotic. If possible, lower the dose of the antipsychotic or discontinue it, which may cause initial worsening of the symptoms of TD.

• Although complete remission of TD following antipsychotic discontinuation is rare, ~30% of patients will improve. However, TD appears to be a risk factor for relapse.

• If the patient's history precludes lowering the dose, then switch to an atypical antipsychotic or add Vitamin E, which often has an antidyskinetic effect, especially in those with a shorter duration of TD.

Standard dosage	Olanzapine, 2.5–10.0 mg
	Risperidone, 2–8 mg
	Clozapine, begin at 12.5 mg and titrate slowly to 300–500 mg.
	Vitamin E, 400 IU (2 tablets) twice daily.
Contraindications	*Clozapine*: myeloproliferative disorders, uncontrolled epilepsy, history of clozapine-induced agranulocytosis or severe granulocytopenia, CNS depression or comatose state; patients taking other agents that can cause agranulocytosis or bone-marrow suppression. Use with caution in those with cardiovascular or pulmonary disease.
	Vitamin E: diarrhea
Main side effects	*Clozapine*: agranulocytosis (1%); seizures (5%); tachycardia, sialorrhea, sedation, weight gain, and neuroleptic malignant syndrome (rare).
	Olanzapine: sedation, mild weight gain, extrapyramidal symptoms at increased doses.
	Risperidone: anxiety, agitation, insomnia, extrapyramidal symptoms at higher doses, headache, constipation, rhinitis.
Main drug interactions	*Clozapine*: bone-marrow suppressants, benzodiazepines (respiratory arrest), highly protein-bound cimetidine, phenytoin, epinephrine.
	Caution should be used with any psychotropic, antihypertensive, anticholinergic drug, or those metabolized by the hepatic cytochrome P450 2D6 subsystem.
Special points	*Clozapine*: has little, if any, risk of producing TD, but this must be weighed against its risk of agranulocytosis, required weekly blood tests, and increased expense.
	Olanzapine and *risperidone*: appear to have a low TD liability if used in doses that do not produce extrapyramidal symptoms; however, greater exposure time is necessary to prove this.

Treatment aims

To reduce or eliminate the symptoms of tardive dyskinesia.
To reduce the risk of TD by using only antipsychotics when indicated at the lowest possible dose for the least amount of time necessary.

Prognosis [2,3,6]

• The course is often fluctuating, and spontaneous remissions are relatively common.
• Up to 30% of patients improve when antipsychotics are discontinued, especially if the patient is younger, employed, and carries a diagnosis other than schizophrenia. However, many relapse into psychosis.
• Although the majority of cases are mild, relapse can have high morbidity.

Other treatments [1,4]

• Decrease or eliminate anticholinergic drugs because these may worsen TD.
• γ-Aminobutyric acid agents (eg, benzodiazepines) may also be helpful.

Follow-up and management [1,3,4]

• Informed consent should be obtained at the initiation of antipsychotic treatment (if the patient is competent) and on a regular basis thereafter.
• Risks versus benefits of continued antipsychotic use should be assessed and documented regularly.
• Presence and severity of TD symptoms should be documented on a regular basis for any patient on antipsychotics.

Key references

1. Tardive dyskinesia: summary of a task force report of the American Psychiatric Association. *Am J Psychiatry* 1980, 137:1163–1172.
2. Latimer PR: Tardive dyskinesia: a review. *Can J Psychiatry* 1995, 40 (suppl 2):S49–S53.
3. Jeste DV, Caliguiri MP: Tardive dyskinesia. *Schizophr Bull* 1993, 19:303–315.
4. Feltner DE, Hertzman M: Progress in the treatment of tardive dyskinesia: theory and practice. hospital and community. *Psychiatry* 1993, 44:25–34.
5. Lohr JB, Caliguiri MP: A double-blind placebo-controlled study of vitamin E treatment of tardive dyskinesia. *J Clin Psychiatry* 1996, 57:167–173.
6. Glazer WM, Morgenstern H, Schooler N, et al.: Predictors of improvement in tardive dyskinesia following discontinuation of neuroleptic medication. *Br J Psychiatry* 1990, 157:585–592.

Diagnosis

DSM-IV diagnostic criteria

1. Both multiple motor and one or more vocal tics are present at some time during the illness, although not necessarily concurrently (a tic is a sudden, rapid, recurrent, nonrhythmic, stereotyped motor movement or vocalization.)

2. The tics occur many times per day (usually in bouts) nearly every day or intermittently throughout a period of more than 1 year, and during this period, there was never a tic-free period of more than 3 consecutive months.

3. The disturbance causes marked distress or significant impairment in social, occupation, or other important areas of functioning.

4. The onset is <18 years of age.

5. The disturbance is not due to the direct physiologic effects of a substance (eg, stimulants) or a general medical condition (eg, Huntington's disease or postviral encephalitis).

Symptoms and signs

Motor tics: these may take many forms, and typically involve the face and head (eg, blinking, mouth opening, grimacing, head shaking, etc.); any other stereotyped behavior involving the body may be classified as a tic; the hallmark of a tic is that it is suppressible for variable periods of time; however, tics are often worse in times of anxiety, fatigue, or other stress.

Vocal tics: virtually any repetitive, stereotyped sound or utterance may be a tic; typical examples include sniffing, throat clearing, humming, and coughing, but more obvious noises (eg, barking and hooting) occur; coprolalia affects a minority of patients.

Echopraxia, pallilalia, and echolalia: often present.

Attention deficit disorder and/or obsessive–compulsive behavior: the family history is almost always significant for the presence of tics and these disorders.

Investigations

Pertinent family, psychosocial, and medical history.

Neurologic examination: should be nonfocal.

Antistreptolysin (ASO) and anti-DNase B (ADB) titers: should be performed in cases suggestive of Sydenham's chorea.

Complications

Significant loss of self-esteem and development of associated social problems: if Tourette syndrome (TS) is undiagnosed; however, in young children, stresses may be more of an issue for the family.

School and/or employment issues: often of major importance, depending on the degree of abnormal behavior.

Differential diagnosis

• Most conditions that may be confused with TS are on the same spectrum (eg, transient tic disorder, chronic tic disorder) and differ from TS with respect to duration of tics or the absence of both motor and vocal tics.

• Conditions in which tics and Tourette-like behaviors may occur include tardive dyskinesia, autism, mental retardation, Wilson's disease, Sydenham's chorea, and Huntington's disease.

Etiology

• Frequency of positive family history indicates a genetic component, but no marker has been identified. Empiric response to pharmacologic manipulation of brain dopamine and serotonin neurochemistry indicate an abnormality of these neurotransmitter systems. Very rare cases have been described subsequent to head trauma.

Epidemiology

• Worldwide prevalence is estimated to be between 0.1–1.0:1000. Expression is influenced by sex, with males more likely to exhibit tics, and females more prone to obsessive–compulsive behaviors or the disorder itself.

Treatment

Diet and lifestyle

• No particular dietary modifications are recommended.

• Stress and anxiety are clearly contributory to exacerbations of tics, and occasionally relaxation strategies are of benefit.

Pharmacologic treatment

• TS is a chronic condition and by definition follows a waxing and waning course. Accurate identification of the most troublesome symptoms guides the therapeutic interventions. The treatments of attention deficit disorder and obsessive–compulsive disorder are discussed elsewhere.

For motor and vocal tics

• Neuroleptics may be beneficial, with efficacy related to the degree of D2 blockade.

• The α-agonist clonidine has also been used to treat tics, but its mechanism of action is unknown.

Standard dosage	Neuroleptics, *eg*, haloperidol, pimozide, fluphenazine, and thiothixene (dosage must be individually titrated in children, and in all patients, it is advisable to start at a low dose).
	Clonidine (dosage must be individually titrated in children, and in all patients, it is advisable to start at a low dose).
Contraindications	*Neuroleptics*: previous sensitivity to neuroleptics (*eg*, neuroleptic malignant syndrome), history of tardive dyskinesia. Pimozide may prolong QT interval on electrocardiography, and it is not recommended in patients with arrhythmogenic conditions.
Main side effects	*Neuroleptics*: lethargy, dysphoria, dystonic reactions, akathisia, tardive dyskinesia.
	Clonidine: lethargy, somnolence, headache, dizziness.
Special points:	*All agents*: the presence of side effects must be weighed against the severity of symptoms.
	Neuroleptics: the risk of developing tardive dyskinesia in children is felt to be remote but must be discussed with patients and their families.

Nonpharmacologic treatment

• Relaxation therapies have been tried, but no consistent responses have been reported.

Treatment aims

To identify what, if any, symptoms require therapy; the diagnosis alone is not sufficient to mandate treatment.
To exhaust every effort to discern what the problematic features are in an individual and to address them appropriately.

Prognosis

• Although a chronic condition, there are relatively fewer adults followed for TS than children. This may represent gradual resolution of the condition or possibly an adaptation to the disorder.

Follow-up and management

• Patients and families should be well informed about the condition, and the education of peers, school, and employment personnel is very important.
• If pharmacologic intervention is undertaken, patients should be monitored for side effects and treatment responses. Periodic attempts to taper medications should be made.

Support groups

Tourette Syndrome Association, Inc.
42-40 Bell Boulevard
Bayside, NY 11361-2874
Phone: 718-224-2999
Fax: 718-279-9596

General references

Cohen DJ, Riddle MA, Leckman JF: Pharmacotherapy of Tourette's syndrome and associated disorders. *Psychiatr Clin North Am* 1992, 15:109–129.

Singer HS: Neurobiological issues in Tourette syndrome. *Brain Dev* 1994, 16:353–364.

Diagnosis

Symptoms and signs

• This paraphilia involves sexual excitement in heterosexual males resulting from recurrent, intense fantasies, urges, or behaviors of dressing in female clothing. Individuals are diagnosed only if 1) there is significant distress or impairment in functioning due to fantasies, urges, or behavior; and 2) symptoms are present for at least 6 months.

• The disorder may occur with or without gender dysphoria: the individual may have discomfort with his gender role.

• Transvestic fetishism is usually evident based on the following signs: 1) although individuals with the disorder attempt to conceal their symptoms, roommates or spouses may find articles of women's clothing hidden in drawers or closets; 2) individuals with transvestic fetishism may request that their sexual partners also participate in cross-dressing to heighten sexual arousal; and 3) commonly arousing items include undergarments, pantyhose, and lingerie.

• Transvestites are generally not effeminate in childhood.

• Transvestites frequently have stereotypical masculine jobs such as truck drivers, construction workers, and businessmen.

• Cross-dressing and anal stimulation are associated with deaths from autoerotic asphyxiation (*see* Sexual sadism). The relationship between the fatal behavior and transvestic fantasy is under debate.

• The definition of transvesic fetishism as a disorder has been questioned. It has been suggested that to qualify as a disorder, the fetish must create distress, disability, and disadvantage.

Investigations

Laboratory investigations: none are indicated.

Penile plethysmography: may offer additional information to establish arousal associated with wearing women's clothing and to assess for arousal associated with other paraphilias; the reliability of this measure is questionable, however, and may result in false-negative information.

Psychologic testing: may offer additional information concerning sexual preferences and psychopathology that may affect the fetish behavior.

Complications

Impairment in social functioning: individuals with this paraphilia tend to withdraw to hide their disorder, which may lead to loneliness.

Impairment in sexual functioning: arousal may be impaired when cross-dressing is not involved, which may be especially disruptive to sexual relationships in which the partner does not enjoy or approve of cross-dressing.

Differential diagnosis

Fetishism: in this disorder, the individual may be aroused by women's clothing, but the focus is on the article of clothing itself, not on wearing the items. Sexual masochism: this disorder may involve cross-dressing, but sexual arousal results from the humiliation of being forced to dress in women's clothing. Transsexualism: transsexual males cross-dress as part of their perceived female identity, but sexual arousal is not associated with the act.

Etiology

• The etiology of transvestic fetishism is unclear. Several theories have been proposed as explanations for the disorder.

Biological theory: temporal lobe epilepsy, seizures, head injury, and damage to the limbic and temporal lobe structures have been associated with transvestic fetishism.

Psychosocial theory: suggests that the thought or behavior of wearing women's clothing has been paired with sexual arousal (classic conditioning) that is reinforcing (operant conditioning); research suggests that the fetish is also associated with anger, hostility, and rejection toward and from women that may further reinforce the fetish.

Epidemiology

• By definition, this fetish only occurs in heterosexual males.
• Homosexual males may, however, engage in transvestic behaviors.
• Age of onset is typically between childhood and mid-adolescence.

Treatment

Pharmacologic treatment
• Treatment is typically based on case studies. A combination of drug treatment and psychotherapy may prove effective.

Antiandrogenic medication
• Medroxyprogesterone acetate and cyproterone acetate (UK) have been used as "chemical castration" to result in lowered sex drive. Too few studies have been completed to determine the efficacy of these medications.

• Surgical castration and psychosurgery are generally reserved for severe, life-threatening cases of transvestic fetishism. The ethics of these procedures is under debate.

Psychotropic medication (antidepressant)
• The following medications have been documented in case studies: buspirone, fluoxetine, clomipramine, desipramine, sertraline, and lithium. Several of these medications are thought to work by treating the obsessional nature of the disorder and taking advantage of the sexual side effect profiles. It is unclear if this is truly the mode of action for these medications.

• Dosage has not been well established and may be similar to that for obsessive-compulsive disorder. Titrate dose until symptoms are lessened or until side effects become too severe.

Standard dosage	Fluoxetine, 20–80 mg/d.
	Paroxetine, 20–60 mg/d.
	Clomipramine, 150–300 mg/d.
	Fluvoxamine, 50–300 mg/d.
	Sertraline, 50–200 mg/d.
	Desipramine, 150–300 mg/d.
	Imipramine, 150–300 mg/d.
Main side effects	*All agents*: agitation, anxiety, sleep disturbance, sexual dysfunction (primarily anorgasmia), and headache.
Main drug interactions	*All agents*: potentially fatal interactions with monoamine oxidase inhibitors; potential fatal interaction with antiar-rythmic medications; serotonergic crisis (hypertension, hyperpyrexia, and seizure) is possible in patients on other serotonergic medications.

Lithium
Standard dosage	0.8–1.2 mEq/L serum range (similar to that for bipolar disorder).
Main side effects	Excessive thirst, polyuria, memory problems, tremor, weight gain, drowsiness, diarrhea.
Special points	Risk to the fetus during pregnancy.

Nonpharmacologic treatment
Behavior therapy.

Covert sensitization.

Orgasmic reconditioning.

Plethysmographic biofeedback.

Satiation.

Challenging distorted thinking and beliefs that contribute and maintain the behavior.

Social skills training, assertiveness training, communication skills training, anger management.

Relapse prevention.

Aversion therapy (pairing deviant arousal stimuli to electrical or chemical punishment.

Treatment aims
To decrease arousal associated with cross-dressing.
To decrease cross-dressing behavior.

Prognosis
• Poor prognosis is associated with low intelligence, poor social supports, poor employment history, and family conflict.

Follow-up and management
• Some individuals benefit from support groups for sexual addictions or paraphilias.
• Sexual therapy may be warranted for individuals with dissatisfying sexual relationships.
• Individual therapy may be indicated for related psychopathology.

General references
Laws DR, O'Donohue W: *Sexual Deviance*. New York: Guilford Press; 1997.

Rubenstein EB: Successful treatment of trans-vestic fetishism with sertraline and lithium. *J Clin Psychiatry* 1996, 57:92.

Travin S, Protter B: *Sexual Perversion: Integrative Treatment Approaches for the Clinician*. New York: Plenum Press; 1993.

Diagnosis

Definition

• Trichotillomania is a disorder characterized by recurrent pulling of one's own hair that results in noticeable hair loss. The behavior is associated with increasing tension before pulling, or when attempting to resist pulling. Pleasure, gratification, or relief are associated with completion of the behavior. The hairpulling causes significant distress or impairment in functioning.

Symptoms and signs [1,2]

• Some individuals tug or twist their hair without noticeable pulling or hair loss.

• Frequent sites of hair pulling include the scalp and head, eyebrows, eyelashes, pubic area, underarm, and

arms and legs.

• Individuals frequently pull from more than one site.

• Pulling is not necessarily associated with stressors. Vulnerable times for the behavior include watching television, boredom, driving, reading, using the telephone, and before bed or sleeping.

• Two "styles" of hairpulling have been identified:

Focused: attention is focused on the current hairpulling behavior; generally the minority of hairpulling occurs in this fashion.

Automatic: occurs with little or no awareness, frequently described as habitual pulling.

• Oral manipulation (eg, mouthing the hair, eating part or all of the hair) occurs among 25%–50% of trichotillomania patients.

DSM-IV criteria

1. Recurrent pulling out of one's hair resulting in noticeable hair loss.

2. Increasing tension prior to pulling hair or when attempting to resist pulling hair.

3. Pleasure, gratification, or relief when pulling out hair.

4. Behavior causes significant distress or impairment in functioning.

• The strictness of criteria has been debated; many individuals deny either tension prior to pulling or relief following pulling.

• It has been hypothesized that trichotillomania has diagnostic, etiologic, and treatment similarities with compulsive skin-picking and nail-biting.

Investigations

Psychologic testing: measures to indicate symptom severity (eg, Massachusetts General Hospital Hairpulling Scale, Yale-Brown Obsessive-compulsive Scale modified for trichotillomania) and other psychological measures may offer additional information concerning additional psychopathology that may affect treatment outcome.

Laboratory studies: dermatological biopsy may be beneficial.

Complications

Potential infection at follicle sites.

Changes in hair texture or color.

Emotional or behavioral consequences of hairpulling: shame, guilt, decreased social activities and relationships, depression, anxiety.

Carpal tunnel syndrome.

Medical concerns: resulting from decreased visits to various health professionals such as the gynecologist and the optometrist or ophthalmologist.

Trichophagy: hair ingestion (may include entire hair or only certain parts of the hair) may result in trichobezoars (hairballs).

Trichobezoars: hair balls resulting from trichophagy; can lead to decreased appetite, stomach pain, obstruction, anemia, and mortality if untreated.

Differential diagnosis

Alopecia.

Psychosis or hallucinations, especially of parasites in hair.

Self-destructive; self-mutilating behavior: frequently associated with borderline personality disorder, dissociative disorders, or affective disorders.

Etiology

• Trichotillomania has been associated with the following etiological theories:

Family dysfunction.

Sexual and nonsexual trauma.

Neurological abnormalities (particularly basal ganglia and frontal lobes).

Serotonin and dopamine system abnormalities.

Disorder of grooming habits (associated with compulsive feather-picking in birds, feline psychogenic alopecia in cats, and acral lick dermatitis in dogs).

Obsessive-compulsive spectrum disorder, including tics and Tourette's syndrome.

Possible iron deficiency associated with trichophagia.

Epidemiology

• Lifetime prevalence rates (LPR) in men and women are estimated at 0.6%.

Using less strict criteria for diagnosis: LPR in men, 1.5%; in women, 3.4%.

For adults, appears to affect substantially more women than men.

Prior to age 18, female-to-male ratio fairly equivalent ~2:1.

Onset generally between late childhood and early adolescence.

Waxing and waning symptoms.

Chronic course without treatment.

Treatment [1,3,4]

Pharmacologic treatment

• Results from case studies and open-trial studies indicate possible efficacy of psychotropic medications. Although very few placebo-controlled, double blind studies have been completed, most fail to demonstrate long-term treatment efficacy.

• Further studies are required to determine the actual efficacy of these agents. Psychotherapy and medication may provide better results than medication alone. It is generally accepted that appropriate medications and their dosages are similar to those prescribed for obsessive-compulsive disorder.

Standard dosage	Clomipramine, 150–300 mg/d (superior results when compared with desipramine treatment).
	Fluoxetine, 20–80 mg/d (not superior over placebo).
	Fluvoxamine, 50–300 mg/d.
	Paroxetine, 20–60 mg/d.
	Sertraline, 50–200 mg/d.
Special points	May report improvement if medication is augmented with other agents such as pimozide, clonazepam, or lithium.
	Relapse frequently occurs upon discontinuation of pharmacological treatment, or after 6 months of treatment.

Nonpharmacologic treatment

• Again, treatment results are generally derived from case studies and therefore provide only partial evidence for treatment efficacy.

• Usually the nonpharmacological therapies are combined with other treatments such as assertiveness training, relaxation training, monitoring, supportive therapy, cognitive therapy, and communication skills training.

Behavioral treatment: habit reversal training generally consists of up to 13 components including a daily monitoring, competing response, and relaxation; generally positive treatment results depend on treatment compliance; considered treatment of choice for normal intelligence patients.

Hypnosis: a few case studies indicate potential efficacy.

Pain sensitivity increase: topical agents designed to increase pain sensation and increase negative consequences associated with pulling; mixed treatment results.

• Most individuals have experimented with various behaviors for self-treatment, including wearing lotions or oils on fingers and hair, gloves, wigs, turbans, hats, and shaving the target areas. These methods usually meet with poor success.

Treatment aims
To decrease hairpulling.
To decrease urge to pull hair.

Prognosis
Better prognosis associated with onset within 6 mo prior to treatment and with younger age.

Follow-up and management
• Other therapeutic issues and modalities may need to be considered, including family therapy, couples or marital therapy, personality characteristics, assertiveness training, communication skills, and relaxation training.
• Continue assessment for other psychiatric concerns such as tics, obsessive-compulsive disorder, other anxiety disorders and affective disorders (eg, depression).

Key references
1. Christenson GA, Crow SJ: The characterization and treatment of trichotillomania. *J Clin Psychiatry* 1996, 57:42–47.
2. Stein DJ, Simeon D, Cohen LJ, Hollander E: et al.: Trichotillomania and obsessive-compulsive disorder. *J Clin Psychiatry* 1995, 56:28–34.
3. Ristvedt SL, Christenson GA: The use of pharmacologic pain sensitization in the treatment of repetitive hair-pulling. *Behav Res Ther* 1996, 34:647–648.
4. Steichenwein SM, Thornby JI: A long-term, double-blind, placebo-controlled crossover trial of the efficacy of fluoxetine for trichotillomania. *Am J Psychiatry* 1995, 152:1192–1196.

Diagnosis

Signs and symptoms

Recurrent or persistent involuntary contraction of the perineal muscles surrounding the outer third of the vagina when penetration with a penis, finger, tampon, or speculum is attempted or anticipated: contraction may vary from mild to severe and painful; genital anatomy is normal; the muscle spasms may occur in anticipation of intercourse, while fantasizing or thinking about intercourse, or during intromission; partners report a feeling like there is an obstruction approximately 1 inch within the vagina.

Investigations [1]

History and confirmation by physical examination: many cases first become evident (to the physician) during routine gynecologic examination; causative physical abnormalities (*eg*, endometriosis, rigid hymen, hemorrhoids, tissue inflammation, infection, or tumor [rare]) should be ruled out.

Psychologic assessment and testing: may reveal characteristics, behaviors, or disorders that may be contributing to the intensity, duration, or frequency of vaginal muscle spasms.

Complications [2]

Relationship problems: can be severe; may cause or result from the difficulty.

Unconsummated marriages: some evidence that this occurs more frequently in non-Western cultures.

Impaired procreation: thought to be one of leading reasons affected individuals seek treatment for this disorder.

Physical injury: may result from "forcing" penetration.

Differential diagnosis [2,3]

• Organic causes should be ruled out by a vaginal exam (under anesthesia, if necessary).

• It is often difficult to distinguish between vaginismus and dyspareunia, hypoactive sexual desire disorder, and sexual aversion disorder. These conditions may be more appropriate diagnoses than vaginismus, or they may be comorbid conditions.

Etiology

• Vaginismus has been viewed as an involuntary reflex due to imagined, anticipated, or real attempt at vaginal penetration.

• Behavioral models suggest that pain (emotional or physical) becomes associated with intercourse and results in the unconditioned response of self-protective muscle tightening. The tightening returns when sexual intercourse is considered or initiated through a means of classical conditioning. The reflexive muscle tightening allows the individual to avoid intercourse, thus avoiding the pain and reinforcing the reflexive action (operant conditioning).

• Factors frequently associated with vaginismus include a history of sexual trauma or abuse, conflicts regarding sexuality, severe relationship problems, the inhibiting influence of religious orthodoxy, and occasionally, a defensive response towards an overly aggressive or insensitive partner.

Epidemiology

• Although considered to be relatively rare, it is likely that vaginismus exists to a far greater degree than is statistically reported. Females usually seek treatment only if 1) it creates marital distress, 2) they want to procreate, or 3) the disorder comes to the attention of the physician who tries to perform a vaginal examination. Some evidence suggests that it is more common in non-Western cultures.

Treatment

Pharmacologic treatment

• Short-acting benzodiazepines taken on an as-needed basis may be helpful but only with a fully willing patient.

• *Note*: Inhibiting the defenses of an individual who is already feeling threatened is contratherapeutic.

Nonpharmacologic treatment

Cognitive-behavioral treatment [1,4]

Cognitive-behavioral treatment will most likely include the following components:

1. Education regarding sexual anatomy and normal sexual function.

2. Enlistment of the partner's cooperation, understanding, and patience.

3. Sex therapy (may include exercises to relieve pelvic floor muscle tension, use of lubricants and anesthetic gels, sensate focus exercises, relaxation therapy, and therapeutic insertion of graduated sizes of vaginal dilators; individuals opposed to the use of dilators have successfully utilized fingers or penile insertion in a graduated manner).

4. Addressing relationship problems and conflicts over intimacy and sexuality.

5. Addressing sexual abuse or sexual trauma (treatment of individuals who have been sexually traumatized or abused is difficult and best undertaken by a clinician who has the experience and time necessary to help the patient safely and successfully resolve these traumatic experiences).

Treatment aims

To increase sexual satisfaction for the individual (and, hopefully, her partner).
To allow individual to attend to routine health needs (eg, gynecologic examinations).
To identify interventions that increase likelihood of impregnation.

Prognosis

• Prognosis is generally considered good, although treatment outcome relies upon several complex issues. Patient motivation is essential; treatment sought only to please the partner has a lower success rate than treatment that is sought to understand and explore the patient's own sexual difficulties. Vaginal penetration should not by the only measure of treatment success.

Key references

1. Shaw J: Treatment of primary vaginismus: a new perspective. *J Sex Marital Ther*, 1994, 20:146–154.

2. Leiblum S, Pervin LLL, Campbell E: The treatment of vaginismus: success and failure. In *Principles and Practices of Sex Therapy*. Edited by Leiblum S, Rosen R; 1989.

3. *Handbook of Sex Therapy*. Edited by LoPiccolo J, LoPiccolo L. New York: Plenum; 1978.

4. Wincze JP, Carey MP: *Sexual Dysfunction: A Guide for Assessment and Treatment*. New York: Guilford Press; 1991.

General references

• *See* General references for Orgasmic disorder, female.

Diagnosis

Definition
• Vascular dementia is caused by multiple strokes (small or large) that can result in cell death; used to be called "hardening of the arteries."

Symptoms
• DSM-IV describes patients as having vascular dementia if they have short-term memory impairment, discrete losses based on the area of the brain that is damaged, and an impaired ability to learn new information or recall previously learned information. In addition, one or more of the following disturbances should be present:

1. Aphasia (language disturbance).

2. Apraxia (impaired ability to carry out motor activities despite intact motor function).

3. Agnosia (failure to recognize or identify objects despite intact sensory function).

4. Disturbance in executive functioning (eg, planning, organizing, sequencing, abstracting).

• Impairments cause significant problems in functioning and represent a decline in functioning.

• Also indicative of vascular dementia are focal neurologic signs and symptoms or laboratory evidence characteristic of cerebrovascular disease that are judged to be etiologically related to the disturbance.

• Deficits do not occur exclusively during the course of a delirium.

Investigation
Thorough history.

Physical examination.

Laboratory assessment: to rule out reversible causes of dementia.

Computed tomography or magnetic resonance imaging scans of the brain.

Electroencephalography: to rule out seizure disorder.

Single photon emission computed tomography scan of the brain.

Neuropsychologic testing: to evaluate memory, mood, concentration, and ability to learn new information.

Complications
Depression: sad mood with disturbance of sleep, memory, concentration, appetite, sex drive, energy, interests, and sometimes thoughts of suicide

Delirium: fluctuating mental status due to infections, medications, metabolic imbalances

Delusions: fixed, false belief.

Hallucinations: can be visual or auditory; patients generally become suspicious.

Etiology
Predisposing factors include the following:
Hypertension.
Heart disease.
Blood clots.
Atherosclerosis (blood vessels close down and prevent blood supply).

Epidemiology
• Between 10%–15% of patients with dementia have vascular dementia, which is the second most common type of dementia.

Treatment

General information

• There is no cure for vascular dementia; it is a progressive and irreversible illness. Once a nerve cell dies, it does not regenerate.

• Patients will eventually need 24-hour supervision in either an assisted-living facility or nursing home due to memory impairment. They will require help with finances and decision-making, and they eventually will be unable to drive.

• Patients should be guarded against exploitation.

Diet and lifestyle

• Blood pressure, diabetes, and heart disease should be controlled. The patient should also discontinue smoking.

Pharmacologic treatment

• Enteric-coated aspirin, Coumadin, or Ticlid should be administered to minimize further damage due to stroke.

• Avoid anticholinergic drugs, antihistamines (*eg*, Benadryl, Vistaril/Atarax; unless there is an allergic reaction), and anticholinergic antidepressants (*eg*, Elavil). These can cause increased confusion and possible hallucinations.

• Cautiously use benzodiazepines

• Any psychiatric medications should be initiated in low doses and increased slowly.

Follow-up and management

• Caregiver support is vital.

• Caregivers are at an increased risk of developing depression.

General references

American Psychiatric Association: *Diagnostic and Statistical Manual of Mental Disorders*, ed 4. Washington, DC: American Psychiatric Association; 1994.

Busse EW, Blazer DG: *Textbook of Geriatric Psychiatry*, ed 2. Washington, DC: American Psychiatric Press, Inc.; 1996.

Diagnosis

Symptoms and signs

• This paraphilia involves the behavior of observing unsuspecting individuals who are naked, disrobing, or engaging in sexual activities. The observing (peeping) is associated with sexual excitement and arousal. Individuals are diagnosed only if 1) there is significant distress or impairment in functioning due to fantasies, urges, or actual voyeuristic behaviors; and 2) symptoms are present for at least 6 months.

• Usually no sexual activity with the observed person is sought, although it may be fantasized.

• Usually the individual being observed is a stranger.

• The disorder is generally associated with poor social relationships.

• Voyeurs may choose jobs that enable them to engage in this behavior (*eg*, telephone repairmen, water meter readers).

• May also experience a variety of other paraphilias or sexual dysfunction.

• Some studies revealed that 37% of voyeurs were involved in rape, 63% in exhibitionism, 11% in sadism.

• It appears that more invasive sex crimes are preceded by acts of voyeurism: several studies indicate that voyeurism is commonplace among rapists.

Investigations

Laboratory investigations: none are indicated.

Psychologic testing: may suggest additional psychiatric disorders that may contribute to the severity of the voyeuristic behavior.

Penile plethysmography: may offer additional information to establish arousal associated with this behavior and assess for arousal associated with other paraphilias; the reliability of this measure is questionable, however, and may result in false-negative information.

• *See* Fetishism for specific psychologic tests.

Complications

Legal implications of behavior: voyeurism is generally not considered a sex crime, and frequently the individual is arrested for trespassing, loitering, vagrancy, disorderly conduct, or illegal entry.

Impaired social or sexual functioning: some individuals may only be able to achieve sexual arousal through voyeuristic activities.

Risk for injuries: physical injuries may result due to falls from precarious viewing positions (*eg*, rooftops, trees, telephone poles).

Differential diagnosis

Normal sexual arousal: diagnosis is not made unless the person being viewed is unsuspecting. Sexual arousal while viewing others naked, disrobing, or engaging in sexual activity is not voyeuristic if all individuals consent (eg, strip bars, adult movies or magazines, three-way interaction).

Psychosis: psychotic individuals may engage in the behavior for reasons other than sexual excitement, and the behavior only exists during the course of the illness.

Etiology

Biologic theory: suggests that men are "wired" to become sexually aroused by viewing women's genitals so that "male reproductive opportunities" will be maximized; another view focuses on abnormal neurochemical functioning that may contribute to poor impulse control and deviant behavior.

Behavioral theory: suggests that the behavior is paired with sexual arousal (classic conditioning) that was inherently a positive experience (reinforcing); the behavior was not paired with guilt, remorse, feelings for the "victim" and therefore was not aversive (punishing); the behavior is further reinforced by masturbatory fantasies involving the voyeurism.

Neuronal model: when an individual is not allowed to complete a desired act, he will experience increasing tension and excitement that leads to his feeling compelled to complete the act; because the voyeur rarely engages in sexual activity with the individual, the act is never complete and therefore the observing becomes a compulsion.

Psychodynamic theory: the perversion is symptomatic of underlying psychopathology and unresolved conflicts; generally focused on his relationship with his mother or his need to humiliate others.

Epidemiology

• Onset occurs generally in those less 15 y of age.

• The prevalence is almost exclusively male (>90% male).

Treatment

General information

• Very little data have been collected regarding treatment modalities or treatment efficacy for voyeurism. Frequently these individuals do not seek treatment themselves but rather are forced into treatment due to legal difficulties. All treatment for voyeurism should be considered experimental.

Pharmacologic treatment

Antiobsessionals

• These medications are thought to work by treating the obsessional nature of the disorder and by taking advantage of their sexual side effect profiles.

• Dosing is hypothesized to be similar to that for obsessive-compulsive disorder, titrating until symptoms are controlled or side effects are intolerable.

Standard dosage	Fluoxetine, 20–80 mg/d.
	Paroxetine, 20–60 mg/d.
	Clomipramine, 150–300 mg/d.
	Fluvoxamine, 50–300 mg/d.
	Sertraline, 50–-200 mg/d.
	Desipramine, 150–300 mg/d.
	Imipramine, 150–300 mg/d.
Main side effects	*All agents:* gastrointestinal upset, diarrhea, vomiting, anorexia, agitation, insomnia, sexual dysfunction.
	Clomipramine: may also be associated with dry mouth, orthostasis, constipation, weight gain, urinary retention, cardiac dysrhythmias, and lowered seizure threshold.
Main drug interactions	*All agents*: potentially fatal interaction with monoamine oxidase inhibitors, potentially fatal interaction with antiarrythmic medications, serotonergic crisis (hypertension, hyperpyrexia, seizures) possible in patients on other serotonergic medications.

Hormonal agents

• Hormonal agents have been shown to be effective in suppressing sexual urges, but they may truncate the individual's sexual life, resulting in decreased compliance with medication.

Standard dosage	Medroxyprogesterone acetate, 500 mg/wk i.m. or 80 mg/d orally.
	Leuprolide acetate, 7.5 mg/mo i.m. or 1 mg/d s.c.
Contraindications	*Medroxyprogesterone acetate*: use cautiously in patients with hyperlipidemia (serum lipoproteins [high-density lipoprotein and low-density lipoprotein]) should be monitored during therapy), thrombophlebitis, thromboembolic disease, asthma, congestive heart failure, nephrotic syndrome or other renal disease, or cardiac disease; may exacerbate major depression, migraine, or seizure disorder; should not be used with bromocriptine (the combination would be counterproductive).
	Leuprolide acetate: patients with urinary tract obstruction may have worsening of symptoms during the first weeks of treatment; flutamide (250 mg orally 3 times daily) should be given concurrently during the first 2 weeks of therapy to prevent a possible transient increase in sex drive; androgens and estrogens are relatively contraindicated and would defeat the purpose of leuprolide therapy.
Main side effects	*All agents*: weight gain, hypertension, lethargy, hot flashes, mood lability (during early treatment), phlebitis (rare), and gynecomastia (rare).

Treatment aims

• Reduce voyeuristic behavior.
• Improve sexual functioning with consenting individuals. (prevent relapse).

Prognosis

• Without treatment, the course of this disorder tends to be chronic. Although the actual behavior may decrease as the patient ages, his fantasies may remain voyeuristic in content.
• Indicators of poor prognosis include early age of onset, no guilt for the behavior, high frequency of engaging in the behavior, and poor sexual and social relationships.

Follow-up and management

• Identify vulnerable situation to prevent relapse.
• Encourage consensual sexual activities.
• Assess need for counseling regarding paraphilias or other psychopathology.

Nonpharmacologic treatment

Cognitive-behavioral therapy

• Treatment may include the following:
Behavior therapy: to reduce inappropriate sexual arousal and increase appropriate sexual arousal.
Challenging distorted thinking and beliefs: especially those concerning justification for the paraphilic behavior.
Social skills training, assertiveness training, communication skills training.
Relapse prevention: to help identify vulnerable thoughts and situations and intervene to prevent or stop the behavior by using various cognitive skills and behavioral skills.
Psychodynamic therapy: generally considered to be an unsuccessful treatment modality.

General references

Diagnostic and Statistical Manual of Mental Disorders, ed 4. Washington, DC: American Psychiatric Association; 1995.

Laws DR, O'Donohue W: *Sexual Deviance*. New York: Guilford Press; 1997.

INDEX

INDEX